Tech1-c6150

AF779470

Platelet Activating Factor and Human Disease

FRONTIERS IN PHARMACOLOGY & THERAPEUTICS

SERIES ADVISORS

R. J. Flower PhD

Professor, Department of Biomedical Pharmacology
St Bartholomew's Hospital Medical College, London

C. F. George BSc, MB, ChB, FRCP

Professor of Pharmacology
University of Southampton

R. G. Hill BPharm, PhD

Director of Pharmacology
Smith, Kline & French Research Ltd, Welwyn

FRONTIERS IN PHARMACOLOGY & THERAPEUTICS

Platelet Activating Factor and Human Disease

edited by

Peter J. Barnes MA, DM, DSc, FRCP
Department of Thoracic Medicine, National Heart and Lung Institute, University of London

Clive P. Page PhD
Department of Pharmacology, King's College, University of London

Peter M. Henson PhD
Department of Pediatrics, National Jewish Center for Immunology and Respiratory Medicine, Denver, Colorado

BLACKWELL SCIENTIFIC PUBLICATIONS
OXFORD LONDON
EDINBURGH BOSTON MELBOURNE

QU
93
P715

© 1989 by
Blackwell Scientific Publications
Editorial offices:
Osney Mead, Oxford OX2 0EL
8 John Street, London WC1N 2ES
23 Ainslie Place, Edinburgh EH3 6AJ
3 Cambridge Center, Suite 208
Cambridge, Massachusetts 02142,
USA
107 Barry Street, Carlton
Victoria 3053, Australia

All rights reserved. No part of this publication may be reproduced, stored in a retrieval system, or transmitted, in any form or by any means, electronic, mechanical, photocopying, recording or otherwise without the prior permission of the copyright owner

First published 1989

Set by Associated Publishing Services Ltd
Petersfield, Hampshire and printed and bound in Great Britain by Cambridge University Press, Cambridge

DISTRIBUTORS

UK
Marston Book Services Ltd
PO Box 87
Oxford OX2 0DT
(*Orders*: Tel: 0865-791155
Fax: 0865-791927
Telex: 837515)

USA
Year Book Medical Publishers
200 North LaSalle Street
Chicago, Illinois 60601
(*Orders*: Tel: (312) 726-9733)

Canada
The C.V. Mosby Company
5240 Finch Avenue East
Scarborough, Ontario
(*Orders*: Tel: (416) 298-1588)

Australia
Blackwell Scientific Publications
(Australia) Pty Ltd
107 Barry Street
Carlton, Victoria 3053
(*Orders*: Tel: (03) 347-0300)

British Library
Cataloguing in Publication Data

Platelet activating factor
and human disease.
1. Man. Blood. Platelets. Biochemistry
I. Barnes, P. J. (Peter John), *1946–*
II. Page, Clive P.
III. Henson, Peter M.
IV. Series
612′ 177

ISBN 0-632-02684-7

Contents

Contributors

Peter J. Barnes *Department of Thoracic Medicine, National Heart and Lung Institute, London SW3 6LY, UK*

René Bourgain *Vrije Universiteit Brussel, Laboratorium voor Fysiologie en Fysiopathologie, B-1090 Brussels, Belgium*

Pierre Braquet *Institut Henri Beaufour Research Laboratories, 17 Avenue Descartes, 92350 Le Plessis-Robinson, France*

Donna Bratton *Department of Pediatrics, National Jewish Center for Immunology and Respiratory Medicine, Denver, Colorado 80206, USA*

Giovanni Camussi *Cattedra di' Nefrologia Sperimentale, Universitá di Napoli, Italy*

K. Fan Chung *Department of Thoracic Medicine, National Heart and Lung Institute, London SW3 6LY, UK*

Fiona M. Cunningham *Department of Veterinary Basic Sciences, The Royal Veterinary College, Hawkshead Lane, North Mymms, Hertfordshire AL9 7TA, UK*

Gordon Dent *Department of Thoracic Medicine, National Heart and Lung Institute, London SW3 6LY, UK*

Yigal H. Ehrlich *CSI/IBR Center for Developmental Neuroscience, The City University of New York at the College of Staten Island, New York 10301, USA*

Juan V. Esplugues *Department of Pharmacology, Wellcome Research Laboratories, Langley Court, Beckenham, Kent BR3 3BS, UK*

Giora Z. Feuerstein *Smith, Kline and French Laboratories, 709 Swedeland Road, King of Prussia, Pennsylvania 19406, USA*

Peter M. Henson *Department of Pediatrics, National Jewish Center for Immunology and Respiratory Medicine, Denver, Colorado 80206, USA*

David Hosford *Institut Henri Beaufour Research Laboratories, 17 Avenue Descartes, 92350 Le Plessis-Robinson, France*

John M. Johnston *Department of Biochemistry, University of Texas Southwestern Medical Centre, 5323 Harry Hines Boulevard, Dallas, Texas 75235-9038, USA*

Elizabeth Kornecki, *Department of Anatomy and Cell Biology, State University of New York, Health Science Center at Brookyln, New York 11203, USA*

Ten-ching Lee *Medical and Health Sciences Division, Oak Ridge Associated Universities, Post Office Box 117, Oak Ridge, Tennessee 37831-0117, USA*

Noriei Maki *Department of Obstetrics-Gynecology, University of Texas Southwestern Medical Centre, 5323 Harry Hines Boulevard, Dallas, Texas 75235-9038, USA*

Giuseppe Montrucchio *Laboratorio di Immunopatologia, Universitá di Torino, Italy*

Joseph T. O'Flaherty *Department of Medicine, Bowman Gray School of Medicine, 300 S. Hawthorne Road, Winston-Salem, North Carolina 27103, USA*

Christopher O'Neill *Human Reproduction Unit, Royal North Shore Hospital of Sydney, St Leonards, 2065 New South Wales, Australia*

Clive P. Page *Department of Pharmacology, King's College, Chelsea Campus, London SW3 6LX, UK*

Marek Rola-Pleszczynski *Faculty of Medicine, University of Sherbrooke, 3001 12th Avenue North, Sherbrooke, Quebec J1H 5N4, Canada*

Gennaro Salvidio *Cattedra di' Nefrologia, Universitá di Genoa, Italy*

Frederick Snyder *Medical and Health Sciences Division, Oak Ridge Associated Universities, Post Office Box 117, Oak Ridge, Tennessee 37831-0117, USA*

Ciro Tetta *Laboratorio di Immunopatologia, Universitá di Torino, Italy*

Dieter Ukena *Abteilung für Pneumologie, Medizinische Universitätsklinik und Poliklinik, 6650 Homburg/Saar, FRG*

B. Boris Vargaftig *Unité de Pharmacologie Cellulaire, Unité Associée Institut Pasteur/INSERM No. 285, 25 Rue du Dr Roux, 75015 Paris, France*

Brendan J. R. Whittle *Department of Pharmacology, Wellcome Research Laboratories, Langley Court, Beckenham, Kent BR3 3BS, UK*

Robert L. Wykle *Department of Biochemistry, Wake Forest University Medical Center, Winston-Salem, North Carolina 27103, USA*

Preface

In 1966 Barbaro & Zvaifler [1] demonstrated release of histamine from rabbit platelets during the acute allergic response. It was later shown that this was caused by release of a soluble factor from leukocytes capable of causing platelet activation [2–5]. The cell source in this system was identified as the sensitized rabbit basophil [2,6], the factor was shown to be released by a calcium- and temperature-dependent process [4] and to involve IgE antibody [6]. Accordingly, the mediator became associated conceptually with allergic reactions and, as a consequence, has long been thought of as a potential contributor to such responses. In 1972, the material was named platelet activating factor (PAF), since it was recognized by its potent ability to stimulate platelet aggregation and secretion [6]. During the 1970s, the material was studied as a factor which could be derived from cells of different species, including man, and which was produced by neutrophils, mononuclear phagocytes and other inflammatory cells. Thus, PAF began to be considered as a likely inflammatory, as well as allergic, mediator.

The structure was elucidated by three independent groups in 1979 [7–9] as 1-alkyl-2(*R*)-acetyl-glycerol-3-phosphocholine (Fig. 1) and was subsequently termed either PAF-acether ('ace' for acetate and 'ether' for the alkyl bond) [7], acetylglyceryletherphosphorylcholine (AGEPC) [8], or anti-hypertensive polar reno-medullary lipid (APRL) [9]. The original nomenclature of PAF is now generally accepted and has been used throughout the book, although it is now clear that PAF has many other biological activities in addition to platelet aggregation.

PAF was partially synthesized in 1979 [7] and total synthesis was achieved in 1980 [10]. The major molecular formation exists naturally and has a hexadecyl (C_{16}) alkyl moiety but several other species of molecule have been demonstrated. However, to date, no major differences in function have been found between these different forms. Ether lipids had long been known as constituents of mammalian cell membranes and pathways for their synthesis had been worked out even though their biological role was largely unknown. With the elucidation of PAF as an ether lipid, synthesis of the molecule, and subsequent demonstration of the wide range of effects of the synthetic PAF, a number of pathophysiological activities for this class of lipids have been described.

Although PAF was discovered in the 1960s, it is only relatively recently that interest in this inflammatory lipid mediator has increased dramati-

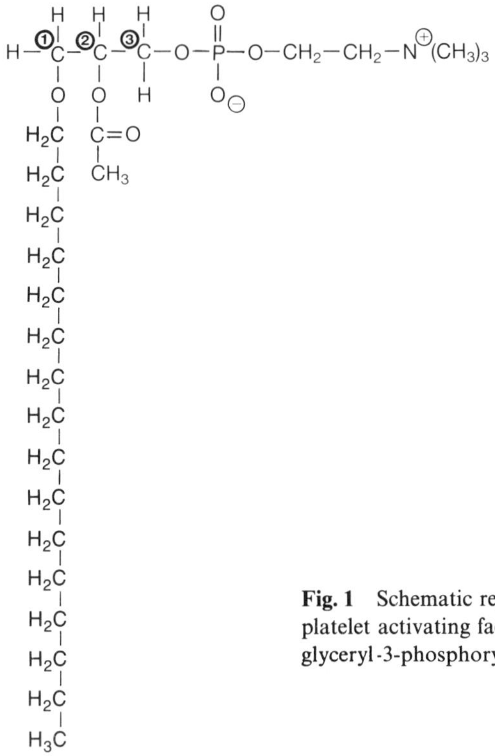

Fig. 1 Schematic representation of the structure of platelet activating factor (PAF), 1-O-alkyl-2-acetyl-*sn*-glyceryl-3-phosphorylcholine.

cally, partly because the attention of the scientific community was focussed on other mediators such as prostaglandins and, more recently, leukotrienes. However, it is now becoming increasingly obvious that PAF has multiple and complex inflammatory effects which may be relevant in many human diseases. One problem which has hampered progress is the difficulty of measuring PAF in biological fluids. Functional assays which measure PAF-like activity may be difficult to interpret in the presence of natural inhibitors or different molecules with the same activity, and radioimmunoassay is not currently possible. Chemical analysis with gas chromatography–mass spectrometry is the only direct measure of PAF, but it is time consuming, expensive and not widely available. In the future, receptor binding competition assays may be the most useful method to adopt.

The recent development of specific PAF antagonists has proved to be a most promising approach and the availability of several drugs of differing chemical structure will greatly advance our understanding of the role of PAF in animal models and in human disease. Of course, it is also likely that these drugs will prove to be useful in the treatment of several inflammatory diseases, including asthma, endotoxic shock, graft rejection and ischaemic diseases. These are all discussed in detail in the various chapters which follow.

PAF may also be involved in physiological processes. Little is yet understood of its function as a local regulator, but it may play a critical role in ovo-implantation and parturition, as is discussed in Chapters 14 and 15. This raises important issues about the long-term effects of PAF antagonists which must be addressed at a later date.

It is likely that, in the future, we will understand much more about the pathways involved in the synthesis and degradation of PAF, and whether or not critical enzymes may be modulated by drugs or in disease states. Advances in molecular techniques and the isolation of the genes which regulate these enzymes will be an important approach. PAF effects appear to be mediated by surface receptors and there is increasing evidence for the existence of sub-types of receptors; receptor cloning will be essential to resolve these issues. Additionally, much of the PAF synthesized in inflammatory cells is retained within the cell, but what effects intra-cellular PAF has on cell function is not yet clear, and further research in this area is important.

With the vast increase in our understanding of PAF and its implication in a whole range of human diseases, we felt that it was timely to bring this wide diversity of information together in a single volume. We hope that this will be helpful for the researcher and also for the clinician. PAF antagonists are now with us and, over the next few years, will be tried in a whole range of diseases. We believe this book might provide a useful framework for their use and provide a stimulus to future research into this fascinating molecule.

Peter J. Barnes *London* *April 1989*
Clive P. Page *London*
Peter M. Henson *Denver*

REFERENCES

1 Barbaro J. F. & Zvaifler, N. J. Antigen induced histamine release from platelets and rabbits producing homologous PCA antibody. *Proc. Soc. Exp. Biol. Med.* (1966), **122**, 1245–1247.

2 Siraganian, R. P. & Osler, A. Destruction of rabbit platelets in the allergic response of sensitized leukocytes: demonstration of a fluid phase intermediate. *J. Immunol.* (1971), **106**, 1244–1251.

3 Siraganian, R. P. & Osler, A. Antigenic release of histamine by rabbit leukocytes. *J Immunol.* (1970), **104**, 1340–1348.

4 Henson, P. M. Role of complement and leukocytes in immunologic release of vasoactive amines from platelets. *Fed. Proc.* (1969), **28**, 1721–1728.

5 Henson, P. M. Release of vasoactive amines from rabbit platelets induced by sensitized mononuclear leukocytes and antigen. *J. Exp. Med.* (1970), **131**, 287–306.

6 Benveniste, J., Henson, P. M. & Cochrane, C. G. Leukocyte dependent histamine release from rabbit platelets: the role of IgE, basophils and a platelet activating factor. *J. Exp. Med.* (1972), **136**, 1356–1377.

7 Benveniste, J., Tence, M., Varenne, P., Bidault, J., Boullet, C. & Polonsky, J. Semi-synthèse et structure proposee du facteur activant les plaquettes (PAF): PAF-acether, un alkyl ether analogue de la lysophosphatidylcholine. *C. Rend. Acad. Sci.* (1979), **289**, 1037–1040.

8 Demopoulos, C. A., Pinckard, R. N. & Hanahan, D. J. Platelet activating factor: evidence for 1-O-alkyl-2-acetyl-*sn*-glyceryl-3-phosphorylcholine as the active component (a new class of lipid chemical mediators). *J. Biol. Chem.* (1979), **254**, 9355–9358.

9 Blank, M. L., Snyder, F., Byers, W. L., Brooks, B. & Muirhead, E. E. Antihypertensive activity of an alkyl ether analog of phosphatidylcholine. *Biochem. Biophys. Res. Comm.* (1979), **90**, 523–534.

10 Godfroid, J. J., Heymans, F., Michel, E., Redeuilh, C., Steiner, E. & Benveniste, J. Platelet activating factor (PAF-acether): total synthesis of 1-O-octadecyl-2-O-acetyl-*sn*-glycero-3-phosphorylcholine. *FEBS Lett.* (1980). **116**, 161–164.

List of abbreviations

ACTH	adrenocorticotrophic hormone
ADP	adenosine diphosphate
AGEPC	acetylglyceryletherphosphorylcholine
AM	alveolar macrophages
AMP	adenosine monophosphate
APRL	anti-hypertensive polar reno-medullary lipid
ARDS	adult respiratory distress syndrome
ATP	adenosine triphosphate
ATPase	adenosine triphosphatase
BHR	bronchial hyper-responsiveness
BSA	bovine serum albumin
cAMP	cyclic adenosine monophosphate
CBF	cerebral blood flow
CDP	cytidine diphosphate
CNS	central nervous system
Con A	concanavalin A
COPD	chronic obstructive pulmonary disease
CRH	corticotropin-releasing hormone
CSA	cyclosporin A
CTL	cytotoxic T-lymphocytes
DHAP	dihydroxyacetonephosphate
DTT	dithiothreitol
ECF	eosinophil chemotactic factor
EDRF	endothelium-derived relaxing factor
EDTA	ethylenediaminetetra-acetic acid
EGTA	ethylene glycol tetra-acetic acid
EPO	eosinophil peroxidase
ETP	epipolythiodioxopiperazine
FABMS	fast-atom bombardment mass spectrometry
fMLP	formyl-methionyl-phenylalanine
GABA	γ-aminobutyric acid
GDP	guanosine diphosphate
GLC	gas-liquid chromatography
GLC/MS	gas-liquid chromatography/mass spectrometry
GMP	glycine monophosphate
GPC	glycerophosphocholine
GPE	glycerophosphorylethanolamine

Gro	glycerol
GTP	guanosine triphosphate
hCG	human chorionic gonadotrophin
HDL	high-density lipoproteins
HEC	human epithelial cells
HES	hypereosinophilic syndrome
HETE	hydroxyicosatetraenoate
HPLC	high-pressure liquid chromatography
5-HT	serotonin (5-hydroxytryptamine)
ICM	inner cell mass
iCRH	immunoreactive corticotropin-releasing hormone
Ig	immunoglobulin
IL	interleukin
INF	interferon
LDL	low-density lipoprotein
LPS	lipopolysaccharide
LT	leukotriene
MDP	muramyl dipeptide
MPO	myeloperoxidase
NADPH	nicotinamide-adenine-dinucleotide phosphate
NKCL	natural killer cytotoxic factor
NMR	nuclear magnetic resonance
PA	phosphatidic acid
PAF	platelet activating factor
PBML	peripheral blood mononuclear leukocytes
PDFG	platelet-derived growth factor
PG	prostaglandin
PGI_2	prostacyclin
PHA	phytohaemagglutinin
PI	phosphatidylinositol
PIP	phosphatidylinositol-4-phosphate
PIP_2	phosphatidylinositol-4,5-bisphosphate
PIP_4	phosphatidylinositol-1,3,4,5-tetraphosphate
PKC	protein kinase C
PL	phospholipase
PLC	phospholipase C
PMA	phorbol-12-myristate-13-acetate
PMN	polymorphonuclear neutrophils
PMNL	polymorphonuclear leukocytes
PMSF	phenylmethanesulfonyl fluoride
PPE	plasma protein extravasation
PRP	platelet-rich plasma
2-PPPC	2-[*N*-palmitoylamino]-propylphosphocholine
3-PPPC	3-[*N*-palmitoylamino]-propylphosphocholine

SHR	spontaneous hypertensive rats
TLC	thin-layer chromatography
TNB	trinitrobenzene sulfonic acid
TNF	tumour necrosis factor
TX	thromboxane
WBC	white blood cells
ZAP	zymosan-activated plasma

Chapter 1
Overview of PAF biosynthesis and catabolism*

Ten-ching Lee and Frederick Snyder

Introduction

Soon after the chemical structure of platelet activating factor (PAF) was described [1–3], the enzymes responsible for catalyzing its synthesis and catabolism were characterized [4]. These and the subsequent studies that led to the complete elucidation of the enzymatic pathways involved in PAF metabolism (Fig. 1.1) were developed from a strong database [5,6]. This was established in the early 1970s from studies of the metabolism of the long-chain alkylacyl and alk-1-enylacyl types of phospholipids that contain choline and ethanolamine polar head groups. In this overview, we cover the following topics related to PAF metabolism: enzymatic pathways, cellular and *in vivo* metabolism, regulatory controls, enzyme inhibitors, and strategies for pharmacological intervention in PAF-related diseases. Emphasis is on work reported during the past several years since earlier studies of PAF metabolism have already been covered in depth [7–14].

* This work was supported by the Office of Energy Research, US Department of Energy (Contract No. DE-AC05-76OR00033), the American Cancer Society (Grant BC-7OT), and the National Heart, Lung, and Blood Institute (Grants HL-27109-08 and HL-35495-03).

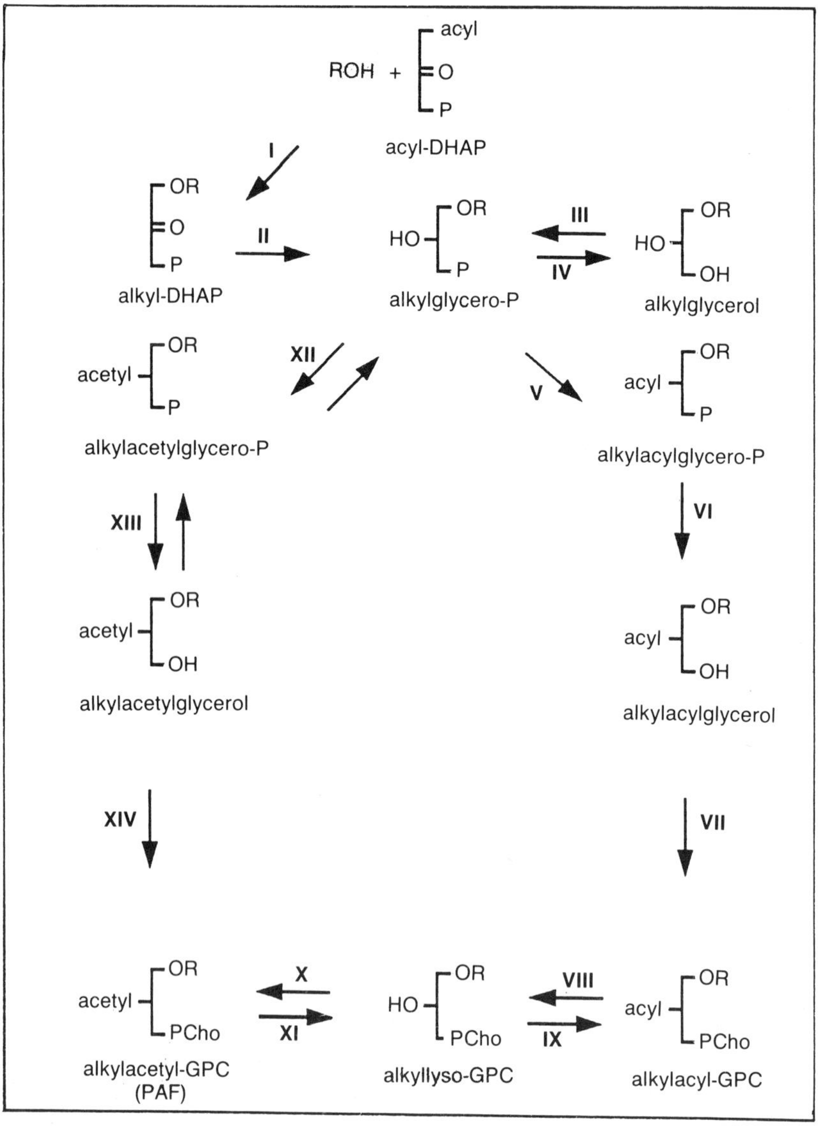

Fig. 1.1 Metabolic pathway for the biosynthesis of O-alkyl phospholipids that contain choline. The Roman numerals refer to the following enzymes: **I** alkyl-DHAP synthase (EC 2.5.1.26); **II** NADPH:alkyl-DHAP oxidoreductase (EC 1.1.1.101); **III** ATP:1-alkyl-*sn*-glycerol phosphotransferase (EC 2.7.1.93), **IV** 1-alkyl-*sn*-glycero-3-P phosphohydrolase; **V** acyl-CoA:1-alkyl-2-lyso-*sn*-glycero-3-P acyltransferase (2.3.1.63); **VI** 1-alkyl-2-acyl-*sn*-glycero-3-P phosphohydrolase; **VII** CDP-choline:1-alkyl-2-acyl-*sn*-glycerol DTT-sensitive cholinephosphotransferase (EC 2.7.8.2); **VIII** phospholipase A_2; **IX** polyenoic acid transacylase; **X** acetyl CoA:1-alkyl-2-lyso-*sn*-glycero-3-phosphocholine acetyltransferase (EC 2.3.1.67); **XI** 1-alkyl-2-acetyl-*sn*-glycero-3-phosphocholine acetylhydrolase (EC 3.1.1.48); **XII** acetyl-CoA:1-alkyl-2-lyso-*sn*-glycero-3-P acetyltransferase; **XIII** 1-alkyl-2-acetyl-*sn*-glycero-3-P phosphohydrolase; and **XIV** CDP-choline:1-alkyl-2-acetyl-*sn*-glycerol DTT-insensitive cholinephosphotransferase. Reproduced with permission from Snyder *et al.* [102].

General pathways of ether lipid metabolism

Formation of the alkyl ether bond in glycerolipids

In order to understand better the only two known routes of PAF biosynthesis, it is essential to have some grasp of the overall pathway of ether lipid metabolism that was originally delineated in the early 1970s. The initial reaction forming the O-alkyl linkage at the *sn*-1 position of the *sn*-glycerol moiety of phospholipids is catalysed by alkyldihydroxyacetone-P (DHAP) synthase; the reaction between acyl-DHAP and fatty alcohols in this step involves the replacement of the entire acyl group of acyl-DHAP with a long-chain fatty alcohol. Alkyl-DHAP synthase is of peroxisomal origin in most cells, but exceptions are known such as Ehrlich ascites cells where peroxisomes appear to be absent. Researchers in the laboratories of Hajra, Friedburg and Snyder made significant contributions leading to our understanding of the reaction catalysed by alkyl-DHAP synthase; the reader is referred to two reviews on this subject that provide referencing to the original publications [5,6].

Two important features of the reaction catalysed by alkyl-DHAP synthase include: (i) an exchange of the pro-R hydrogen at C-1 of the DHAP moiety of acyl-DHAP with water but without any change in the stereochemical configuration at this position; and (ii) the complete cleavage of the RCOO-group of acyl-DHAP before the RO-group of the fatty alcohol is added. Kinetic data implicate a 'ping-pong' type of reaction with a DHAP–enzyme complex proposed as an intermediate. This mechanism is substantiated by the fact that either fatty acids or fatty alcohols can react with the proposed enzyme–DHAP intermediate to produce acyl-DHAP or alkyl-DHAP, respectively. It has also been clearly documented that both oxygens of the acyl group in acyl-DHAP end up with the fatty acid product formed in the cleavage step and that the oxygen of the ether bond is derived from the substituted fatty alcohol. Furthermore, experiments done with a highly purified preparation of alkyl-DHAP synthase have shown this enzyme does not possess any intrinsic acyl-DHAP hydrolase activity as originally thought.

Surprisingly, alkyl-DHAP synthase has a broad range of substrate specificities despite the fact that native alkyl chains exhibit limited carbon chain lengths (mainly 16:0, 18:0 and 18:1) and virtually no polyunsaturation. O-alk-1-enyl chains in plasmalogens mirror the native alkyl chains found in alkylacylglycerophosphoethanolamines, their immediate precursors. The reason for the narrow range of ether-linked aliphatic moieties encountered in nature appears to be due to the high degree of specificity of the acyl-CoA reductase that catalyses the conversion of acyl-CoAs to the fatty alcohols, the precursor of the O-alkyl moiety.

Conversion of alkyl-DHAP to alkylacylglycerophosphocholines

Alkyl-DHAP is converted to a membrane phospholipid constituent (Fig. 1.1) through a reaction sequence involving: (i) the reduction of the ketone group by an NADPH-oxidoreductase to form the lyso-alkyl analogue of phosphatidic acid; (ii) acylation of this lyso intermediate to the alkyl analogue of phosphatidic acid by an acyl-CoA acyltransferase; (iii) dephosphorylation of the alkyl phosphatidate by a phosphohydrolase to an alkylacylglycerol product; and (iv) a final step catalysing the transfer of the phosphocholine moiety from CDP-choline to alkylacylglycerol to form alkylacylglycerophosphocholine by a DTT-sensitive cholinephosphotransferase. All of the enzymes in these reactions are membrane-bound. Alkylacylglycerophosphocholines, the final product of this sequence of steps, have a dual function since they serve as an important membrane constituent in many cells, as well as being a stored precursor of two bioactive lipids, PAF and arachidonic acid mediators, in the remodelling pathway (see below).

PAF biosynthesis

Stored precursors

PAF is synthesized by either remodelling or *de novo* pathways. The stored precursor for the remodelling pathway is alkylacyl-GPC (see below), while alkyllysoglycero-P is the direct precursor for the *de novo* route (see below). No information is available about the pool size of precursors in the *de novo* synthetic route. On the other hand, considerable data are available on the

Table 1.1 Alkylacyl-GPC content in mammalian cells that synthesize PAF*

Cell types	Reference	Alkylacyl-GPC (pmol/10^6 cells)	Percentage of total diradyl-GPC
Fibroblasts	[98]	0.7	N.A.
Platelets	[20,101]	5.5–70	4.5–18.0
Endothelial cells	[99]	N.A.	4.6
Monocytes	[20,101]	400	N.A.
PMN	[20,101]		
peritoneal		860–910	16–46
blood		1110–1630	44–50
Macrophages	[20,101]	2600–7400	14–35
Eosinophils	[100]	2900	76

* Results are summarized from the recent reviews by Lee [20] and Sugiura & Waku [101] unless otherwise stated.
N.A. = Not available.

Table 1.2 Alkylarachidonoyl-GPC content of mammalian cells that synthesize PAF*

Cell types	Alkylarachidonyl-GPC (pmol/10^6 cells)	Percentage of *sn*-2-acyl groups as 20 : 4
Platelets		
rabbit	5	20.9
human	6	43.7
PMN		
rabbit (peritoneal)	12	1.3
human (blood)	156	10.4
rat (peritoneal)	N.A.	26.4
guinea pig (peritoneal)	18	2.1
Macrophages		
rabbit (alveolar)	2850	38.6–51.5
guinea pig (peritoneal)	75	2.9

* Data are compiled from reviews by Lee [20] and Snyder *et al.* [102].
N.A. = Not available.

content of alkylacyl-GPC in cells that synthesize PAF through the remodelling pathway (Table 1.1). Since alkylarachidonoyl-GPC is converted to PAF in human polymorphonuclear leukocytes (PMNL) stimulated with calcium ionophore [15] and PAF synthesis is inhibited in PMNL depleted of arachidonic acid [16], alkylarachidonoyl-GPC has been proposed as the necessary precursor of PAF (see the discussion below on regulatory controls). Table 1.2 shows there is a wide range in the concentrations of total alkylacyl-GPC, including alkylarachidonoyl-GPC, in different cell types. Noticcably, rabbit alveolar macrophages and human eosinophils have the highest alkylacyl-GPC content of all cells studied so far. It is likely that the total amount of PAF synthesized through the remodelling pathway is directly related to the pool size of alkylacyl-GPC/alkylarachidonoyl-GPC in a particular cell type.

Remodelling route

Biosynthesis of PAF through the remodelling route involves the hydrolysis of a long-chain acyl group from alkylacyl-GPC by a phospholipase A_2 to form alkyllyso-GPC, followed by the acetylation of alkyllyso-GPC by alkyllyso-GPC:acetyl-CoA acetyltransferase to produce PAF. Even though ample indirect evidence suggests a role of phospholipase A_2 in the formation of PAF, no unique phospholipase A_2 responsible for catalysing the specific hydrolysis of the *sn*-2 fatty acyl group of alkylacyl-GPC has yet been identified. On the other hand, considerable information has been gathered about alkyllyso-GPC: acetyl-CoA acetyltransferase.

Alkyllyso-GPC:acetyl-CoA acetyltransferase was first characterized in rat spleen microsomes [17]. Subsequently, substrate specificity [18] and partial purification [19] of this enzyme have been reported. The activity of acetyltransferase increases in parallel with enhanced production of PAF in different cell types stimulated with a variety of agonists. Cells that can be stimulated by agonists to produce PAF and activate acetyltransferase activity have been summarized [20]. In general, most inflammatory agents induce PAF production and increase acetyltransferase activity in certain blood cell types. Recently, an increase in PAF formation along with acetyltransferase activity was also demonstrated in ionophore A23187-stimulated chick retina [21], carbamoylcholine-treated guinea-pig parotid glands [22], tumour necrosis factor-stimulated rat peritoneal macrophages, rat PMNL and human endothelial cells [23], interleukin 1α-treated human endothelial cells [24], and PAF-treated rat PMNL [25].

Activation of acetyltransferase by some of the agonists is achieved through the phosphorylation of the enzyme, with the dephosphorylated form of the enzyme being inactive [22,26–28]. In addition, Gomez-Cambronero *et al.* [19] demonstrated that a serine residue of 30-kDa protein in a partially-purified acetyltransferase preparation from rat spleen microsomes is phosphorylated by cyclic AMP-dependent protein kinase *in vitro* with increased enzyme activity. However, increase in the acetyltransferase activity in tumour necrosis factor-treated human endothelial cells was thought to be due to net synthesis of the enzyme rather than to its activation, because the increase in acetyltransferase activity could be blocked by pretreatment of human endothelial cells with cycloheximide; also PAF synthesis in response to tumour necrosis factor was inhibited by cycloheximide and actinomycin D [24].

De novo route

The *de novo* pathway, beginning with alkyl-DHAP as the starting point (see above), requires the participation of four enzymes: NADPH:alkyl-DHAP oxidoreductase, alkyllyso-GP:acetyl CoA acetyltransferase, alkyl-acetyl-GP phosphohydrolase and dithiothreitol-insensitive alkylacetyl-glycerol:CDP-choline cholinephosphotransferase. Initially, NADPH: alkyl-DHAP oxidoreductase catalyses the formation of alkyllyso-GP from alkyl-DHAP [5,6]. Alkyllyso-GP is an important branch point intermediate in the *de novo* biosynthesis of PAF and ether-containing lipids with a long-chain acyl group at the *sn*-2 position of glycerol. It is not clear at present whether the same enzyme can catalyse both the acetylation or acylation of alkyllyso-GP. However, it appears that alkyllyso-GP: acetyl-CoA acetyltransferase differs from the acetyltransferase responsible for the transfer of acetate from acetyl-CoA to alkyllyso-GPC to form PAF in the remodelling pathway [29]. Likewise, the activity of alkylacetyl-GP phosphohydrolase can be distinguished from the activity of a non-specific phosphomonoesterase or phosphatidate phosphohydrolase [30] and the cholinephosphotransferases catalysing the formation of PAF and phosphatidylcholine appear to be two separate enzymes [31,32].

The notion that the *de novo* pathway is important for the production of PAF at basal physiological levels comes from the following observations: (i) in leukocytes [33] or rabbit platelets [34], the dithiothreitol-insensitive cholinephosphotransferasc is not affected by inflammatory stimuli, while the alkyllyso-GPC:acetyl-CoA acetyltransferase is increased several-fold by these agents; (ii) [^{3}H] alkylacetylglycerol can be converted into PAF in intact rabbit platelets [35,36] and rat glomerular mesangial cells [37], and (iii) the specific activities of enzymes involved in the *de novo* pathway are high in most tissues and the activity of alkyllyso-GPC:acetyl-CoA acetyltransferase, the remodelling enzyme, is very low in rat kidneys [32] and glandular mucosa [38] tissues, which maintain a basal level of PAF.

A branch of the *do novo* pathway can also lead to the synthesis of alkylacetylacylglycerols, conceivably a neutral storage form of acetylated lipids [39]. This enzyme activity, which has been observed both in microsomal preparations and in intact cells, has a preference for acylating linoleic acid at the *sn*-3 position of glycerol. The acyltransferase that catalyses the acylation of alkylacetylglycerols exhibits different properties from those of the acyltransferase that utilizes long-chain diacylglycerols as substrates.

Enzyme inhibitors

Known inhibitors of enzymes involved in the *de novo* pathway of PAF biosynthesis are limited. However, there are several reports regarding inhibitors of alkyllyso-GPC:acetyl-CoA acetyltransferase, the acetylating enzyme in the remodelling pathway. Ketotifen, a prophylactic anti-asthma drug, inhibits the antigen-induced formation and release of PAF, release of granular contents, stimulation of alkyllyso-GPC:acetyl-CoA acetyltransferase and Ca^{2+} entry in mast cells derived from mouse bone marrow [40]. However, the ionophore A23187-induced Ca^{2+} influx and acetyltransferase stimulation were not inhibited by ketotifen. These results suggested that ketotifen acts at a very early stage of immunological activation, i.e. Ca^{2+} entry, instead of on acetyltransferase *per se*.

Alkyllyso-GPC:acetyl-CoA acetyltransferase from rat spleen microsomes, after solublization in 25% glycerol, was markedly inhibited by *p*-chloromercuribenzenesulfonic acid and *N*-ethylmaleimide; these results indicate that the enzyme requires an -SH group for activity [41]. In addition, palmitoyllyso-GPC is a competitive inhibitor in the reaction with respect to the concentration dependence of alkyllyso-GPC [18]; 2-methyl-lyso-PAF, which can serve as substrate in the acetyltransferase assay system and be acetylated, also inhibits alkyllyso-GPC:acetyl-CoA acetyltransferase reaction [42]. *p*-Bromophenacyl bromide, Triton X-100, or pre-incubation of the microsomes with diisopropylfluorophosphate also inhibit the remodelling acetyltransferase activity [17].

Two amphipathic compounds, 2-[*N*-palmitoylamino]-propylphosphocholine (2-PPPC) and 3-[*N*-palmitoylamino]propylphosphocholine (3-PPPC), inhibit PAF synthesis in intact mouse peritoneal leukocytes stimulated with ionophore A23187. When these inhibitors were incubated with microsomal acetyltransferase from rat spleen, IC_{50} values of 5 μM were obtained. However, a similar structural analogue, *N*-palmitoylaminoethylphosphocholine, inhibited both acetyltransferase and phospholipase A_2. Therefore, 2-PPPC and 3-PPPC do not appear to be very specific inhibitors of acetyltransferase and they may also inhibit phospholipase A_2 activities [43].

PAF catabolism

Intact cells

Catabolism of PAF has been studied in a variety of cell types. In human leukemia HL-60 cells [44], Madin Darby canine kidney cells [44], rabbit platelets [45,46] and rabbit [47] and human [48] neutrophils, the major metabolite from PAF is alkylacyl-GPC, with only a small amount of alkyllyso-GPC appearing as a transient intermediate. On the other hand, alkylacyl-GPC and alkyllyso-GPC are the major metabolites in human platelets [49], human endothelial cells [50], rat alveolar macrophages [51] and rat glomerular mesangial cells [37]; alkyllyso-GPC accumulates mainly in the media, whereas alkylacyl-GPC is predominantly associated with cellular lipids [50,51]. In addition, alkylacyl-GPC formed from PAF is highly enriched in polyenoic acids ($\geqslant$4 double bonds) in both rabbit [45] and human [52] platelets, human neutrophils [48], rat alveolar macrophages [51] and neonatal rat myocytes [53]. However, dienoic fatty acids (55 %) are the major fatty acids incorporated into the *sn*-2 position of alkylacyl-GPC in rabbit neutrophils [47]. When human leukemia HL-60 cells [44] and rabbit platelets [45,54] were incubated with [^{3}H]PAF in the presence of unlabelled alkyllyso-GPC, the formation of [^{3}H]alkylacyl-GPC was decreased with a concomitant build-up of [^{3}H]alkyllyso-GPC. Furthermore, the molecular species composition of [^{3}H]alkylacyl-GPC derived from PMNL incubated with [^{3}H]PAF was identical to that obtained from PMNL incubated with [^{3}H]alkyllyso-GPC [47,48]. These data indicate that PAF is inactivated (via acetylhydrolase) to form alkyllyso-GPC, which is subsequently converted to alkylacyl-GPC (via transacylase) (also see below).

In cultured rat hepatocytes, a significant amount of PAF was converted into alkylglycerols with alkylacyl-GPC, alkyllyso-GPC, and fatty aldehydes as minor products [55]. These authors proposed that the de-acetylation–re-acylation step is not the main metabolic pathway of PAF in these cells, but instead a lysosomal phospholipase C, which hydrolyses the phosphocholine from alkyllyso-GPC, is responsible for the generation of alkylglycerols. Alkylglycerols were also detected in cultured neonatal myocytes, but at a higher concentration of PAF or alkyllyso-GPC ($\geqslant 2 \times 10^{-7}$M) [53] than those used by Okayasu *et al.* [55]. Sodium fluoride, a phosphatase inhibitor, partially blocked the conversion of alkyllyso-GPC to alkylglycerol with a concomitant accumulation of alkyllyso-GP; these data suggest that the accumulation of alkylglycerols generated from alkyllyso-GPC in neonatal rat myocytes is due to the combined actions of lysophospholipase D and a phosphatase.

Enzymes

Alkylacetyl-GPC acetylhydrolase

Alkylacetyl-GPC acetylhydrolase catalyses the inactivation of PAF by removal of the acetate moiety from PAF to form alkyllyso-GPC which is biologically inactive. Two forms of acetylhydrolase, one intracellular [56] and the other in plasma [57–61], have been described. Both types of acetylhydrolase do not require Ca^{2+} for activity and since they are not inhibited by the addition of EDTA or phosphatidylcholine, both forms of the acetylhydrolase are thought to be distinctly different from typically reported phospholipase A_2 activities. Also, both acetylhydrolases are severely inhibited by diisopropylfluorophosphate [56,60].

There are subtle biochemical differences between tissue and plasma acetylhydrolases. For example, tissue acetylhydrolase has a broad pH optimum, between 7.5 and 8.5 [56], and is sensitive to trypsin, pronase and subtilisin treatments, while rat plasma acetylhydrolase has a pH optimum of 7.4 and is insensitive to proteases [57]. However, pH optimum for 500-fold purified acetylhydrolase from human serum and 25 000-fold purified acetylhydrolase from human plasma was 6.2 [61] and 7.5 [59], respectively. Human serum acetylhydrolase is pronase- and trypsin-sensitive, but papain-resistant [61]. In addition, the molecular weight of the cytosolic acetylhydrolase from rat kidney cortex has been reported to be 100 000 [5], whereas the acetylhydrolase from human plasma has a molecular weight of 43 000 [60].

Acetylhydrolase exhibits low substrate specificity for the *sn*-1 position of PAF since the enyzme is not markedly dependent on the type of bond, i.e. ester versus ether at the *sn*-1 position [56,60,61]. With an acyl chain at the *sn*-1 position, the carbon chain length has to be >10 in order to be a substrate [61]. In contrast, the acetylhydrolase shows a strong specificity for the residue at the *sn*-2 position. Hydrolysis is maximal with the acetyl group and decreases 18-fold when the acyl chain is extended by a single methylene group; activity becomes minimal when the acyl group is increased to six carbons [60,61]. Moreover, the enzyme has an absolute requirement for an ester linkage at the *sn*-2 position of the glycerol backbone, since alkylethyl-GPC, at concentrations up to 40 μM, did not inhibit the hydrolysis of its ester analogue of PAF [60]. Acetylhydrolase can also act on PAF analogues with modified polar head groups [56,60], except one report did indicate alkylacetyl-GPE could not serve as a substrate [61].

Plasma acetylhydrolase activity is found exclusively in lipoprotein fractions, with two-thirds associated with the low-density lipoproteins (LDL) and one-third with the high-density lipoproteins (HDL) [62]. The LDL-associated activity accounts for all of the PAF degradation that occurs in plasma, *ex vivo*, whereas the HDL-associated enzyme is inactive. Nevertheless, the PAF-acetylhydrolase activity can be transferred between apo-B containing LDL to apo-E containing HDL in a pH-dependent manner.

Recently, Suzuki *et al.* [63] reported that cellular acetylhydrolase was released into the supernatant after treating bovine platelets with 0.1–10 nM PAF; maximal release was attained at 10 nM PAF with 80% of total cellular acetylhydrolase being secreted into the media. The activity of released acetylhydrolase was not affected by Ca^{2+} or EDTA, but was inhibited by the PAF antagonists CV-3988 and ONO-6240 with K_i values of 1.17 μM and 0.84 μM, respectively. The release of acetylhydrolase was also detected when the platelets were stimulated with ADP and thrombin. These data suggested that the structure of the active PAF-binding site in acetylhydrolase might be similar to that of PAF receptors. In addition, the acetylhydrolase release from the aggregated platelets may cooperate with the plasma acetylhydrolase in controlling the physiological levels of PAF in blood.

Acylation and transacylation of alkyllyso-GPC

Three different mechanisms have been described for the acylation of alkyllyso-GPC to produce alkylacyl-GPC with membrane or microsomal preparations. These include: (i) an acyl-CoA dependent acylation [64–68]; (ii) a CoA-dependent transacylation [66–69]; and (iii) a CoA-independent transacylation [52,66–69]. Experiments conducted with the addition of only CoA (CoA-dependent transacylation), CoA plus ATP/Mg^{2+} (acyl-CoA acyltransferase), or no cofactors (CoA-independent transacylation) to microsomal preparations along with exogenous alkyllyso-GPC have demonstrated that the molecular species composition of alkylacyl-GPC formed by the three different acylation pathways differ. CoA-independent transacylation produces a high percentage of polyunsaturated molecular species, i.e. 16:0–22:6, 16:0–22:5 ($n-3$) and 16:0–20:4; acyl-CoA dependent acylation generates the least polyunsaturated molecular species; and CoA-dependent transacylation gives intermediate values of unsaturation [66,68,70]. In CoA-independent transacylations, the polyunsaturated groups (22:6, 22:4, 20:5 ($n-3$), 20:4) for the acylation of alkyllyso-GPC are derived from diacyl-GPC [69,71,72], with the transfer rates of 16:0, 18:0 and 18:1 from diacyl-GPC to alkyllyso-GPC being very slow [69].

In intact cells, CoA-independent transacylase probably plays an important role in contributing to the formation of alkylacyl-GPC, because alkylacyl-GPC generated from PAC inactivation in most cells is highly enriched with polyenoic fatty acids (see above). Diacyl-GPC is the source of the arachidonic acid used to acylate the alkyllyso-GPC intermediate formed when PAF is inactivated by rabbit whole platelets [45].

Phospholipase C

A phospholipase C which catalyses the hydrolysis of PAF to alkylacetyl-Gro (glycerol) and phosphocholine was purified to near homogeneity from rabbit liver lysosomes [73]. This enzyme consisted of two forms, having a p*I* of 4.7 and 5.8 with an apparent molecular weight of 33 000 and 75 000, respectively. It differed from the rat liver lysosomal phospholipase C described by Matsuzawa & Hostetler [74] in that the rabbit liver lysosomal phospholipase C had an alkaline optimum pH (8.2–8.5); also it was inhibited by EDTA and restored to the original level upon addition of Ca^{2+}. Furthermore, the PAF-related enzyme from rabbit liver lysosomes appeared to be relatively specific for ether-linked lipids. Other phospholipids (i.e. phosphatidyl-choline, -ethanolamine, -serine and -inositol; sphingomyelin, phosphatidic acid and alkyllyso-GPC) are hydrolyzed at about 20–30% of the rate found for PAF. However, it is not clear at present whether this phospholipase C is the same as the one that converts alkyllyso-GPC to alkylglycerol in rat hepatocytes as proposed by Okayasu *et al.* [55].

Lysophospholipase D and phosphohydrolase

An alternative route for the generation of alkylglycerols from alkyllyso-GPC as reported in neonatal rat myocytes [53] is through the combined actions of lysophospholipase D and a phosphohydrolase. Lysophospholipase D catalyses the hydrolysis of choline from alkyllyso-GPC to form alkyllyso-GP which is subsequently dephosphorylated to produce alkylglycerols by a phosphohydrolase [75].

Lysophospholipase D acts specifically on ether-containing lysophospholipids [76,77]. This enzyme only hydrolyzes ethanolamine or choline from alkyl(alk-1-enyl)lyso-GPE or alkyllyso-GPC, respectively, but does not utilize acyllyso-GPC(-GPE) or alkylacylphospholipids as substrates. There are two types of lysophospholipase D based on metal requirements: the Mg^{2+}-dependent lysophospholipase D with a pH optimum at 7.2 [75] is the major activity in rat tissues, whereas a Ca^{2+}-dependent enzyme with optimal activity at pH 8.4 is predominant in rabbit tissues [78].

Phosphohydrolases that utilize alkyllyso-GP as the substrate are present in microsomal preparations from rat brain and mouse preputial gland tumours and lysosomes from rat liver [5]. These activities can be maximally inhibited by NaF at concentrations > 40 mM; other properties of the enzyme have not been characterized in detail.

Pte·H$_4$-dependent alkyl monooxygenase

The only report suggesting that a Pte·H_4-dependent alkyl monooxygenase (Pte = pteridine) might play a role in the catabolism of PAF in intact cells was by Okayasu *et al.* [55] who showed that fatty aldehydes were one of the metabolic products formed when PAF was incubated with rat hepatocytes. Tietz *et al.* [79] were the first to demonstrate that alkylglycerols can be degraded by a Pte·H_4-dependent alkyl monooxygenase in the microsomes of rat livers to generate free glycerol and fatty aldehydes. Subsequently, this enzyme was purified to near homogeneity with an apparent molecular weight of 45 000 daltons, a pH optimum of 8.5, and a requirement for reduced glutathione and phospholipids for the full expression of enzyme activity [80]. Results on the Pte·H_4 requirement, tissue distribution, and responses to thermal inactivation and inhibitors indicate that the same enzyme is also responsible for the cleavage of alkyllyso-GPC to form fatty aldehyde and glycero-3-phosphocholine [81]. Therefore, it is possible the fatty aldehydes detected in rat hepatocytes could be derived from PAF by the alkyl monooxygenase utilizing either alkyllyso-GPC and/or alkylglycerol as the substrates.

Regulatory controls

Whereas some progress has been made in our understanding of the regulation of the enzyme responsible for the metabolism of PAF and related ether-linked lipids, there is still a paucity of information on this subject. To a large extent this is due to the fact that most of the PAF-related enzymes are membrane-associated, and therefore, purification for the detailed characterization of their properties and regulatory features has been difficult to achieve. However, some success has been made in sorting out the rate-limiting steps in the biosynthesis of PAF and in identifying factors that can influence the metabolism of PAF either by direct effects on specific PAF enzymes or through their influence on intermediary steps in the overall ether lipid pathway.

Calcium (Ca^{2+}) is of major importance in controlling PAF metabolism since it can modulate the activities of most of the enzymes involved in the biosynthesis of PAF, in addition to affecting the formation of some PAF precursors and PAF catabolic enzymes. This divalent cation inhibits all of the enzymes in the *de novo* pathway of PAF biosynthesis [29,30,32], whereas it is required in the remodelling route [82–84]. In addition, Ca^{2+} also is a potent inhibitor of the DTT-sensitive cholinephosphotransferase [85]. Moreover, Ca^{2+} can affect the activity of enzymes involved in the catabolism of PAF metabolites; for example, lysophospholipase D in rabbit tissues has an absolute requirement for Ca^{2+} [78], whereas the de-acetylation and transacylation steps [86] as well as the Pte·H_4-dependent alkyl cleavage enzyme [87] are inhibited by Ca^{2+}. Obviously, small changes in the micro-environment of Ca^{2+} levels in cells could have a profound influence on most of the enzymes that control the intracellular concentrations of PAF.

Factors others than Ca^{2+} are also important in the regulation of PAF metabolism. Enzymatic studies have clearly shown that thiol compounds influence the cholinephosphotransferase in the *de novo* pathway [32] and that pH optima for the enzymes in the *de novo* [29,30,32] and remodelling routes differ [17]. Compartmentalization of PAF enzymes must also be of significance in governing PAF metabolism; however, very little is known about the precise organelle distribution or the membrane orientation of the enzymes and the lipid precursors they utilize. In addition, endogenous inhibitors of PAF-induced responses must be considered in the context of regulatory controls. Such inhibitors have been found in the liver [88] and uterus of rats [89]. In the latter report, acyllyso-GPC, alkyllyso-GPC and *N*-acyl-sphingo-4-enyl-phosphocholine [89] were shown to suppress biological activities of PAF. The presence of endogenous inhibitors can especially complicate the interpretation of PAF-induced biological responses since such lipids often have chromatographic mobilities similar to PAF and, therefore, when PAF is isolated in some chromatography systems for biological testing, endogenous inhibitors might also be present in the same preparation.

Catabolic enzymes are obviously of a vital importance in PAF regulation; this is especially true for acetylhydrolase, the enzyme that inactivates PAF by catalysing the hydrolysis of the acetate moiety. Detailed studies regarding the regulatory significance of acetylhydrolase have not been conducted but it is apparent that this enzyme is important in controlling PAF levels in both the plasma and intracellular compartments. Other catabolic enzymes such as lysophospholipase D [75–78] and the Pte·H_4-dependent alkyl cleavage enzyme [81] can be important in regulating the PAF precursor pool of ether-linked phospholipids in membranes since their combined activities can effectively decrease the total cellular levels of ether-linked lipid precursors of PAF. However, any effect on the pool size of PAF precursors due to these latter enzymes would only appear to be relevant over a sustained period.

Enzyme activation provides an important regulatory mechanism of PAF biosynthesis in the PAF cycle. The acetyltransferase in the remodelling pathway must first be phosphorylated to be catalytically active and inactivation occurs through dephosphorylation by a phosphohydrolase [19,22,26–28,90]. Although the precise biochemical mechanism for this activation is unknown, it appears that the phosphorylation requires a cAMP dependent kinase in some systems [27,90] and in others a calcium-calmodulin dependent protein kinase has been implicated [22]. The phosphorus label in [γ^{32}P]ATP is thought to be transferred to a serine residue in the acetyltransferase [19].

McIntyre *et al.* [91] have also proposed that an activation step is required for the expression of phospholipase A_2 activity in the remodelling pathway. Their studies suggest protein kinase C might be responsible since long-chain amine inhibitors of protein kinase C do not alter acetyltransferase activity in the remodelling pathway but they do inhibit PAF production when cells are stimulated with calcium ionophore. Furthermore, the inhibition of PAF production under these conditions can be reversed if protein kinase C is activated by phorbol-12-myristate-13-acetate (PMA) even though direct activation of protein kinase C with PMA does not increase PAF synthesis. The conclusion reached from these results is that protein kinase C activity is required for coupling a rise in intracellular Ca^{2+} to the initiation of the synthesis of PAF and eicosanoid mediators.

Rate-limiting steps in the *de novo* pathway are thought to be catalysed by the cytidylyltransferase that provides the precursor (CDP-choline) of the polar head group of PAF [92] and the acetyltransferase [29] responsible for catalysing the initial step to formation of the lipid moiety (alkylacetylglycerol) of PAF in this pathway. Evidence for the *de novo* acetyltransferase step being rate limiting is based on the fact that it exhibits the lowest reaction rates of all the enzymes in the *de novo* pathway [29]. The rate-limiting reaction catalysed by cytidylyltransferase has been documented in experiments that have shown when this enzyme is activated through translocation of its activity from the cytosol to microsomal membranes (induced by oleic acid), a 7- to 8-fold increase in PAF synthesis occurs [92]. Also studies done with permeabilized rabbit platelets (saponin-treated) have demonstrated that the addition of exogenous CDP-choline to incubations containing the permeabilized cells significantly increases the amount of PAF synthesized when compared to control values (unpublished). PMA has also been reported to stimulate PAF biosynthesis via the *de novo* pathway [93] and this also is undoubtedly explained in terms of the ability of PMA to activate cytidylyltransferase [94]. It has been known from earlier work [94] that cytidylytransferase also catalyses the rate-controlling reaction in the biosynthesis of phosphatidylcholine. Thus, cytidylyltransferase plays a major role in controlling both the production of phospholipid membrane constituents, as well as phospholipid cell mediators.

Conclusions from several laboratories based on data obtained with HL-60 cells and neutrophils as models have indicated that phospholipase A_2 catalyses the rate-limiting reaction in the remodelling pathway and that arachidonic acid is an important regulator of the remodelling route. First, results by Billah & co-workers [95] have shown differentiated HL-60 cells can produce PAF when stimulated with calcium ionophore, whereas undifferentiated HL-60 cells are unable to synthesize PAF even though the acetyltransferase activities in the undifferentiated and differentiated HL-60 cells are the same. Secondly, Ramasha & Pickett [16] found that when rat polymorphonuclear leukocytes are depleted of arachidonic acid, they are unable to produce PAF upon stimulation with calcium ionophore. These investigators suggested the defect might be explained on the basis of a phospholipase A_2 that is highly selective for arachidonoyl species of the alkylacyl-GPC precursor of PAF. Finally, more detailed follow-up studies by Kawasaki *et al.* [96] with 20:4-depleted and 20:4-supplemented HL-60 cells (after differentiation into a granulocytic form) demonstrated the supplementation of these cells with arachidonic acid-stimulated PAF production 3- to 5-fold over unsupplemented or 18:1-supplemented control cells. PAF production in these experiments was assessed by stimulating the cells with ionophore A23187 and then measuring the incorporation of [^{3}H]acetate into the PAF produced. Cyclooxygenase and lipoxygenase inhibitors had very little effect on the increased production of PAF in the 20:4-supplemented cells, whereas phospholipase A_2 inhibitors caused up to a 95% reduction in the formation of PAF [97]. The inhibitor data strongly suggest an arachidonoyl-specific phospholipase A_2 is responsible in the initiating step of the remodelling pathway of PAF biosynthesis; moreover, the results obtained with cells depleted of arachidonic acid further indicate this reaction can be rate limiting.

Potential metabolic targets for pharmacological intervention in PAF-related diseases

The excessively high levels of PAF produced in the remodelling pathway of PAF biosynthesis have been implicated as a contributing factor in a variety of diseases. Thus, therapeutic strategies to date have led to the development of a variety of antagonists [7] that are capable of blocking receptor-mediated responses of PAF. In clinical investigations these receptor antagonists have shown considerable promise in the treatment of asthma (see Chapter 7). However, an alternative approach in the treatment of PAF-related diseases is to inhibit the biosynthesis of the excessive amounts of PAF formed through biosynthesis via the remodelling pathway in cells exposed to inflammatory stimuli, i.e. block a crucial enzymatic step in the formation of PAF. Such an approach seems pragmatic since the specific enzyme activities in the *de novo* and remodelling routes appear to be catalysed by distinctly different proteins and these enzymes also differ from all others known to be involved in the metabolism of lipids (see the above discussion on PAF biosynthesis).

Obviously, the development of a selective inhibitor for the initial phospholipase A_2 step in the remodelling route could be of major importance, particularly if the arachidonoyl species of alkylacyl-GPC are the primary precursor of PAF, since such an inhibitor would not only decrease PAF production but it would also inhibit the release of arachidonic acid from the PAF precursor pool. Acetyltransferase, the other potential enzyme target for an inhibitor in the remodelling route, could also be used to manipulate the excessive production of PAF via the remodelling pathway. Such blocks would be very effective in controlling PAF levels without affecting the *de novo* synthesis of PAF required for essential physiological functions.

Success in developing highly specific enzyme inhibitors as anti-PAF drugs would provide much more selective control of PAF activities than the PAF-receptor antagonists that are currently under investigation. Moreover, inhibitors for specific enzymatic steps in PAF metabolism would also serve as useful probes for evaluating the significance of the *de novo* versus remodelling pathways in both physiological and pathophysiological processes.

References

1 Demopoulos, C. A., Pinckard, R. N. & Hanahan, D. J. Platelet-activating factor. Evidence for 1-O-alkyl-2-acetyl-*sn*-glyceryl-3-phosphorylcholine as the active component (a new class of lipid chemical mediators). *J. Biol. Chem.* (1979), **254**, 9355–9358.

2 Blank, M. L., Snyder, F., Byers, L. W., Brooks, B. & Muirhead, E. E. Antihypertensive activity of an alkyl ether analog of phosphatidylcholine. *Biochem. Biophys. Res. Commun.* (1979), **90**, 1194–1200.

3 Benveniste, J., Tence, M., Varenne, P., Bidault, J., Boullet, C. & Polonsky, J. Semi-synthèse et structure proposee du facteur activant les plaquettes (PAF); PAF-acether, un alkyl ether analogue de la lysophosphatidylcholine. *C.R. Acad. Sci. (D) (Paris)* (1979), **289**, 1037–1040.

4 Renooij, W., Wykle, R. L., Blank, M. L., *et al.* Metabolism of 1-alkyl-2-acetoyl-*sn*-glycero-3-phosphocholine, and antihypertensive phospholipid. *Fed. Proc.* (1980), **39**, 2187 (Abstract 3059).

5 Snyder, F., Lee, T-c. & Wykle, R. L. Ether-linked glycerolipids and their bioactive species: enzymes and metabolic regulation. In Martonosi, A. (ed.) *The Enzymes of Biological Membranes*, 2nd edn (1985), pp. 1–58. Plenum Press, New York.

6 Hajra, A. K. Biosynthesis of O-alkylglycerol ether lipids. In Mangold, H. K. & Paltauf, F. (eds) *Ether Lipids: Biochemical and Biomedical Aspects* (1983), pp. 85–106. Academic Press, New York.

7 Braquet, P., Touqui, L., Shen, T. Y. & Vargaftig, B. B. Perspectives in platelet-activating factor research. *Pharmacol. Rev.* (1987), **39**, 97–145.

8 Hanahan, D. J. Platelet activating factor: a biologically active phosphoglyceride. *Annu. Rev. Biochem.* (1986), **55**, 483–509.

9 Lee, T-c. & Snyder, F. Function, metabolism, and regulation of platelet activating factor and related ether lipids. In Kuo, J. F. (ed.) *Phospholipids and Cellular Regulation* (1985), pp. 1–39. CRC Press, Boca Raton, FL.

10 O'Flaherty, J. T. & Wykle, R. L. Mediators of anaphylaxis. *Clin. Lab. Med.* (1983), **3**, 619–643.

11 Pinckard, R. N., McManus, L. M., Demopoulos, C. A. *et al.* Molecular pathobiology of acetyl glyceryl ether phosphorylcholine: evidence for the structural and functional identity with platelet-activating factor. *J. Reticuloendothel. Soc.* (1980), **28**, 95S–103S.

12 Snyder, F. Chemical and biochemical aspects of 'platelet activating factor', a novel class of acetylated ether-linked choline phospholipids. *Med. Res. Rev.* (1985), **5**, 107–140.

13 Snyder, F. Historical aspects of alkyl lipids and their biologically active forms (ether lipids, platelet-activating factor and antihypertensive renal lipids). In Snyder, F. (ed.) *Platelet-Activating Factor and Related Lipid Mediators* (1987), pp. 1–5. Plenum Press, New York.

14 Snyder, F. Biochemistry of platelet activating factor: a unique class of biologically active phospholipids. *Proc. Exp. Biol. Med.* (1989), **190**, 125–135.

15 Chilton, F. H., Ellis, J. M., Olson, S. C. & Wykle, R. L. 1-O-alkyl-2-arachidonoyl-*sn*-glycero-3-phosphocholine, a common source of platelet-activating factor and arachidonate in human polymorphonuclear leukocytes. *J. Biol. Chem.* (1984), **259**, 12 014–12 019.

16 Ramesha, C. S. & Pickett, W. C. Platelet-activating factor and leukotriene biosynthesis is inhibited in polymorphonuclear leukocytes depleted of arachidonic acid. *J. Biol. Chem.* (1986), **261**, 7592–7596.

17 Wykle, R. L., Malone, B. & Snyder, F. Enzymatic synthesis of 1-alkyl-2-acetyl-*sn*-glycero-3-phosphocholine, a hypotensive and platelet-aggregating lipid. *J. Biol. Chem.* (1980), **255**, 10 256–10 260.

18 Lee, T-c. Biosynthesis of platelet activating factor: substrate specificity of 1-alkyl-lyso-2-*sn*-glycero-3-phosphocholine:acetyl-CoA acetyltransferase in rat spleen microsomes. *J. Biol. Chem.* (1985), **260**, 10 952–10 955.

19 Gomez-Cambronero, J., Mato, J. M., Vivanco, F. & Sanchez Crespo, M. Phosphorylation of partially purified 1-O-alkyl-2-lyso-*sn*-glycero-3-phosphocholine: acetyl-CoA acetyltransferase from rat spleen. *Biochem. J.* (1987), **245**, 893–898.

20 Lee, T-c. Enzymatic control of the cellular levels of platelet activating factor. In Snyder, F. (ed.) *Platelet-Activating Factor and Related Mediators* (1987), pp. 115–133. Plenum Press, New York.

21 Bussolino, F., Gremo, F., Tetta, C., Pescarmona, G. P. & Camussi, G. Production of platelet-activating factor by chick retina. *J. Biol. Chem.* (1986), **261**, 16 502–16 508.

22 Domenech, C., Machado-De Domenech, E. & Soling H.-D. Regulation of acetyl-CoA:1-alkyl-*sn*-glycero-3-phosphocholine O^2-acetyltransferase (lyso-PAF-acetyltransferase) in exocrine glands. Evidence for an activation via phosphorylation by calcium/calmodulin-dependent protein kinase. *J. Biol. Chem.* (1987), **262**, 5671–5676.

23 Camussi, G., Bussolino, F., Salvidio, G. & Baglioni, C. Tumor necrosis factor/cachectin stimulates peritoneal macrophages, polymorphonuclear neutrophils, and vascular endothelial cells to synthesize and release platelet-activating factor. *J. Exp. Med.* (1987), **166**, 1390–1404.
24 Bussolino, F., Camussi, G. & Baglioni, C. Synthesis and release of platelet-activating factor by human vascular endothelial cells treated with tumor necrosis factor or interleukin 1α. *J. Biol. Chem.* (1988), **263**, 11 856–11 861.
25 Doebber, T. W. & Wu, M. S. Platelet-activating factor (PAF) stimulates the PAF-synthesizing enzyme acetyl-CoA:1-alkyl-*sn*-glycero-3-phosphocholine O^2-acetyl transferase and PAF synthesis in neutrophils. *Proc. Natl. Acad. Sci. (USA)* (1987), **84**, 7557–7561.
26 Lenihan, D. J. & Lee, T-c. Regulation of platelet activating factor synthesis: modulation of 1-alkyl-2-lyso-*sn*-glycero-3-phosphocholine:acetyl-CoA acetyltransferase by phosphorylation and dephosphorylation in rat spleen microsomes. *Biochem. Biophys. Res. Commun.* (1984), **120**, 834–839.
27 Gomez-Cambronero, J., Velasco, S., Mato, J. M. & Sanchez Crespo, M. Modulation of lyso-platelet activating factor: acetyl-CoA acetyltransferase from rat splenic microsomes. The role of cyclic AMP-dependent protein kinase. *Biochim. Biophys. Acta* (1985), **845**, 516–519.
28 Ninio, E., Joly, F., Hieblot, C., Bessou, G., Menica-Huerta, J. M. & Benveniste, J. Biosynthesis of PAF-acether. IX. Role for a phosphorylatic-dependent activation of acetyltransferase in antigen-stimulated mouse mast cells. *J. Immunol.* (1987), **139**, 154–160.
29 Lee, T-c., Malone, B. & Snyder, F. A new *de novo* pathway for the formation of 1-alkyl-2-acetyl-*sn*-glycerols, a precursor of platelet activating factor. Biochemical characterization of 1-alkyl-2-lyso-*sn*-glycero-3-P:acetyl-CoA acetyltransferase. *J. Biol. Chem.* (1986), **261**, 5373–5377.
30 Lee, T-c., Malone, B. & Snyder, F. Formation of 1-alkyl-2-acetyl-*sn*-glycerols via *de novo* biosynthetic pathway for platelet activating factor. Characterization of 1-alkyl-2-acetyl-*sn*-glycero-3-phosphate phosphohydrolase in rat spleens. *J. Biol. Chem.* (1988), **263**, 1755–1760.
31 Renooij, W. & Snyder, F. Biosynthesis of 1-alkyl-2-acetyl-*sn*-glycero-3-phosphocholine (platelet activating factor and a hypotensive lipid) by choline-phosphotransferase in various rat tissues. *Biochim. Biophys. Acta* (1981), **663**, 545–556.
32 Woodard, D. S., Lee, T-c. & Snyder, F. The final step in the *de novo* biosynthesis of platelet activating factor. Properties of a unique CDP-choline:1-alkyl-2-acetyl-*sn*-glycerol cholinephosphotransferase in microsomes from the renal inner medulla of rats. *J. Biol. Chem.* (1987), **262**, 2520–2527.
33 Alonso, F., Gil, M. G., Sanchez Crespo, M. & Mato, J. M. Activation of 1-alkyl-2-lyso-glycero-3-phosphocholine. Acetyl-CoA transferase during phagocytosis in human polymorphonuclear leukocytes. *J. Biol. Chem.* (1982), **257**, 3376–3378.
34 Snyder, F., Lee, T-c., Blank, M., Malone, B., Woodard, D. & Robinson, M. Platelet activating factor (PAF): Alternate pathways of biosynthesis, the mechanism of inactivation, and the reacylation of lyso-PAF with arachidonate. *Adv. Prost. Thromb. Leuk. Res.* (1985), **15**, 693–696.
35 Blank, M. L., Lee, T-c., Cress, E. A., Malone, B., Fitzgerald, V. & Snyder, F. Conversion of 1-alkyl-2-acetyl-*sn*-glycerols to platelet activating factor and related phospholipids by rabbit platelets. *Biochem. Biophys. Res. Commun.* (1984), **124**, 156–163.
36 Satouchi, K., Oda, M., Saito, K. & Hanahan, D. J. Metabolism of 1-O-alkyl-2-acetyl-*sn*-glycerol by washed rabbit platelets: formation of platelet activating factor. *Arch. Biochem. Biophys.* (1984), **234**, 318–321.

37 Lianos, E. A. & Zanglis, A. Biosynthesis and metabolism of 1-O-alkyl-2-acetyl-*sn*-glycero-3-phosphocholine in rat glomerular mesangial cells. *J. Biol. Chem.* (1987), **262**, 8990–8993.

38 Fernandez-Gallardo, S., Gijon, M. A., Garcia, M. d-C., Cano, E. & Sanchez-Crespo, M. Biosynthesis of platelet-activating factor in glandular gastric mucosa. Evidence for the involvement of the *de novo* pathway and modulation by fatty acids. *Biochem. J.* (1988), **254**, 707–714.

39 Kawasaki, T. & Snyder, F. Synthesis of a novel acetylated neutral lipid related to platelet-activating factor by acyl-CoA:1-O-alkyl-2-acetyl-*sn*-glycerol acyltransferase in HL-60 cells. *J. Biol. Chem.* (1988), **263**, 2593–2596.

40 Joly, F., Bessou, G., Benveniste, J. & Ninio, E. Ketotifen inhibits PAF-acether biosynthesis and β-hexosaminidase release in mouse mast cells stimulated with antigen. *Eur. J. Pharmacol.* (1987), **144**, 133–139.

41 Seyama, K. & Ishibashi, T. Biochemical characterization of acetyl-CoA:1-alkyl-2-lyso-*sn*-glycero-3-phosphocholine acetyltransferase in rat spleen microsomes. *Lipids* (1987), **22**, 185–189.

42 Bittman, R., Witzke, N. M., Lee, T-c., Blank, M. L. & Snyder, F. Synthesis and biochemical studies of analogs of platelet-activating factor bearing a methyl group at C2 of the glycerol backbone. *J. Lipid Res.* (1987), **28**, 733–738.

43 Shen, T. Y., Hwang, S. B., Doebber, T. W. & Robbins, J. C. The chemical and biological properties of PAF agonists, antagonists and biosynthetic inhibitors. In Snyder, F. (ed.) *Platelet-Activating Factor and Related Lipid Mediators* (1987), pp. 153–190. Plenum Press, New York.

44 Cabot, M. C., Blank, M. L., Welsh, C. J., Horan, M. J., Cress, E. A. & Snyder, F. Metabolism of 1-alkyl-2-acetyl-*sn*-glycero-3- phosphocholine by cell cultures. *Life Sci.* (1982), **31**, 2891–2898.

45 Malone, B., Lee, T-c & Snyder, F. Inactivation of platelet activating factor (PAF) by rabbit platelets: lyso-PAF as a key intermediate with phosphatidylcholine as the source of arachidonic acid in its conversion to a tetraenoic acylated product. *J. Biol. Chem.* (1985), **260**, 1531–1534.

46 Pieroni, G. & Hanahan, D. J. Metabolic behaviour of acetyl glyceryl ether phosphorylcholine on interaction with rabbit platelets. *Arch. Biochem. Biophys.* (1983), **224**, 485–493.

47 Chilton, F. H., O'Flaherty, J. T., Ellis, J. M., Swendsen, C. L. & Wykle, R. L. Metabolic fate of platelet-activating factor in neutrophils. *J. Biol. Chem.* (1983), **258**, 6357–6361.

48 Chilton, F. H., O'Flaherty, J. T., Ellis, J. M., Swendsen, C. L. & Wykle, R. L. Selective acylation of lyso platelet activating factor by arachidonate in human neutrophils. *J. Biol. Chem.* (1983), **258**, 7268–7271.

49 Alam, I. & Silver, M. J. Metabolism of 1-alkyl-2-acyl-GPC in human platelets in response to stimulation by thrombin. *Thromb. Res.* (1987), **45**, 311–322.

50 Blank, M. L., Spector, A. A., Kaduce, T. L., Lee, T-c & Snyder, F. Metabolism of platelet activating factor (1-alkyl-2-acetyl-*sn*-glycero-3-phosphocholine) and 1-alkyl-2-acetyl-*sn*-glycerol by human endothelial cells. *Biochim. Biophys. Acta* (1986), **876**, 373–378.

51 Robinson, M. & Snyder, F. Metabolism of platelet activating factor by rat alveolar macrophages: Lyso-PAF as an obligatory intermediate in the formation of alkylarachidonyl glycerophosphocholine species. *Biochim. Biophys. Acta* (1985), **837**, 52–56.

52 Kramer, R. M., Patton, G. M., Pritzker, C. R. & Deykin, D. Metabolism of platelet-activating factor in human platelets: Transacylase-mediated synthesis of 1-O-alkyl-2-arachidonoyl-*sn*-glycero-3-phosphocholine. *J. Biol. Chem.* (1984), **259**, 13 316–13 320.

53 Qian, C., Lee, T-c. & Snyder, F. Metabolism of platelet activating factor (PAF) and related ether lipids by neonatal rat myocytes. *J. Lipid Mediators* (1989), **1**, 113–123.
54 Touqui, L., Jacquemin, C. J., Dumarey, C. & Vargaftig, B. B. 1-O-alkyl-acyl-*sn*-glycero-3-phosphocholine is the precursor of platelet-activating factor in stimulated rabbit platelets. Evidence for an alkylacetyl-glycerophosphorylcholine cycle. *Biochim. Biophys. Acta* (1985), **833**, 111–118.
55 Okayasu, T., Hoshii, K., Seyama, K., Ishibashi, T. & Imai, Y. Metabolism of platelet-activating factor in primary cultured adult rat hepatocytes by a new pathway involving phospholipase C and alkyl monooxygenase. *Biochim. Biophys. Acta* (1986), **876**, 58–64.
56 Blank, M. L., Lee, T-c., Fitzgerald, V. & Snyder, F. A specific acetylhydrolase for 1-alkyl-2-acetyl-*sn*-glycero-3-phosphocholine (a hypotensive and platelet-activating lipid). *J. Biol. Chem.* (1981), **256**, 175–178.
57 Blank, M. L., Hall, M. N., Cress, E. A. & Snyder, F. Inactivation of 1-alkyl-2-acetyl-*sn*-glycero-3-phosphocholine by a plasma acetylhydrolase: higher activities in hypertensive rats. *Biochem. Biophys. Res. Commun.* (1983), **113**, 666–671.
58 Farr, R. S., Cox, C. P., Wardlow, M. L. & Jorgensen, R. Preliminary studies of an acid-labile factor (ALF) in human sera that inactivates platelet-activating factor (PAF). *Clin. Immunol. Immunopathol.* (1980), **15**, 318–330.
59 Farr, R. S., Wardlow, M. L., Cox, C. P., Meng, K. E. & Greene, D. E. Human serum acid-labile factor is an acylhydrolase that inactivates platelet-activating factor. *Fed. Proc.* (1983), **42**, 3120–3122.
60 Stafforini, D. M., Prescott, S. M. & McIntyre, T. M. Human plasma platelet-activating factor acetylhydrolase. Purification and properties. *J. Biol. Chem.* (1987), **262**, 4223–4230.
61 Wardlow, M. L., Cox, C. P., Meng, K. E., Greene, D. E. & Farr, R. S. Substrate specificity and partial characterization of the PAF-acylhydrolase in human serum that rapidly inactivates platelet activating factor. *J. Immunol.* (1986), **136**, 3441–3446.
62 Stafforini, D. M., Mcintyre, T. M., Carter, M. E. & Prescott, S. M. Human plasma platelet-activating factor acetylhydrolase. Association with lipoprotein particles and role in the degradation of platelet-activating factor. *J. Biol. Chem.* (1987), **262**, 4215–4222.
63 Suzuki, Y., Miwa, M., Harada, M. & Matsumoto, M. Release of acetylhydrolase from platelets on aggregation with platelet-activating factor. *Eur. J. Biochem.* (1988), **172**, 117–120.
64 Waku, K. & Nakazawa, Y. Regulation of the fatty acid composition of alkyl ether phospholipid in Ehrlich ascites tumor cells. *J. Biochem.* (1977), **82**, 1779–1784.
65 McKean, M. L. & Silver, M. J. Phospholipid biosynthesis in human platelets. The acylation of lyso-platelet-activating factor. *Biochem. J.* (1985), **225**, 723–729.
66 Robinson, M., Blank, M. L. & Snyder, F. Acylation of lysophospholipids by rabbit alveolar macrophages: Specificities of CoA-dependent and CoA-independent reactions. *J. Biol. Chem.* (1985), **260**, 7889–7895.
67 Cornic, M., Breton, M & Colard, O. Acylation of 1-alkyl- and 1-acyl-lysophospholipids by rat platelets. *Pharmacol. Res. Commun.* (1986), **18**, 43–49.
68 Ojima, A., Nakagawa, Y., Sugiura, T., Masuzawa, Y. & Waku, K. Selective transacylation of 1-O-alkylglycerophosphoethanolamine by docosahexaenoate and arachidonate in rat brain microsomes. *J. Neurochem.* (1987), **48**, 1403–1410.
69 Sugiura, T., Masuzawa, Y., Nakagawa, Y. & Waku, K. Transacylation of lyso platelet-activating factor and other lysophospholipids by macrophage microsomes. Distinct donor and acceptor selectives. *J. Biol. Chem.* (1987), **262**, 1119–1205.

70 Lee, T-c., Blank, M. L., Fitzgerald, V. & Snyder, F. Mechanisms of acylation for alkyllysophospholipids. *Fed. Proc.* (1987), **46**, 2126.
71 Sugiura, T., Masuzawa, Y. & Waku, K. Transacylation of 1-O-alkyl-*sn*-glycero-3-phosphocholine (lyso platelet activating factor) and 1-O-alkyenyl-*sn*-glycero-3-phosphoethanolamine with docosahexaenoic acid (22: 6ω3). *Biochem. Biophys. Res. Commun.* (1985), **133**, 574–580.
72 Sugiura, T. & Waku, K. CoA-independent transfer of arachidonic acid from 1,2-diacyl-*sn*-glycero-3-phosphocholine to 1-O-alkyl-*sn*-glycero-3-phosphocholine (lyso platelet-activating factor) by macrophage microsomes. *Biochem. Biophys. Res. Commun.* (1985), **127**, 384–390.
73 Nishihira, J & Ishibashi, T. A phospholipase C with a high specificity for platelet-activating factor in rabbit liver light mitochondria. *Lipids* (1986), **21**, 780–785.
74 Matsuzawa, Y. & Hostetler, K. Y. Properties of phospholipase C isolated from rat liver lysosomes. *J. Biol. Chem.* (1980), **255**, 646–652.
75 Wykle, R. L. & Schremmer, J. M. A lysophospholipase D pathway in the metabolism of ether-linked lipids in brain microsomes. *J. Biol. Chem.* (1974), **249**, 1742–1756.
76 Wykle, R. L., Kraemer, W. F. & Schremmer, J. M. Studies of lysophospholipase D of rat liver and other tissues. *Arch. Biochem. Biophys.* (1977), **184**, 149–155.
77 Wykle, R. L., Kraemer, W. F. & Schremmer, J. M. Specificity of lysophospholipase D. *Biochim. Biophys. Acta* (1980), **619**, 58–67.
78 Kawasaki, T. & Snyder, F. The metabolism of lyso-platelet-activating factor (1-O-alkyl-2-lyso-*sn*-glycero-3-phosphocholine) by a calcium-dependent lysophospholipase D in rabbit kidney medulla. *Biochim. Biophys. Acta* (1987), **920**, 85–93.
79 Tietz, A., Lindberg, M. & Kennedy, E. P. A new pteridine-requiring enzyme system for oxidation of glyceryl ethers. *J. Biol. Chem.* (1964), **239**, 4081–4090.
80 Ishibashi, T. & Imai, Y. Affinity purification of alkylglycerol monooxygenase from rat liver microsomes by chimyl alcohol–Sepharose 4B column chromatography. *J. Lipid Res.* (1985), **26**, 393–395.
81 Lee, T-c. Blank, M. L., Fitzgerald, V. & Snyder, F. Substrate specificity in the biocleavage of the O-alkyl bond: 1-alkyl-2-acetyl-*sn*-glycero-3-phosphocholine (a hypotensive and platelet-activating lipid) and its metabolites. *Arch. Biochem. Biophys.* (1981) **208**, 353–357.
82 Gomez-Cambronero, J., Inarrea, P., Alonso, F. & Sanchez Crespo, M. The role of calcium ions in the process of acetyltransferase activation during the formation of platelet-activating factor (PAF-acether). *Biochem. J.* (1984), **219**, 419–424.
83 Lee, T-c., Lenihan, D. J., Malone, B., Roddy, L. L. & Wasserman, S. I. Increased biosynthesis of platelet-activating factor in activated human eosinophils. *J. Biol. Chem.* (1984), **259**, 5526–5530.
84 Ludwig, J. C., McManus, L. M., Clark, P. O., Hanahan, D. J. & Pinckard, R. N. Modulation of platelet-activating factor (PAF) synthesis and release from human polymorphonuclear leukocytes (PMN): role of extracellular Ca^{2+}. *Arch. Biochem. Biophys.* (1984), **232**, 102–110.
85 Kennedy, E. P. & Weiss, S. B. The function of cytidine coenzymes in the biosynthesis of phospholipids. *J. Biol. Chem.* (1956), **222**, 193–214.
86 Touqui, L., Shaw, A. M., Dumarey, C., Jacquemin, C. & Vargaftig, B. B. The role of Ca^{2+} in regulating the catabolism of PAF-acether (1-O-alkyl-2-acetyl-*sn*-glycero-3-phosphocholine) in rabbit platelets. *Biochem. J.* (1987), **241**, 555–560.
87 Soodsma, J. F., Piantadosi, C. & Snyder, F. Partial characterization of the alkylglycerol cleavage enzyme system of rat liver. *J. Biol. Chem.* (1972), **247**, 3923–3929.

88 Miwa, M., Hill, C., Kumar, R., Sugantani, J., Olson, M. S. & Hanahan, D. J. Occurrence of an endogenous inhibitor of platelet-activating factor in rat liver. *J. Biol. Chem.* (1987), **262**, 527–530.

89 Nakayama, R., Yasuda, K. & Saito, K. Existence of endogenous inhibitors of platelet-activating factor (PAF) with PAF in rat uterus. *J. Biol. Chem.* (1987), **262**, 13 174–13 179.

90 Nieto, M. L., Velasco, S. & Sanchez Crespo, M. Modulation of acetyl-CoA:1-alkyl-2-lyso-*sn*-glycero-3-phosphocholine (lyso-PAF) acetyltransferase in human polymorphonuclears. The role of cyclic AMP-dependent and phospholipid sensitive calcium-dependent protein kinases. *J. Biol. Chem.* (1988), **263**, 4607–4611.

91 McIntyre, T. M., Reinhold, S. L., Prescott, S. M. & Zimmerman, G. A. Protein kinase C activity appears to be required for the synthesis of platelet-activating factor and leukotriene B_4 by human neutrophils. *J. Biol. Chem.* (1987), **262**, 15 370–15 376.

92 Blank, M. L., Lee, Y. J., Cress, E. A. & Snyder, F. Stimulation of the *de novo* pathway for the biosynthesis of platelet activating factor (PAF) via cytidylyltransferase activation in cells with minimal endogenous PAF production. *J. Biol. Chem.* (1988), **263**, 5656–5661.

93 Nieto, M. L., Velasco, S. & Sanchez Crespo, M. Biosynthesis of platelet-activating factor in human polymorphonuclear leukocytes. Involvement of the cholinephosphotransferase pathway response to the phorbol esters. *J. Biol. Chem.* (1988), **263**, 2217–2222.

94 Pelech, S. L., Paddon, H. B. & Vance, D. E. Phorbol esters stimulate phosphatidylcholine biosynthesis by translocation of CTP:phosphocholine cytidylyltransferase from cytosol to microsomes. *Biochim. Biophys. Acta* (1984), **795**, 447–451.

95 Billah, M., Eckel, S., Myers, R. & Siegel, M. Metabolism of platelet-activating factor (1-O-alkyl-2-acetyl-*sn*-glycero-3-phosphocholine) by human promyelocytic leukemic HL60 cells. *J. Biol. Chem.* (1986), **261**, 5824–5831.

96 Kawasaki, T., Blank, M. L. & Snyder, F. Arachidonic acid (AA) regulates platelet activating factor (PAF) synthesis in HL-60 cells. *FASEB J.* (1988), **2,** A1376.

97 Suga, K., Kawasaki, T., Blank, M. L. & Snyder, F. Phospholipase A_2 (PLA_2) regulates the increases of platelet activating factor (PAF) synthesis in arachidonic acid (AA)-supplemented differentiated HL-60 cells. *FASEB J.* (1989), **3**, A1224.

98 Michel, L., Denizot, Y., Thomas, Y. *et al.* Biosynthesis of PAF-acether factor-acether by human skin fibroblasts *in vitro*. *J. Immunol.* (1988), **141**, 948–953.

99 Blank, M. L., Spector, A. A., Kaduce, T. L. & Snyder, F. Composition and incorporation of [^{3}H]arachidonic acid into molecular species of phospholipid classes by cultured human endothelial cells. *Biochim. Biophys. Acta* (1986), **877**, 211–215.

100 Ojima-Uchiyama, A., Masuzawa, Y., Sugiura, T. *et al.* Phospholipid analysis of human eosinophils: high levels of alkylacylglycerophosphocholine (PAF precursor). *Lipids* (1988), **23**, 815–817.

101 Sugiura, T. & Waku, K. Composition of alkyl ether-linked phospholipids in mammalian tissues. In Snyder, F. (ed.) *Platelet Activating Factor and Related Lipid Mediators* (1987), pp. 55–85. Plenum Press, New York.

102 Snyder, F., Lee, T-c. & Blank, M. L. Metabolism of ether analogs of phosphatidylcholine, including platelet activating factor. In Vance, D. E. (ed.) *Phosphatidylcholine Metabolism* (1989). CRC Press, Boca Raton, FL, in press.

Chapter 2
Cellular origins of PAF

Donna Bratton and Peter M. Henson

Introduction

The list of cells capable of synthesizing platelet-activating factor (PAF, Paf, PAF-acether, AGEPC) has expanded tremendously since the identification in 1972 of the basophil as the source in rabbit blood of the recently-described mediator that stimulated platelets [1] and its subsequent chemical identification in 1979 [2]. Indeed as the list continues to grow, a role for PAF in physiological as well as patho-physiological processes must be entertained. While it appears that ether phospholipids, the precursors of PAF, may be identified in diverse organisms spanning the animal kingdom, PAF has been best characterized from a variety of mammalian sources. Significant differences have been noted between species with regard to the cells that synthesize PAF. However, on closer analysis, many of these differences may turn out to be methodological. Herein, in order to relate the observations to the issues of clinical involvement of the mediator, the production of PAF from human cells will be the primary subject for consideration.

Any discussion of the cellular origins of PAF must take into account the technical issues of detection and identification of this unique lipid mediator, and such concerns are outlined in the following section. Additionally, in reviewing the data presented here and throughout the literature the reader is alerted to the phrase 'PAF release' as opposed to 'PAF synthesis' or 'PAF production'. In many investigations, particularly in earlier studies, only the cell incubation medium (supernatant) was tested for the presence of released PAF. As a lipid mediator which in many cases remains cell associated, and may have an intracellular role in cell functions, the lack of release does not constitute the lack of synthesis, nor the amount of released material necessarily reflect the amount synthesized.

Determination of the cell types that synthesize (and secrete) PAF is of critical importance in gaining an overall understanding of the role that the mediator plays in physiological and pathological processes. Despite its myriad potential biological activities in stimulating cell functions, the real importance of PAF is yet to be determined. Unfortunately, demonstrating that a given cell type can produce PAF may lead to inappropriate emphasis on its involvement in particular types of reactions. Thus the early finding of IgE and basophil involvement in PAF generation in rabbit blood led to the concept of PAF as a mediator of allergic reactions. Similarly, the current attention placed on PAF as a mediator of inflammatory processes derives in large part from the observations that neutrophils, eosinophils and mononuclear phagocytes make large quantities of the molecule. While it may well be true that PAF is a critical mediator in such reactions, definitive demonstration is still lacking. Moreover, these circulating inflammatory cells are easy to isolate and stimulate and thus many more studies have been carried out with these than with tissue cells. Were a given tissue cell (e.g. the alveolar type II, epithelial cell or a neuronal cell) shown to make and secrete large quantities of PAF, new possibilities for its function in the body would have to be entertained.

Detection and measurement of PAF

Much of what has been said about the synthesis of PAF from various cell sources must be examined with regard to a few important technical concerns. Briefly, the characterization of PAF from cell sources has frequently relied on a variety of biological assays, most frequently rabbit platelet aggregation [1] and/or release of 5-hydroxytryptamine [3], sometimes without rigorous attention to isolation and identification of the active principle. The use of such biological assays are not only fraught with uncontrolled variables by their very nature but also may be selectively sensitive to certain PAF species while insensitive to others [4,5]. Minimal standards for attributing biological activity to PAF must include first isolation and then identification of the active agent as PAF which can be done by a variety of schemes. Isolation can be accomplished by extraction of the lipid from biological samples using a system of organic solvents generally by a modification of the method by Bligh & Dyer [6]. This is followed by separation by one of several chromatographic schemes which have recently been reviewed in depth by Blank *et al.* [7]. Thin-layer chromatography is perhaps the easiest and most widely used to isolate PAF and is probably adequate for radiolabelled biological samples. Generally, plates are developed in a solvent system of chloroform, methanol with varying amounts of water, acetic acid or ammonium hydroxide. Typically losses of PAF (probably due to sticking to glass plates) are substantial making quantification of material from biological samples difficult [8]. Separation of PAF from other lipids with similar R_f (phosphatidylinositol, phosphatidylserine, the ester analogue, acylacetyl-PC and sphingomyelin) is generally not accomplished. Subsequent bioassay of samples contaminated with large amounts of the ester analogue (acylacetyl-GPC) [9] in particular, is a problem in that it is active in some biological assays at approximately 200-fold less than PAF [2]. Alternatively, several phospholids from biological sources [10,11] exhibiting PAF-like chromatographic characteristics have been shown to have inhibitor activity in bioassay systems. Thus inability to separate PAF from other lipids which exert either stimulatory or inhibitory activity in bioassay systems limits both detection and quantitation.

Normal phase HPLC is also frequently used but likewise presents difficulty in detection of PAF where non-radiolabelled samples are used. Blank *et al.* [7] have used unsaturated lysophosphatidylcholine detected by UV absorption as a 'marker' of PAF which elutes between it and sphingomyelin. Quantification is again difficult because of sticking of PAF to the columns and must be monitored with known standards. The use of benzoate derivatives of PAF allow detection and separation of different diradyl species when present at less than microgram quantities [7]. Future use of derivatized PAF to an UV-absorbing, fluorescent or electrically-active diglyceride would vastly expand the current utilization of HPLC in the detection of PAF [12]. Reversed-phase HPLC has been used to discriminate several species of PAF differing in the length of the alkyl chain [13,14].

Once isolated, material suspected to be PAF may be further characterized by its pattern of degradation by various phospholipases and acetylhydrolase. The products of degradation can then be identified physiochemically or assayed for biological activity. Typically, samples are subjected to hydrolysis by PLA_2 or PLC (both obtained from a variety of biological sources) which upon cleavage of the 2-position acetyl group or polar head respectively, abolishes bioactivity of the sample. Similarly, treatment of test samples with acetylhydrolase obtained from serum [15–17] results in the formation of lyso-PAF and in the loss of biological activity. In contrast, treatment of test samples by PLA_1 (likewise obtained from a variety of biological sources) results in no loss of bioactivity as the enzyme is unable to cleave to the *sn*-1 ether linkage.

Where precise identification and quantification issues become important, the use of mass spectrometry is unsurpassed in sensitivity and specificity and surely represents the gold standard [18]. The combined use of gas–liquid chromotography and mass spectrometry has brought the limit of detection to the picomolar range. The main disadvantage of this technique is the requirement for degrading and derivatizing PAF so that it is rendered volatile and may be analysed in the gaseous state and detected as a ionic species with a specific mass-to-charge ratio (m/z). Generally this involves removal of the polar head group of PAF to form the diglyceride followed by derivatization of the primary alcohol to either an ether or ester. Contaminants introduced during degradation and derivatization (either chemical or enzymatic) must be removed prior to analysis. Sample processing is considerable and the main shortcoming of this methodology.

The newer evolving technology of fast-atom bombardment eliminates the requirement of volatility and allows for the analysis of underivatized PAF as an ionized molecule. PAF from samples must first be purified from other isobaric contaminants (C_{18}-lyso-PAF versus C_{16}-PAF) by thin-layer chromatography followed by HPLC [18]. Test samples are analysed dissolved in a matrix and can then be recovered, subjected to specific chemical alteration/degradation and re-analysed to further confirm specificity of the original material as PAF. In this way numerous species of PAF differing in alkyl chain length and degree of saturation have been identified from the human polymorphonuclear leukocyte [19], the existence of which would not have been recognized in biological assays. Application of this technique for quantification of PAF in biological samples requires use of deuterated standards and can measure to the level of a few nanograms. Technical problems with this method include interference of ionization by salts present in extracts of biological samples. These require meticulous removal prior to analysis.

Recent literature attests to the popular use of detecting synthesis of PAF utilizing radiolabelled precursors, either alkyl lysophosphatidylcholine or acetate followed by isolation of labelled PAF. Where radiolabelled precursors are used, one has to bear in mind particularly the shortcoming that data generated are only representative of potentially non-equilibrium precursor 'pools'. Such radiolabelled data estimating the relative amounts of PAF synthesized and secreted may be very misleading if not correlated with quantification of material produced, either by bioassay or preferably by GLC/MS or FABMS [20].

When questioning whether a certain cell type is capable of PAF biosynthesis, catabolism of PAF must always be considered hand in hand with synthesis of PAF. The frequent presence of acetylhydrolase (see Chapter 1) in plasma [15–17], and a variety of cells and tissues [21,22] may obscure production of this unique lipid by rapid hydrolysis to the biologically inactive product lyso-PAF. For example, Touqui *et al.* [23] have shown in human platelets stimulated with thrombin that inhibition of the acetylhydrolase with a serine-hydrolase inhibitor, phenylmethanesulfonyl fluoride (PMSF) allows one to detect 10–12 times more PAF synthesis. Furthermore, Roubin *et al.* [24] have suggested that alterations in catabolism accompanying zymosan challenge of immuno-stimulated

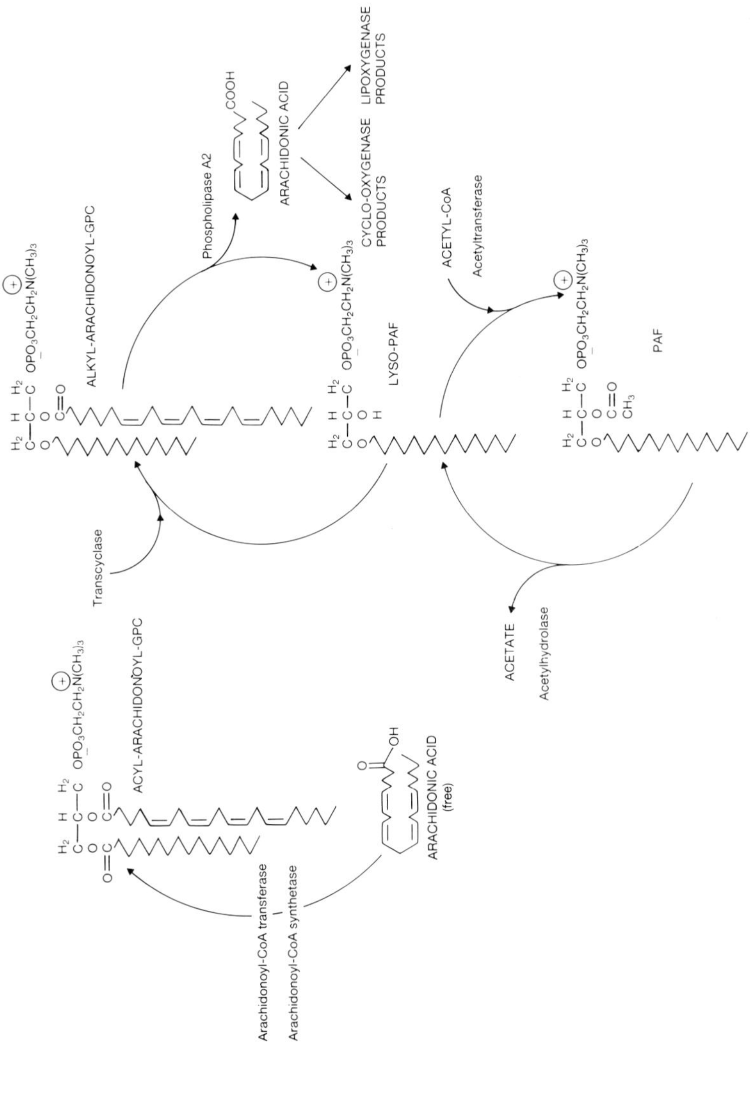

Fig. 2.1 The 'remodelling pathway' of PAF synthesis. Reproduced with permission from *J. Biol. Chem.* (1986), **261**, p. 7776 [130].

(activated) mouse peritoneal macrophages results in diminished PAF accumulation when compared to that seen in zymosan-challenged resident macrophages.

Among technical concerns must be the misassignment of a particular cell as the source of PAF when PAF has been identified either in a relatively impure cell preparation where a few contaminating cells that are avid producers of PAF may lead to an erroneous conclusion, or when PAF is identified in a tissue which is closely composed of numerous cell types that are potential sources. Such a controversy exists concerning the human basophil which cannot be completely isolated from other blood cells (monocytes and neutrophils) which can produce large quantities of PAF [25–29].

Recently, the release of lyso-PAF (considered to be both a precursor and a metabolite of PAF (see Fig. 2.1) [30–34] and the potential use of it as substrate for PAF synthesis by other cells [35] (Fig. 2.2) has made the detection of lyso-PAF synthesis and release of growing importance. To date, four basic techniques for the detection and measurement of lyso-PAF have been devised but have not been widely employed or verified. Lyso-PAF from biological samples can be acetylated to PAF and identified and quantitated by bioassay [36] or alternatively acetylated with radiolabelled acetate and detected after purification [37]. Using acetate of known specific activity in this latter method allows quantification of material isolated as PAF. Both methods assume acetylation proceeds reproducibly to a reasonable yield. However, estimates of completeness of acetylation

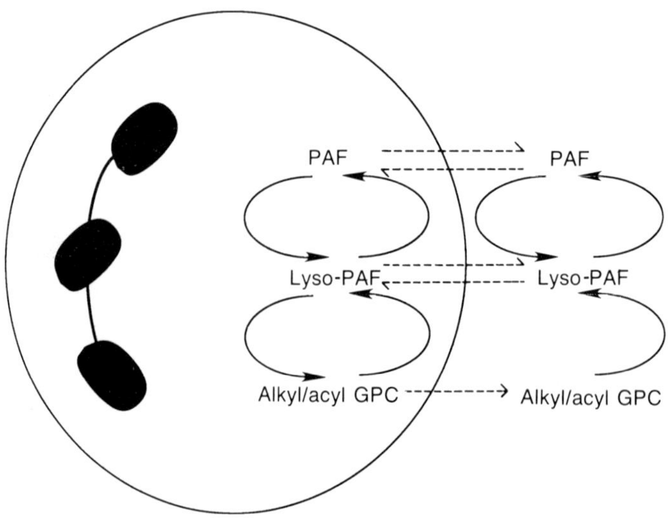

Fig. 2.2 Potential intracellular and extracellular pathways of PAF metabolism.

range from 50% (K. L. Clay, unpublished) to 80% [38]. Specificity is another shortcoming of both acetylation methods as other molecular species of PAF may be acetylated (i.e. acyl, acetyl-GPC) and detected with radiolabel or exhibit agonist or antagonist activity in biological assays. More recently, gas-liquid chromatography/mass spectrometry (GLC/MS) and fast-atom bombardment mass spectrometry have been applied to the detection and measurement of lyso-PAF synthesis by stimulation of human neutrophils [39]. Sensitivity ranged from the picomolar range for GLC/MS and the nanomolar range for FABMS.

Synthesis and secretion of PAF

Proposing a mediator role for PAF in numerous physiological or pathophysiological processes likely necessitates that it be released from the cell of origin to stimulate the specific receptors of the target cell. The finding of PAF in body fluids (urine [40,41]; blood [42]; amniotic fluid [40]) substantiates that at least in some cases, PAF could potentially exert effects either physiologically or patho-physiologically, on even more distant target cells/tissues. From the data shown in Table 2.1 it can be seen that a wide variety of cells secrete PAF where cell-free supernatants have been examined for the presence of PAF (or as in the older studies, biologically-active PAF-like material). It should be noted that cell-associated PAF was not examined or quantified in the majority of these studies (designed only to examine secretion), so that unless noted by a comment or as a percentage in Table 2.1 the relative proportion of PAF released to that synthesized is unknown. In some studies as noted, it appears that only a small proportion of PAF was released as demonstrated for the neutrophil [28,43–45] endothelial cell [46,47] and monocyte [48] regardless of agonist used [28], dose of agonist [28,43], cell-isolation technique [28], albumin concentration [43,44], presence of plasma [28], or cell 'priming' [43]. Furthermore, low amounts of PAF in supernatants cannot be simply attributed to extracellular inactivation (metalbolism) of PAF nor solely to cellular re-absorption of PAF [28].

The fact that large amounts of PAF can be produced and retained, has led to hypotheses regarding an intracellular role for PAF in addition to its mediator functions [43,45,49]. Alternatively, cell-to-cell recognition of PAF without actual release of the mediator, would allow stimulation of nearby cells in a paracrine fashion. Though this possibility has not been thoroughly investigated, it may be envisioned from data where the treatment of intact cells with phospholipases has demonstrated that PAF located on the cell membrane outer leaflet is accessible to enzymatic cleavage and possibly may interact with cells in contact with the source [46,50]. Recognition of endothelial cell-associated PAF by neutrophils may cause neutrophil adherence in the absence of detectable release

Table 2.1 Cellular origins of PAF

Cell	Stimulus[1]	Released[2]	Reference
Neutrophil	A23187	+	[64]
		49%	[48]
		10–20%	[28]
		1–10%	[43]
	A23187 + cyto B	+/−	[44]
	Opsonized zymosan	+	[64]
		+	[153]
		2–6%	[28]
		1–10%	[43]
	Zymosan	+	[27]
	FMLP	1–10%	[43]
	FMLP + cyto B	+	[64]
		33%	[28]
		30–40%	[63]
		30–40%	[53]
	C5a	+	[64]
		+	[25]
	C5a des arg	+	[25]
	Aggregated IgG	+	[64]
		+	[27]
	Immune complexes	+	[27]
		+	[25]
	Neutrophil cationic protein	+	[25]
	Neutrophil cationic protein des arg	+	[25]
	Chymotrypsin	+	[129]
	Elastase	+	[129]
	Cathepsin G	+	[129]
	Complement-activated baker's yeast spores	+	[25]
	IgG ± C3 coated RBC	+	[64]
	pH 10.6	+	[25]
	NaF	+	[64]
	PMA	+	[64]
		+	[154]
	LPS	−	[45]
	IL-1	+	[129]
	TNF	+	[129]
Monocyte	A23187	+	[27]
		+	[25]
		+	[123]
		37%	[48]
		67%	[62]
	Immunoglobulin aggregates	+	[27]
	Opsonized zymosan	+	[27]

Table 2.1 Cellular origins of PAF (*Continued*)

Cell	Stimulus[1]	Released[2]	Reference
		+	[48]
		49 %	[62]
	Zymosan	+	[27]
		+	[123]
		+	[48]
	PMA	32 %	[62]
	C3d–baker's yeast spores	+	[25]
		+	[79]
	C3b–baker's yeast spores	+	[25]
		+	[79]
	IgG–baker's yeast spores	+	[79]
	Bacteria	+	[123]
	Immune complexes	+	[27]
		+	[25]
		+	[123]
	pH 10.6	+	[25]
		+	[79]
	IL-1-β	biphasic release:	[69]
	TNF	< 15 % early;	[69]
	IFN-γ	> 70 % late	[69]
Alveolar macrophage	A23187	+	[81]
		+	[30]
	Anti-IgE	+	[30]
	Specific antigen[3]	+	[30]
Monocyte-derived macrophage	A23187	+	[62]
	PMA	+	[62]
	Opsonized zymosan	+	[62]
Eosinophil	A23187	+	[66]
	FMLP	+	[66]
	ECF-A	+	[66]
	C5a	+	[66]
Mast cell (pulmonary)	Anti-IgE	–	[85]
		–	[155]
Basophil[4] (see text)	A23187	+	[25]
	Synacthen	+	[25]
	Complement-coated baker's yeast spores	+	[25]
	C3a	+	[26]
	C5a	+	[25]

Table 2.1 Cellular origins of PAF (*Continued*)

Cell	Stimulus[1]	Released[2]	Reference
	Neutrophil cationic protein	+	[26]
		+	[25]
	DNA[5]	+	[156]
	Anti-IgE	+	[25]
	pH 10.6	+	[25]
Endothelial cell	A23187	+	[65]
	Angiotension II	+	[65]
	Anti-human factor VIII	+	[65]
	IL-1	25 %	[157]
		30 %	[157]
	Leukotrienes C_4 and D_4	2–3 %	[46]
	Thrombin	N.A.	[92]
		–	[50]
	H_2O_2	–	[47]
		N.A.	[121]
	Clostridial θ toxin	N.A.	[121]
	Melittin	N.A.	[121]
	Membrane attack complex of complement	N.A.	[121]
	Vasopressin	+	[65]
	Histamine	–	[50]
	Bradykinin	–	[50]
	ATP	–	[50]
	TNF	+	[74]
		30%	[95]
	LPS	4–5%	[28]
	Elastase	+	[129]
Platelet	Thrombin	N.A.	[23]
		N.A.	[82]
	A23187	N.A.	[122]
		N.A.	[22]
Large granular lymphocytes (natural killer cells)	Immobilized anti-Fc receptor	+	[91]
	A23187	+	[91]
Transformed or neoplastic cells			
HL-60:			
neutrophil-like[6]	A23187	N.A.	[80]
	FMLP	N.A.	[80]
macrophage-like[7]	pH 9.5	+	[158]
	C3b–baker's yeast spores	+	[158]
	C3d–baker's yeast spores	+	[158]

Table 2.1 Cellular origins of PAF (*Continued*)

Cell	Stimulus[1]	Released[2]	Reference
basophilic leukaemia	A23187	+	[86]
T-cell ALL	A23187 + acetyl CoA ± PHA	+	[90]
common ALL	A23187 + acetyl CoA ± PHA	+	[90]
CLL (B-cell)	A23187 + acetyl CoA ± PHA	+	[90]
CML	A23187 + acetyl CoA ± PHA	+	[90]
AML	A23187 + acetyl CoA ± PHA	+	[90]
T-cell leukaemia cell lines	A23187 ± PHA/ ± acetyl CoA	+	[89]
B-cell leukaemia cell lines	A23187 ± PHA/ ± acetyl CoA	+	[89]
EBV transformed lymphoblastoid cell lines	A23187 ± PHA/ ± acetyl CoA	+	[89]
Fibroblasts (human skin)	A23187	50 %	[38]

[1] *Abbreviations*: A23187, calcium ionophore; cyto B, cytochalasin B; FMLP, *N'*-formyl-methionyl-leucyl-phenylanine; PMA, phorbol-12-myristate-13-acetate; LPS, lipopolysaccharide; TNF, tumour necrosis factor; IL-1, interleukin-1; IFN, interferon; ECF-A, eosinophil chemotactic factor of anaphylaxis; DNA, deoxyribonucleic acid; ATP, adenosine triphosphate; PHA, phytohaemagglutinin.
[2] PAF released: +, detectable PAF release; −, no detectable PAF release; N.A., PAF release not assessed.
[3] Cells from atopic asthmatics or following passive sensitization of cells from normal patients.
[4] Basophil-enriched buffy coat.
[5] In cells from patients with systemic lupus erythematosus.
[6] Differentiated toward neutrophil-like cells with dimethylsulfoxide (DMSO).
[7] Differentiated toward macrophage-like cells with tetradodecanoylphorbol acetate (TPA).

[46,51]. Furthermore, macrophages may be activated by PAF incorporated into liposomes [52]. These findings suggest that PAF embedded in the plasma membrane of a source cell may be recognized and stimulate an adjacent target cell.

The mechanisms by which PAF is released are poorly understood. From several sources it appears that release is dependent on the presence of albumin in the extracellular medium [1,53]. The ability of albumin to bind PAF and other phospholipids and lysophospholipids has long been known, though to date its interaction with PAF is not well quantitated. Albumin has been shown to solubilize PAF in aqueous media [54] and PAF added exogenously to plasma co-elutes with the fraction containing albumin and other plasma proteins [53]. Albumin appears to compete with cells and cell membranes for PAF as it inhibits binding of PAF to human neutrophil membranes [55] and inhibits secretion and aggregation of platelets [56,57]. Other proteins, intracellular and extracellular (in plasma) may also bind PAF. A PAF-specific transport protein(s) has/have been isolated from bovine and rabbit lung macrophages [58] and rat lung [59] which can transfer PAF between lipid bilayers. A PAF-binding protein found in human serum has also been described that apparently can bind PAF more tightly than albumin [60]. From such data it is clear that albumin and possibly other proteins bind to PAF that is released from cells. The mechanism of actual release of PAF is as yet unknown but may proceed in a monomeric fashion, or via an exocytotic process (as in secretion of surfactant phospholipids from alveolar Type-II cells), or from shed membranes of disrupted or lysed cells. As cells do not appear to make PAF in sufficient quantity to exceed the critical micellar concentration of PAF (1.1 μM) [54,61], it is unlikely that PAF is released as micelles. Whether albumin or other proteins essentially extract PAF from the cell surface, or whether PAF is released by one of the above mechanisms and then becomes protein-bound, is unclear. Finally, whether release is a passive process or whether it is an active process is not known [62].

While extracellular calcium appears to be essential for the production of PAF by the remodelling pathway in response to most physiological and pharmacological stimuli (see the section on modulation of synthesis) [63–65], its role in release of PAF is less clear. Ludwig *et al.* [63] demonstrated that in the absence of extracellular Ca^{2+}, while synthesis of PAF was limited to 10–30% of that seen in optimal conditions, release of PAF was undetectable. The dependence of PAF synthesis and secretion on the presence of extracellular Ca^{2+} and albumin [53,63] have led these authors to propose a synthesis–release coupling mechanism for the human neutrophil. They suggest that albumin and extracellular Ca^{2+} are required for release of PAF and that release triggers further synthesis of PAF. In this way, release of newly-synthesized PAF abrogates feedback inhibition of PAF on PAF synthesis. In contrast to this hypothesis are the data of Elstad *et al.* [62] who demonstrated that while both synthesis and release were dependent on albumin concentration in the media, the optimal concentration for release was less than that for optimal synthesis, thus dissociating these phenomena. Against a generalized hypothesis of synthesis–release coupling are the findings of several laboratories. Sisson *et al.* [43] noted that total synthesis of PAF in adherent PMN is decreased when compared to that of PMN in suspension while the amount released is independent of state of adherence. Synthesis was also dissociated from release of PAF in the work of Lynch & Henson [28] who noted that while neutrophils stimulated with FMLP (and cytochalasin B) produced far less PAF than PMN stimulated with calcium ionophore or opsonized zymosan, the relative proportion of PAF released was greatest following FMLP stimulation.

Additional factors appearing to affect PAF release are cell type [62], and species differences [28], with further modulation by agonist in neutrophils [28,54], eosinophils [66] and monocytes [62] cell density [29,64,67] dynamic removal of media [68], pH of the medium [67], state of adherence versus suspension [43,62] or 'phase of response' [69]. Clearly the relationship of PAF synthesis and release may not be straightforward, and confounding variables will likely explain current controversies.

Stimulation of inflammatory cells to produce PAF

Most notable among the human cells synthesizing PAF which are listed in Table 2.1 are the cells involved in inflammatory reactions. Most studies indicate that these cells do not synthesize significant levels of PAF in the baseline, non-stimulated state. Upon stimulation however, large amounts of the molecule are synthesized. Snyder [70] has suggested the presence of two pathways for PAF generation and that the *de novo* pathway involving cholinephosphotransferase leads to low levels of endogenous, non-stimulated production (see Chapter 1). Stimulation then initiates the remodelling pathway (outlined in the previous section) to generate the large amounts of mediator noted. Common to each of these cells is a relative enrichment in their content of ether-linked phospholipids. For example, in the human polymorphonuclear leukocytes > 50% of choline glycerophospholipids appear to be ether-linked in the *sn*-1 position [71]. Adequate amounts of ether-linked substrate (alkylacyl-GPC), the precursor for subsequent PAF synthesis, have been documented in neutrophils [14,44,48,72], platelets [73], human monocytes [48], and in human fibroblasts [38] (also see Chapter 1).

Of all human inflammatory cell sources of PAF, the neutrophil is the most remarkable in amounts of PAF produced (Table 2.2). Stimulation with the calcium ionophore A23187 under optimal conditions has been shown to produce in the range of 10–100 pmol/10^6 cells [28,44,48] (see Table 2.2). The neutrophil also responds with the synthesis of PAF to a variety of stimuli types that act through cell-surface receptors (see Table 2.1). These include complete secretagogues, specific granule secretagogues and phagocytic particles. Differing reports of the ability of phorbol esters to initiate synthesis [43,54,64] raise questions as to the role of protein kinase C in the stimulus–synthesis pathway. Notably, neutrophils have been reported not to respond with detectable production of PAF to a variety of stimuli, some of which are known to initiate other responses in

Table 2.2 Comparison of potential for PAF synthesis and release by human cells*

Cell	PAF synthesis (pmol/10^6 cells)	PAF release (pmol/10^6 cells)	Stimulus	Reference
Neutrophil	100	49	A23187 (9.5 μM)	[48]
	42	4	A23187 (1.9 μM)	[28]
	10	2	A23187 (2.5 μM)	[44]
Monocyte	44	21	A23187 (9.5 μM)	[48]
Macrophage (alveolar)	?	10	A23187 (1.9–9.5 μM)	[159]
Mast cell	3	N.D.	Anti-IgE (2 μg/ml)	[85]
Eosinophil	?	0.0012	A23187 (1 μM)	[66]
Platelet	0.0035	?	A23187 (2.5 μM)	[8]
Lymphocyte	1	0.25	A23187 (9.5 μM)	[48]
Endothelial cell	100–170	N.D.	Thrombin (2 U/ml)	[92]
	153	?	A23187 (1 μM)	[94]
Fibroblast	0.7	0.34	A23187 (2 μM)	[38]

N.D. = Not detectable.
* Values must be considered only as estimates of PAF synthesis and release as there is no uniformity with regard to assay conditions or methods of detection.

the cell, including PAF itself, LTB_4, LTC_4, LTD_4, LTE_4, zymosan-activated serum, platelet-derived growth factor, epinephrine, bradykinin, histamine, thrombin, adenosine triphosphate, vasopressin or fibrinogen [43]. Response to tumour necrosis factor is controversial [43,74]. The issue of neutrophil stimulation is also complicated by the process of priming, whereby exposure of the cell to an agent that itself does not initiate a response nevertheless causes the cell to become much more responsive to a second stimulus. Thus prior exposure to bacterial lipopolysaccharide (priming) significantly increased the amounts of PAF that were synthesized by neutrophils stimulated with the tripeptide FMLP [45]. Similarly, and perhaps identically, adherent cells may exhibit different responses to those in suspension [43]. If, in the various investigations of PAF production by neutrophils, the cells had been inadvertently primed during preparation (a number of agents, including PAF itself are candidates), the subsequent PAF synthesis could have been considerably affected.

The rank order of potency for PAF synthesis in the neutrophil of commonly used stimuli is A23187 > opsonized zymosan > FMLP with or without cytochalasin B as determined by bioassay [28] or by incorporation of labelled acetate [43]. As implied above, it has been possible to dissociate other cellular events from production of PAF by differing time courses or pharmacological modulators. These include secretion of granules [53,63,64], phagocytosis [27], superoxide production [64], aggregation and surface adhesion [43]. On the other hand, production of LTB_4 appears to be closely associated with that of PAF [43]. This is likely due to liberation of arachidonate from the same alkylacyl-GPC that serves as the precursor for PAF [75,76]. Coordinate production of arachidonate metabolites and PAF has been noted in other cell types and has led to the suggestion that the same phospholipid serves as the precursor for both groups of mediators (see below). Additionally however, PAF synthesized by neutrophils may in turn stimulate these same cells to make LTB_4 as a secondary event [77,78] thereby complicating analysis of such data. Because of the amount of PAF produced by neutrophils (and monocytes, see below) contamination of other isolated cell preparations with relatively few neutrophils is clearly a problem when determining the capacity of a given cell type to produce PAF.

The human blood monocyte synthesizes PAF in response to several stimuli as depicted in Table 2.1. On a per-cell basis, it appears to make less PAF than the human neutrophil in some studies with approximately 44 pmol produced per million cells stimulated with A23187 [48] (see Table 2.2). Similar to the neutrophil, the human monocyte appears to respond to the stimuli A23187 > opsonized zymonsan > PMA with production of PAF [62]. Some investigators suggest that release of PAF may be greater on a per-cell basis for the monocyte than the PMN [25,62] Several stimuli for PAF release in the neutrophil (C5a, C5a des arg, neutrophil cationic protein or neutrophil cationic protein des arg) [25,29], and from endothelial cells (rabbit anti-human factor VIII, angiotension II or vasopressin) [65] do not stimulate PAF release from monocytes. As with the neutrophil, the state of adherence may modulate the amount of PAF produced by monocytes though reports are conflicting as to whether synthesis is increased [79] or decreased [62] and may signify a state of activation or priming [27]. Also in similarity to the neutrophil, secretion of lysozyme and phagocytosis are cellular events that can be dissociated from the release of PAF [79]. Recently, Valone & Epstein [69] have reported a novel biphasic PAF biosynthetic response in human monocytes to three cytokines, IL-1-β, TNF, INF-γ. These authors noted that while PAF was largely retained intracellularly during the early peak at 1–2 h of stimulation, it was largely secreted (70%) during the late peak at 6–8 h. Furthermore, the late peak induced by INF-γ was inhibited by specific antibodies to TNF or IL1-β suggesting a role for these monocyte-derived cytokines in stimulated PAF production. Additionally, cycloheximide was found to inhibit the late peak of PAF synthesis suggesting that this phase requires new protein synthesis.

The state of cellular differentiation can alter PAF biosynthesis. While cell lysates of the undifferentiated human pro-myelocytic cell line HL-60 cells appear to have PLA_2 and acetyltransferase, yet PAF synthesis does not occur by the remodelling pathway until cellular differentiation [80].

Differentiation of monocytic cells to alveolar macrophages is also associated with some diminished capacity to produce PAF [62]. Arnoux *et al.* [81] reported release of PAF from human alveolar macrophages in response to A23187 but not to phagocytosis of opsonized zymosan. This finding contrasted with results from alveolar macrophages of other species and led the authors to suggest that the overall state of activation may modulate (production) release. In the case of cells from asthmatics, very small amounts were produced in response to anti-IgE and specific allergen [30], and this was undetectable following treatment of patients with theophylline or theophylline in combination with corticosteroids. The studies outlined above point out the difficulties of determining whether mononuclear phagocytes from a given site are, in fact, synthesizing and releasing PAF. Not only do the enzymes involved in synthesis and degradation of PAF vary with maturational state of the cells, but, in addition, the cells themselves may alter that state upon removal from the *in vivo* environment. The determination of appropriate stimuli for the cells represents but an additional complication. Suffice it to say that the mononuclear phagocyte can produce PAF and may constitute a significant source in both inflammatory and non-inflammatory processes. Studies suggest that human alveolar macrophages also produce and release considerable quantities of lyso-PAF following stimulation with ionophore or, in the cases of cells from asthmatics, specific antigen [30]. Release of lyso-PAF, the immediate precursor and catabolic product of PAF, may place this cell in a unique position to participate in transcellular biosynthesis of PAF by supplying other cells with the immediate precursor of PAF (see following section).

Relative to other cells, the human platelet has been shown to produce small quantities of PAF, 3.5 fmol/10^6 cells in response to A23187 [8] (Table 2.2) and approximately 2–4.8 fmol/10^6 cells for thrombin stimulation [23,82]. This cell seems relatively deficient in acetyltransferase and while it makes little PAF, it may release lyso-PAF that can be in turn utilized by other cells to result in heightened PAF production via transcellular biosynthesis [35]. Additionally, studies suggest that thrombin-stimulated platelets produce 10–12 times more PAF when the degradative acetylhydrolase is inhibited [23]. Whether these cells represent a significant source of the molecule during inflammatory or thrombotic events has yet to be determined.

Eosinophils have been shown to produce PAF though the amount produced by the eosinophil has not been documented. However, these studies of eosinophils have generally utilized blood from patients with a variety of disease states, characterized by eosinophilia in which prior activation (and or priming) of eosinophils as part of the disease state is quite possible. Accordingly, Lee *et al.* [83] have demonstrated heightened activity of several enzymes involved in PAF metabolism in cells from patients with eosinophilia when compared to normal individuals.

While PAF synthesis has been demonstrated in mast cells isolated from animal sources [84], the difficulty in isolating human mast cells (which demonstrate heterogeneity in themselves) from various tissue sources has left the question of the human mast cell as a source of PAF largely open. In mast-cell preparations from human lung tissue purified to 97% or greater, PAF is produced in response to anti-IgE though release of PAF into the media was undetectable [85] (Table 2.2).

Human basophils isolated in crude buffy coat preparations have been accorded the capability of synthesizing PAF in response to a variety of stimuli (see Table 2.1). Additionally PAF synthesis has been detected from human basophil leukemia cells in response to A23187 [86]. Subsequent studies, however, have raised questions concerning the attribution of PAF release to the basophil. In contrast to the rabbit basophil which appears to synthesize and release considerable quantities of PAF in response to anti-IgE or calcium ionophore [1,28,29], the human basophil in enriched fractions or in whole leukocyte preparations appears not to release PAF in response to anti-human IgE, neutrophil cationic protein, C5a, calcium ionophore, opsonized zymosan or protein A [27–29]. A very real possibility is that the human basophil can make PAF perfectly well but is inefficient at releasing it to the exterior. In mixed-cell populations then, it would be difficult to demonstrate this when the proportion of basophils in the populations is generally so low. The use of basophil-specific stimuli in mixed-cell populations to implicate the human basophil as a producer of PAF [25], unfortunately, does not eliminate the presence of secondary signals and other complex cell–cell interactions which could result in PAF production from contaminating cells. The difficulty with current technology in isolating purified human basophils will leave open for now the question of the human basophil as a source of PAF. The development of antibodies and specific probes for the enzymes involved in the synthesis will, in the future, allow a demonstration of at least the potential for this cell type to produce PAF.

To date, there is evidence that human lymphocytes produce little, if any, detectable PAF although a number of investigators including ourselves have looked at this (whether the right stimuli were used always remains a question) and the cell seemingly lacks acetyltransferase activity [48]. To definitively demonstrate that a cell such as the lymphocyte does not, and cannot, synthesize the molecule it will be necessary to show that it either does not make the enzymes required, does not activate them or lacks the precursor phospholipid. There is emerging evidence that PAF can modify a variety of lymphocyte responses via a receptor-mediated process(es) [87,88] and thus unlike the cells listed above, which appear to both produce PAF and be a target for PAF, lymphocytes appear to respond in a paracrine rather than autocrine fashion. Of note, cells isolated from patients with several different types of lymphocytic leukaemias have been shown to produce PAF (Table 2.1) [89,90]. Presumably, the ability to produce PAF is lost with ultimate differentiation along the lymphocytic lineage.

Human natural killer cells found in the rather diverse population of circulating cells, known by their phenotypic appearance as large granular lymphocytes, appear to be capable of synthesis and release of PAF in response to stimulation by A23187 or the Fc receptor (which in this cell is thought to be similar to that found in the human neutrophil) [91]. Any role that PAF may play in the natural killer cell's cytotoxic repertoire is at this time speculative.

Endothelial cells obtained from human vascular beds including the umbilical cord vein [46,50,92], iliac vein [93] and microvasculature [28] appear to make PAF in response to a variety of stimuli (Table 2.1). Most studies have not quantitated the amounts of PAF produced but available estimates range from 100 to 170 pmol/10^6 cells [92,94] (see Table 2.2). These very high amounts have not been found by all investigators but do suggest that the endothelial cell under certain conditions may make remarkable quantities of PAF. Unlike the response to most physiological stimuli which stimulate PAF synthesis to peak and decay within the first hour of stimulation in most cells, PAF synthesis by endothelial cells in response to stimulation with LTC_4 and LTD_4 was prolonged over 2 h [46] while that with IL-1 and TNF stimulation was considerably delayed [95]. Onset of PAF synthesis in response to the latter two stimuli was at 2 h and peak production at 8–12 h. Inhibition of this delayed, prolonged response to cytokines by treatment of cells with cycloheximide and actinomycin D led Bussolino *et al.* [95] to suggest that in endothelial cells, *de novo* synthesis of acetyltransferase may be responsible for the delayed response. However, the situation must be more complicated since increased amounts of acetyltransferase alone would not expected to initiate PAF synthesis. Some activation of the phospholipase A_2 would also be required and it, too, presumably follows the above-mentioned time course. Inhibition of cyclooxygenase has been reported to result in increased production of PAF by endothelial cells in response to thrombin [65], IL-1 and TNF [95] suggesting the possibility of prostanoid regulatory effects on PAF synthesis in these cells. Release of PAF from endothelial cells appears to be variable. In studies by McIntyre *et al.* [46] and Zimmerman *et al.* [51], PAF synthesized in response to LTC_4 and thrombin remained exclusively cell-associated. These investigators have suggested that the PAF is available on the endothelial cell surface to activate passing leukocytes and initiate their adhesion to the endothelium. [46,50].

Transcellular biosynthesis of PAF

Considerable interest has emerged in recent years in the possibilities of cooperation between cells in the synthesis, and/or metabolism of lipid mediators. First shown in the transcellular synthesis of prostaglandins by platelets and endothelial cells [96], the phenomenon has now been extended to a wide variety of mediators, including sulfidopeptide leukotrienes and LTB_4 [97–98]. Three types of cellular interaction that are potentially involved in the production or modulation of lipid mediators have been defined: (i) *transcellular biosynthesis* involves the release of an intermediate (usually unstable) from one cell and its uptake and conversion into the final mediator by another; (ii) *transcellular metabolism* describes the further metabolism (usually to inactive metabolites) by one cell of a mediator first produced by another cell; and (iii) *transcellular stimulation* implies the stimulation of synthesis of a mediator in one cell by a different mediator produced by another cell. The possiblity that neutrophil-derived PAF (particularly if it remained cell-associated) can initiate synthesis of thromboxane by adherent platelets would constitute an example of (iii).

The synthesis and release of lyso-PAF as the immediate precursor of PAF synthesis or its immediate catabolic product, from alveolar macrophages from humans [30–32] and rats [31,32], platelets [33], human endothelial cells [34] and its presence in amniotic fluid [40] raises the possibility that PAF also can be synthesized in a transcellular fashion. Cells such as neutrophils can take up lyso-PAF [48,75] and can metabolize this into other phospholipids. If the acetyltransferase is active it seems reasonable to expect the synthesis of PAF and in fact, such a transcellular process has been described [35]. Furthermore, in the case of neutrophils, the availability of lyso-PAF appears to be a limiting factor in PAF synthesis [48]. Fibroblasts have also been reported to utilize exogenous lyso-PAF to enhance PAF synthesis [38] suggesting that other tissues/cells if supplied with the immediate precursor may have enhanced biosynthetic capability. In the environment of the inflammatory reaction, with multiple-cell types in close contact (both inflammatory and tissue cells), exchange of intermediates would not be unexpected. The presence of albumin from the increased vascular permeability would only serve to enhance this exchange by stabilizing the lipids during the transfer process.

Other cellular sources of PAF

PAF has been found in a variety of body fluids in pathological states. Nasal washing [99] and skin blisters [100] from allergic patients challenged with antigen, sputa from patients with asthma and COPD [101], lung lavage from infants with bronchopulmonary dysplasia [102], blood from patients with cold urticaria undergoing cold challenge [103], blood and ascitic fluid in cirrhotics [104], and psoriatic scales [105] have been reported to contain detectable PAF. The cellular sources of the molecule under these circumstances remains obscure, but inflammatory cells can, in most cases, be suggested to be the most likely candidates.

By contrast, the presence of PAF in body fluids under normal conditions, blood [42], urine [40,41], saliva [106], and amnoitic fluid [40], has led to the very reasonable suggestion that PAF may play a role in normal physiology. Here, however, a note of caution should be raised. While it seems intuitively valid to suggest that the presence of a complicated pathway to synthesize a highly- and broadly-active mediator such as PAF implies a critically important biological role, this role has certainly not yet been determined. A detailed combination of physiological and pharmacological studies, probably combined with some 'accidents of nature' will be required to answer this question. Unfortunately, the sensitivity of cells to stimulation cannot always preclude the possibility that the isolation procedure itself has contributed to the levels of PAF reported in 'normal' biological fluids. Furthermore, the presence of a little inflammation could always account for any PAF detected. For example, the PAF found in saliva could perhaps have been derived from neutrophils emigrating through the gingival crevice. The actual cellular sources synthesizing PAF in these body fluids is yet to be determined. Likely possibilities include mesangial cells [107,108], Type-II cells [109,110], keratinocytes [111], hepatocytes [11], and fibroblasts [38]. At this point, studies suggesting the ability of tissue cells such as these to synthesize PAF have largely been carried out using cells from non-human sources.

It seems possible that most cell types can, under the right conditions of stimulation, produce PAF. In fact, as discussed below, there is a distinct possibility that ether-PC turnover, and even perhaps the production of PAF, may play a role in normal cell physiology, let alone in processes involving whole organs and tissues. Critical to considering PAF as a mediator therefore, will be the determination of when, *in vivo*, the molecule is synthesized and just as critically, when it is released from the cell of origin.

Modulation of synthesis and catabolism of PAF

As a role for PAF in pathological processes is defined, two possible approaches to abrogation of PAF-induced responses can be ultimately explored. One is the use of PAF antagonists, a diverse group of agents (discussed in Chapter 4) utilized to block the effect of PAF on a target cell or tissue. The second possibility is modulation of PAF metabolism, either down-regulation of synthesis or up-regulation of catabolism. While the pathways for PAF biosynthesis and a detailed discussion of the regulation of synthesis and degradation as currently understood are outlined in Chapter 1, a few mechanisms whereby PAF synthesis can be modulated will be discussed here.

While little or no PAF is detectable in the inflammatory cells listed in Table 2.1 without stimulation, the presence of a specific stimulus in the extracellular milieu results in biosynthesis of PAF. Data suggest that both the first and second steps in the remodelling pathway (Fig. 2.1), the cleaving of the long-chained acyl group from the *sn*-2 position of alkyl, acyl-GPC by phospholipase A_2 [112,113] and the transfer of an acetyl group to the *sn*-2 position by alkyl lyso-GPC:acetyl-CoA acetyltransferase [48,66,114] appear to be enhanced with cell stimulation. In the work of Doebber & Wu [115] PAF itself as a stimulus has been shown to augment acetyltransferase activity in human neutrophils suggesting that in some circumstances it may participate in stimulating its own synthesis. Circulating eosinophils of subjects with hypereosinophilia are thought to be 'activated' by several measures and have been shown to demonstrate enhanced acetyl transferase activity [83]. Finally, studies suggest that a post-translational modification of the inactive acetyltransferase results in a quantitative increase in the active enzyme [116,117] and recent data from mouse bone-marrow mast cells [117], rat spleen microsomes [118,119] and rat exocrine gland [120] suggest that phosphorylation of the acetyl transferase by a kinase (as yet undefined) is responsible for heightened activity. In endothelial cells, Bussolino *et al.* [95] have suggested that there is *de novo* synthesis of the acetyltransferase involved in the slow appearance of PAF after stimulation with TNF or IL-1.

In addition to the presence of specific stimuli, other factors in the extracellular milieu also modulate PAF biosynthesis. The presence of extracellular Ca^{2+} is largely required for the synthesis of PAF by human neutrophils [63,64], endothelial cells [121], alveolar macrophages [81], platelets [122] and monocytes [79]. Both enzymatic steps in the biosynthesis of PAF, that catalysed by PLA_2 [112,113] and acetyltransferase [63,64,123] appear to be enhanced under conditions of increased intracellular Ca^{2+} (see Chapter 1). An increase in Ca^{2+} flux from the extracellular medium occurs following stimulation with a variety of physiological stimuli such as FMLP, which opens Ca^{2+} channels by a receptor-driven mechanism. Alternatively, a variety of pharmacological agents (calcium ionophore, melittin in endothelium) which permeablize cell membranes to allow the influx of Ca^{2+} [121] result in PAF synthesis. Accordingly, ketotifen was shown to block Ca^{2+} entry and PAF synthesis into mouse mast cells stimulated with antigen [124] and the Ca^{2+} channel blocker, nifedipine could partially inhibit release/synthesis of PAF from human neutrophils [125]. Similarly, the calmodulin antagonists, trifluoperazine and *N*-(6-aminohexyl)-5-chloro-1-naphthalenesulfonamide inhibited formation of PAF by ionophore-stimulated human neutrophils [126]. Conversely, the small amounts of PAF produced in neutrophils in response to PMA are not dependent on extracellular calcium [54]. Finally, in contrast to the stimulatory effect of calcium on PAF synthesis, increased intracellular Ca^{2+} appears to be inhibitory to the enzymes of PAF degradation [127] thus further contributing to the overall production of PAF.

Other factors in the extracellular milieu also appear to affect synthesis of PAF. Dependence of biosynthesis on the presence of albumin has been demonstrated for the neutrophil [53] and rabbit buffy coat leukocytes [1] and suggests a synthesis–release coupling mechanism (see above). Data from Ninio *et al.* [128] suggest that the complex interaction of albumin with PAF, lyso-PAF (the immediate precursor and degradation product), and other phospholipid analogues may influence acetyltransferase activity by removing end-product feedback inhibition. In lysates of calcium ionophore-treated human neutrophils activity of this final enzyme in the remodelling pathway were shown to be inhibited by high concentrations of lyso-PAF or PAF itself, while low concentrations of lyso-PAF (or lyso-PC), and increased albumin concentrations were protective of enzymatic activity [128]. Other components in plasma may also be important in PAF synthesis as suggested by the work of Camussi *et al.* [129] who showed that the presence of serum anti-proteinases inhibit PAF synthesis in PMN and endothelial cells. This finding led the authors to hypothesize that PAF synthesis and release would be localized to cellular contact areas where plasma proteins are excluded and thereby direct and limit the inflammatory response.

Further regulation of PAF biosynthesis may be possible by limiting substrate availability. Because the liberation and re-incorporation of arachidonic acid has been closely linked to PAF synthesis and catabolism [75,130–132] (see the discussion on interaction of PAF, below), an alternative approach to inhibiting cellular synthesis involves depletion of alkylarachidonoyl-GPC. The supplementation of marine fish oils to inflammatory cells in culture or to whole animals has been associated with increased incorporation of the supplied fatty acid, a decrease in arachidonate release in some studies, and a shift in the yield of leukotrienes and prostaglandins to less potent analogs upon inflammatory cell stimulation [133–136]. A decrease in biosynthesis of PAF has been demonstrated by several laboratories following arachidonic acid depletion. Codde *et al.* [137] found a decrease in whole blood PAF and lyso-PAF in human subjects fed a diet enriched in fish oils. Kawasaki *et al.* [138] demonstrated decreased PAF production in arachidonic acid-deficient HL-60 cells differentiated to granulocytic-type cells and stimulated with calcium ionophore. Furthermore, PAF synthesis was restored following supplementation with arachidonic acid or its precursor. Similar findings were demonstrated in arachidonate-deficient rat polymorphonuclear leukocytes [139].

In much of this preliminary work directed at decreasing substrate availability, it is unclear whether arachidonate depletion to any degree as measured for whole cells or tissues is reflective of limiting substrate in specific precursor pools utilized in PAF biosynthesis. The concept that substrate pools and subcellular locations may restrict substrate availability is unproven but attractive. Actually, little is known of the subcellular localization of enzymes and substrates involved in synthesis and degradation of PAF [114,140,141]. As more is learned of the intracellular topography of these events, perhaps the means to modulate PAF synthesis will be identified.

Alternatively, pharmacological inhibition of the enzymatic steps involved in the biosynthesis of PAF holds some promise. The inhibitors of phospholipase A_2, bromophenacyl bromide and mepacrine (although not necessarily specific for this enzyme), have been shown to inhibit release of PAF from human blood monocytes [79], and synthesis and release from rat alveolar macrophages [32]. Treatment of human subjects with corticosteroids has been associated with decreased PAF biosynthesis from alveolar macrophages of atopic asthmatics [30] as did corticosteroid treatment of colonic biopsy specimens of patients with active ulcerative colitis [142]. Similar findings in guinea-pig lung [143] and rat inflammatory neutrophils [144] have been demonstrated with decreased detectable PAF after treatment with corticosteroids. Additionally, hydrocortisone and partially-purified macrocortin were shown to inhibit release of lyso-PAF from rat peritoneal macrophages stimulated with zymosan [145] suggesting that, as in other studies, corticosteroids may act at the level of PLA_2 rather than at the acetylation step in PAF biosynthesis. Other activities of corticosteroids, such as ATPase, cGMP and phosphodiesterase inhibition have not been systematically examined.

Increases in cellular cAMP may modulate PAF biosynthesis in some cells. Camussi *et al.* demonstrated that isoproterenol, dibutyrl-cAMP, PGE_2, and PGI_2 decreased PAF synthesis in monocytes [79], and similarly PGI_2 in endothelial cells [65], while treatment of atopic asthmatics with theophylline likewise decreased PAF synthesis from isolated alveolar macrophages [30]. Recent data have suggested that the effect of increased cAMP on PAF biosynthesis in stimulated neutrophils was not due to inhibition of Ca^{2+} mobilization, acetyltransferase activity or increased catabolism, but rather to its effect on PLA_2 [146].

Inhibition of acetyltransferase activity has been accomplished with a variety of non-specific agents, sulfhydryl reagents [147], diisopropylfluorophosphate, bromophenacyl bromide [148] and several amphipathic phosphocholines [70,149]. The mechanism of the pharmacological agents, salazopyrine and 5-aminosalicyclic acid [142], in inhibiting PAF synthesis has not been clearly elucidated.

Interaction of PAF with other lipid mediator synthesis

Data from several laboratories suggest that alkylacyl-GPC, the preformed precursor of PAF, is in part comprised specifically of alkylarachidonoyl-GPC (see Chapter 1) [75,139]. This finding has led to the hypothesis that the first step of PAF synthesis, the cleaving of arachidonate from alkylarachidonoyl-GPC would in essence liberate two important precursor molecules, lyso-PAF and arachidonic acid, which depending on the cell type (or in transcellular biosynthesis, on neighbouring cells), could then be metabolized to PAF and lipoxygenase and/or cyclooxygenase products [76,130,139,150]. To date, study of mediator synthesis of several cell types has furnished data suggesting that this may be the case. Perhaps the best studied examples are the concurrent synthesis of PAF and LTB_4 (a lipoxygenase product) in human PMN and PAF and PGI_2 (a cyclooxygenase product) in human endothelial cells. Data linking this type of concurrent synthesis are outlined below.

The recognition that the human neutrophil produces and releases 5-lipoxygenase products of arachidonic acid, particularly LTB_4, and PAF in response to similar stimuli [78,136,151] prompted studies to examine whether dual synthesis of these mediators was linked. Sisson *et al.* [43] found that the two mediators were tightly coupled in time course over 30 min for both adherent and suspended PMN stimulated with ionophore. Additional data linking these two mediators from the common precursor alkylacyl-GPC comes from Chilton [152] who showed that the human neutrophil can utilize arachidonate derived specifically from ether-linked phospholipids for leukotriene synthesis. Complicating this schema is the finding that PAF is itself a stimulus for LTB_4 synthesis in the neutrophil [77,78] while LTB_4 does not apparently stimulate PAF synthesis [43].

Similar to the data above linking eicosanoid and PAF production in the neutrophil, various stimuli of PAF synthesis in the human endothelial cell have been shown to also produce PGI_2. These include LTC_4, LTD_4, histamine, bradykinin and ATP [46,50]. Of the leukotrienes, each appeared to have identical agonist activity in the production of PAF and PGI_2 with the rank order of potency being $LTC_4 > LTD_4 \gg LTB_4 = LTE_4$ [46]. Furthermore, production of both PAF and PGI_2 by stimulation with histamine and bradykinin was shown to be linked through activation specifically of the histamine H_1 and bradykinin B_2-receptor sub-types, respectively. Time courses of initiation of synthesis of the two mediators appear to be closely linked while duration of synthesis (7.5–15 min for PGI_2 and >40 min for PAF) were widely divergent. Also in contrast were the fates of the two mediators, PGI_2 being almost entirely released while PAF was not released to the medium.

In theory, linkage of PAF and eicosanoid biosynthesis would dictate that the inhibition of PAF synthesis by pharmacological agents at the level of the PLA_2 would be accompanied by inhibition of synthesis of eicosanoids. Such circumstantial evidence that the two pathways are linked and can be concomitantly inhibited has been demonstrated in rat neutrophils treated with dexamethasone [144] and in recent studies by Chilton *et al.* [146] who treated human neutrophils with isoproterenol and were able to inhibit synthesis of both PAF and LTB_4. Finally, inhibition of both PAF and LTB_4 synthesis was demonstrated in arachidonic acid-deficient rat polymorphonuclear leukocytes and raises the possibility of modifying the activity of both pathways by depletion of the common precursor molecule, alkylarachidonoyl-GPC, through dietary manipulation [139].

To date, while data linking tandem PAF and eicosanoid biosynthesis in several cell types are available, pin-pointing the actual source of these mediators from a common precursor molecule is yet to be established. Conclusive proof of such tandem biosynthesis and its relative contribution to cellular biosynthesis of these mediators, awaits refinement in detection methods and effective dual labelling of precursor pools to a high degree of specific activity.

Conclusions

In summary, PAF is synthesized and frequently secreted in response to a variety of stimuli from numerous cells, particularly those involved in inflammation. While this fact is undisputed, the role of PAF in pathological processes is far from clear. Proof of such a role requires detection of PAF *in vivo* and abrogation of its effects with specific modulation of its synthesis/release or by specific blockade by antagonists. The lack, to date, of fully established criteria for any inflammatory process attests to the difficulty of this task. Furthermore, as more is learned about cell–cell interactions in sites of inflammation, the degree of complexity with regard to transcellular signalling, the interplay of multiple mediators and transcellular biosynthesis/alteration of mediators appears to increase exponentially.

A homeostatic role for PAF in human physiological processes likewise awaits proof of the mediator synthesis by cells under unstimulated conditions and its effects on target cells. Because PAF under many circumstances appears to remain largely cell-associated, an intracellular role for PAF is an intriguing possibility. Answers to these questions will likely need technical advances to allow refinement in the ability to detect PAF and to modulate its synthesis, release and effects.

References

1 Benveniste, J., Henson, P. M. & Cochrane, C. G. Leukocyte-dependent histamine release from rabbit platelets—the role of IgE, basophils and a platelet-activating factor. *J. Exp. Med.* (1972), **136**, 1356–1377.

2 Demopoulos, C. A., Pinckard, R. N. & Hanahan, D. J. Platelet-activating factor. Evidence for 1-O-alkyl-2-acetyl-*sn*-glyceryl-3-phosphorylcholine as the active component (a new class of lipid chemical mediators). *J. Biol. Chem.* (1979), **254**, 9355–9358.

3 Lynch, J.M, Lotner, G. Z., Betz, S. J. & Henson, P. M. The release of a platelet-activating factor by stimulated rabbit neutrophils. *J. Immunol.* (1979), **123**, 1219–1226.

4 Surles, J. R., Wykle, R. L., O'Flaherty, J. T. *et al.* Facile synthesis of platelet-activating factor and racemic analogues containing unsaturation in the *sn*-1-alkyl chain. *J. Med. Chem.* (1985), **28**, 73–78.

5 Satouchi, K, Pinckard, R. N. & Hanahan, D. J. Influence of alkyl ether chain length of acetyl glyceryl ether phosphorylcholine and its ethanolamine analog on biological activity toward rabbit platelets. *Arch. Biochem. Biophys.* (1981), **211**, 683–688.

6 Bligh, E. G. & Dyer, W. J. A rapid method of total lipid extraction and purification. *Can. J. Biochem. Physiol.* (1959), **37**, 911–917.

7 Blank, M. L., Robinson, M. & Snyder, F. Chromatographic analyses of ether-linked lipids involved in PAF metabolism. In Snyder, F. (ed.) *Platelet-Activating Factor and Related Lipid Mediators* (1987) pp 33–52. Plenum Press, New York.

8 Alam, I., Smith, J. B. & Silver, M. J. Human and rabbit platelets form platelet-activating factor in response to calcium ionophore. *Thomb. Res.* (1983), **30**, 71–9.

9 Satouchi, K., Oda, M., Yasunaga, K. & Saito, K. Evidence for production of 1-acyl-2-acetyl-*sn*-glyceryl-3-phosphorylcholine concomitantly with platelet-activating factor. *Biochem. Biophys. Res. Commun.* (1985), **128**, 1409–1417.

10 Nakayama, R., Yasuda, K & Saito, K. Existence of endogenous inhibitors of platelet-activating factor (PAF) with PAF in rat uterus. *J. Biol. Chem.* (1987), **262**, 13 174–13 179.

11 Miwa, M., Hill, C., Kumar, R., Sugatani, J., Olson, M. S. & Hanahan, D. J. Occurence of an endogenous inhibitor of platelet-activating factor in rat liver. *J. Biol. Chem.* (1987), **262**, 527–530.

12 Murphy, R. C. & Clay, K. L. Measurement of platelet-activating factor by physio-chemical techniques. *Am. Rev. Resp. Dis.* (1987), **136**, 207–210.

13 Pinckard, R. N., Jackson, E. M., Hoppens, C., Weintraub, S. T., Ludwig, J. C., McManus, L. M. & Mott, G. E. Molecular heterogeneity of platelet-activating factor produced by stimulated human polymorphonuclear leukocytes. *Biochem. Biophys. Res. Commun.* (1984), **122**, 325–332.

14 Mueller, H. W., O'Flaherty, J. T. & Wykle, R. L. The molecular species distribution of platelet-activating factor synthesized by rabbit and human neutrophils. *J. Biol. Chem.* (1984), **259**, 14 554–14 559.

15 Wardlow, M. L., Cox, C. P., Meng, K. E., Greene, D. E. & Farr, R. S. Substrate specificity and partial characterization of the PAF-acylhydrolase in human serum that rapidly inactivates platelet-activating factor. *J. Immunol.* (1986), **136**, 3441–3446.

16 Farr, R. S., Cox, C. P., Wardlow, M. L. & Jorgensen, R. Preliminary studies of an acid-labile factor (ALF) in human sera that inactivates platelet-activating factor (PAF). *Clin. Immunol. Immunopathol.* (1980), **15**, 318–330.

17 Stafforini, D. M., Prescott, S. M. & McIntyre, T. M. Human plasma platelet-activating factor acetylhydrolase. *J. Biol. Chem.* (1987), **262(9)**, 4223–4230.

18 Murphy, R. C. & Clay, K. L. Chemical synthesis and mass spectrometry of PAF. In Snyder, F. (ed.) *Platelet-Activating Factor and Related Lipid Mediators* (1987), pp. 9–31. Plenum Press, New York.

19 Clay, K. L., Murphy, R. C., Andres, J. L., Lynch, J. & Henson, P. M. Structure elucidation of platelet activating factor derived from human neutrophils. *Biochem. Biophys. Res. Commun.* (1984), **121**, 815–825.

20 Chilton, F. H. & Connell, T. R. 1-Ether-linked phosphoglycerides: Major endogenous sources of arachidonate in the human neutrophil. *J. Biol. Chem.* (1988), **263**, 5260–5265.

21 Blank, M. L., Lee, T-c, Fitzgerald, V. & Snyder, F. A specific acetylhydrolase for 1-alkyl-2-acetyl-*sn*-glycero-3-phosphocholine (a hypotensive and platelet-activating lipid). *J. Biol. Chem.* (1981), **256**, 175–178.

22 Alam, I., Smith, J. B. & Silver, M. J. Metabolism of platelet-activating factor by blood platelets and plasma. *Lipids* (1983), **18**, 534–538.

23 Touqui, L., Hatmi, M. & Vargaftig, B. B. Human platelets stimulated by thrombin produce platelet-activating factor (1-O-alkyl-2-acetyl-*sn*-glycero-3-phosphocholine) when the degrading enzyme acetylhydrolase is blocked. *Biochem. J.* (1985), **229**, 811–816.

24 Roubin, R., Dulioust, A., Haye-Legrand, I., Ninio, E. & Benveniste, J. Biosynthesis of PAF-acether. VIII. Impairment of PAF-acether production in activated macrophages does not depend upon acetyltransferase activity. *J. Immunol.* (1986), **136**, 1796–1802.

25 Camussi, G., Aglietta, R., Coda, T., Bussolino, F., Piacibello, W. & Tetta, C. Release of platelet-activating factor (PAF) and histamine. II. The cellular origin of human PAF: monocytes, polymorphonuclear neutrophils and basophils. *Immunology* (1981), **42**, 191–199.

26 Camussi, G., Mencia-Huerta, J. M. & Benveniste, J. Release of platelet-activating factor and histamine. I. Effect of immune complexes, complement and neutrophils on human and rabbit mastocytes and basophils. *Immunology* (1977), **33**, 532–534.

27 Sanchez Crespo, M., Alonso, F. & Egido, J. Platelet-activating factor in anaphylaxis and phagocytosis. I. Release from human peripheral polymorphonuclears and monocytes during the stimulation by ionophore A23187 and phagocytosis but not from degranulating basophils. *Immunology* (1980), **40**, 645–655.

28 Lynch, J. M. & Henson, P. M. The intracellular retention of newly synthesized platelet-activating factor. *J. Immunol.* (1986), **137**, 2653–2661.

29 Betz, S. J., Lotner, G. Z. & Henson, P. M. Generation and release of platelet-activating factor (PAF) from enriched preparations of rabbit basophils; failure of human basophils to release PAF. *J. Immunol.* (1980), **125**, 2749–2755.

30 Arnoux, B., Joseph, M., Simoes, M. H. *et al.* Antigenic release of PAF-acether and β-glucuronidase from alveolar macrophages of asthmatics. *Bull. Euro. Physiopathol. Resp. (Oxford)* (1987), **23**, 119–124.

31 Robinson, M. & Snyder, F. Metabolism of platelet-activating factor by rat alveolar macrophages: lyso-PAF as an obligatory intermediate in the formation of alkylarachidonoyl glycerophosphocholine species. *Biochim. Biophys. Acta* (1985), **837**, 52–56.

32 Albert, D. H. & Snyder, H. F. Biosynthesis of 1-alkyl-2-acetyl-*sn*-glycero-3-phosphocholine (platelet-activating factor) from 1-alkyl-2-acyl-*sn*-glycero-3-phosphocholine by rat alveolar macrophages. *J. Biol. Chem.* (1983), **258**, 97–102.

33 Chignard, M., Coeffier, E., Le Couedic, J. P. & Benveniste, J. An unusual PAF-acether: lyso PAF-acether ratio in activated platelets. In *Proceedings of Second International Conference on Platelet-Activating Factor and Structurally Related Alkyl Ether Lipids* (1986), Gatlinburg, Tennessee, p. 70.

34 Blank, M. L., Spector, A. A., Kaduce, T. L., Lee, T-c. & Snyder, F. Metabolism of platelet activating factor (1-alkyl-2-acetyl-*sn*-glycero-3-phosphocholine) and 1-alkyl-2-acetyl-*sn*-glycerol by human endothelial cells. *Biochim. Biophys. Acta* (1986), **876**, 373–378.

35 Coeffier, E., Delautier, D., Le Couedic, J.-P., Chignard, M. & Benveniste, J. Cooperation between platelets and neutrophils for PAF-acether formation. In *Proceedings of Second International Conference on Platelet-Activating Factor and Structurally Related Alkyl Ether Lipids* (1986), Gatlinburg, Tennessee, p. 124.

36 Polonsky, J., Tence, M., Varenne, P., Das, B. C., Lunel, J. & Benveniste, J. Release of 1-O-alkylglyceryl-3-phosphorylcholine, O-deacetyl platelet-activating factor, from leukocytes: chemical ionization mass spectrometry of phospholipids. *Proc. Nat. Acad. Sci. (USA)* (1980), **77**, 7019–1023.

37 Wientzek, M., Arthur, G., Man, R. Y. K. & Choy, P. C. A sensitive method for the quantitation of lysophosphatidylcholine in canine heart. *J. Lipid Res.* (1985), **26**, 1166–1169.

38 Michel, L., Denizot, Y., Thomas, Y. *et al.* Biosynthesis of PAF-acether factor-acether by human skin fibroblasts *in vitro*. *J. Immunol.* (1988), **141**, 948–953.

39 Haroldsen, P. E., Clay, K. L. & Murphy, R. C. Quantitation of lyso-platelet activating factor molecular species from human neutrophils by mass spectrometry. *J. Lipid Res.* (1987), **28**, 42–49.

40 Billah, M. M. & Johnston, J. M. Identification of phospholipid platelet-activating factor (1-O-alkyl-2-acetyl-*sn*-glycero-3-phosphocholine) in human amniotic fluid and urine. *Biochem. Biophys. Res. Commun.* (1983), **113**, 51–58.

41 Sanchez Crespo, M., Inarrea, P., Alvarez, V., Alonso, F., Egido, J. & Hernando, L. Presence in normal human urine of a hypotensive and platelet-activating phospholipid. *Am. J. Physiol.* (1983), **244**, F706–F711.

42 Caramelo, C., Fernandez-Gallardo, S., Marin-Cao, D. Presence of platelet-activating factor in blood from humans and experimental animals; its absence in anephric individuals. *Biochem. Biophys. Res. Commun.* (1984), **120**, 789–796.

43 Sisson, J. H., Prescott, S. M., McIntyre, T. M. & Zimmerman, G. A. Production of platelet-activating factor by stimulated human polymorphonuclear leukocytes. *J. Immunol.* (1987), **138**, 3918–3926.

44 Oda, M., Satouchi, K., Yasunaga, K. & Saito, K. Molecular species of platelet-activating factor generated by human neutrophils challenged with ionophore A23187. *J. Immunol.* (1985), **134**, 1090–1093.

45 Worthen, G. S., Seccombe, J. F., Clay, C. L., Guthrie, L. A. & Johnston, Jr, R.B. The priming of neutrophils by lipopolysaccharide for production of intracellular platelet-activating factor. *J. Immunol.* (1988), **140**, 3553–3559.

46 McIntyre, T. M., Zimmerman, G. A. & Prescott, S. M. Leukotrienes C_4 and D_4 stimulate human endothelial cells to synthesize platelet-activating factor and bind neutrophils. *Proc. Nat. Acad. Sci. (USA)* (1986), **83**, 2204–2208.

47 Lewis, M. S., Whatley, R. E., Cain, P., McIntyre, T. M., Prescott, S. M. & Zimmerman, G. A. Hydrogen peroxide stimulates the synthesis of platelet-activating factor by endothelium and induces endothelial cell-dependent neutrophil adhesion. *J. Clin. Invest.* (1988), **82**, 2045–2055.

48 Jouvin-Marche, E., Ninio, E., Beaurain, G., Tence, M., Niaudet, P. & Benveniste, J. Biosynthesis of PAF-acether (platelet-activating factor). VII. Precursors of PAF-acether and acetyl-transferased activity in human leukocytes. *J. Immunol.* (1984), **133**, 892–898.

49 Henson, P. M. Extracellular activities of PAF. In Snyder, F. (ed.) *Platelet-Activating Factor and Related Lipid Mediators* (1987), pp. 255–271. Plenum Press, New York.

50 McIntyre, T. M., Zimmerman, G. A., Satoh, K. & Prescott, S. M. Cultured endothelial cells synthesize both platelet-activating factor and prostacyclin in response to histamine, bradykinin, and adenosine triphosphate. *J. Clin. Invest.* (1985), **76**, 271–80.

51 Zimmerman, G. A., McIntyre, T. M. & Prescott, S. M. Thrombin stimulates the adherence of neutrophils to human endothelial cells *in vitro*. *J. Clin. Invest.* (1985), **76**, 2235–2246.

52 Hayashi, H., Kudo, I., Inoue, K., Nomura, H. & Nojima, S. Macrophage activation by PAF incorporated into dipalmitoyl-phosphatidylcholine-cholesterol liposomes. *J. Biochem.* (1985), **97**, 1255–1258.

53 Ludwig, J. C., Hoppens, C. L., McManus, L. M., Mott, G. E., & Pinckard, R. N. Modulation of platelet-activating factor (PAF) synthesis and release from human polymorphonuclear leukocytes (PMN): role of extracellular albumin. *Arch. Biochem. Biophys.* (1985), **241**, 337–347.

54 Ludwig, J. C., McManus, L. M. & Pinckard, R. N. Synthesis–release coupling of platelet activating factors (PAF) from stimulated human neutrophils. *Adv. Inflammation Res.* (1986), **11**, 111–125.

55 Valone, F. H. Platelet-activating factor binding to specific cell membrane receptors. In Snyder, F. (ed.) *Platelet-Activating Factor and Related Lipid Mediators* (1987), pp. 137–151. Plenum Press, New York.

56 Tokumura, A., Yoshida, J.-I., Maruyama, T., Fukuzawa, K. & Tsukatani, H. Platelet aggregation induced by ether-linked phospholipids. I. Inhibitory actions of bovine serum albumin and structural analogues of platelet activating factor. *Thromb. Res.* (1987), **47**, 51–63.

57 Hoppens, C. M., Ludwig, J. C., Castillo, R., McManus, L. M. & Pinckard, R. N. Albumin modulation of rabbit platelet activation by 1-O-hexadecyl-2-acetyl-*sn*-glyceryl-3-phosphorylcholine (AGEPC). *Fed. Proc.* (1983), **42**, 693 (Abstract).

58 Banks, J. B., Wykle, R. L., O'Flaherty, J. T. & Lumb, R. H. Evidence for protein-catalyzed transfer of platelet activating factor by macrophage cytosol. *Biochim. Biophys Acta* (1988), **961**, 48–52.

59 Lumb, R. H., Pool, G. L., Bubacz, D. G., Blank, M. L. & Snyder, F. Spontaneous and protein-catalyzed transfer of 1-alkyl-2-acetyl-*sn*-glycero-3-phosphocholine (platelet-activating factor) between phosholipid bilayers. *Biochim. Biophys. Acta* (1983), **750**, 217–22.

60 Matsumoto, M. & Miwa, M. Platelet-activating factor-binding protein in human serum. *Adv. Prost. Thromb. Leuk. Res.* (1985), **15**, 705–706.

61 Kramp, W., Pieroni, G., Pinckard, R. N. & Hanahan, D. J. Observations on the critical micellar concentration of 1-O-alkyl-2-acetyl-*sn*-glycero-3-phosphocholine and a series of its homologs and analogs. *Chem. Phys. Lipids* (1984), **35**, 49–62.

62 Elstad, M. R., Prescott, S. M., McIntyre, T. M. & Zimmerman, G. A. Synthesis and release of platelet-activating factor by stimulated human mononuclear phagocytes. *J. Immunol.* (1988), **140**, 1618–1624.

63 Ludwig, J. C., McManus, L. M., Clark, P. O., Hanahan, D. J. & Pinckard, R. N. Modulation of platelet-activating factor (PAF) synthesis and release from human polymorphonuclear leukocytes (PMN): role of extracellular Ca^{2+}. *Arch. Biochem. Biophys.* (1984), **232**, 101–110.

64 Betz, S. J. & Henson, P. M. Production and release of platelet-activating factor (PAF); dissociation from degranulation and superoxide production in the human neutrophil. *J. Immunol.* (1980), **125**; 2756–2763.

65 Camussi, G., Aglietta, M., Malavasi, F., *et al.* The release of platelet-activating factor from human endothelial cells in culture. *J. Immunol.* (1983), **131**, 2397–2403.

66 Lee, T-c., Lenihans, D. J., Malone, B., Roddy, L. L. & Wasserman, S. I. Increased biosynthesis of platelet-activating factor in activated human eosinophils. *J. Biol. Chem.* (1984), **259**, 5526–5530.
67 Leyravaud, S. & Benveniste, J. Release of PAF-acether from human neutrophils depends on extracellular pH and cell concentration. *FASEB J.* (1989), **3**, A1223 (Abstract).
68 Cluzel, M., Undem, B. J., Chilton, F. H. & Lichtenstein, L. Platelet-activating factor (PAF) is released from neutrophils in a dynamic system. *FASEB J.* (1989), **3**, A1088.
69 Valone, F. H. & Epstein, L. B. Biphasic platelet-activating factor synthesis by human monocytes stimulated with IL-1β, tumor necrosis factor, or IFN-γ. *J. Immunol.* (1988), **141**, 3945–3950.
70 Snyder, F. Enzymatic pathways for platelet-activating factor, related alkyl glycerolipids and their precursors. In Snyder, F. (ed.) *Platelet-Activating Factor and Related Lipid Mediators* (1987), pp. 89–113. Plenum Press, New York.
71 Sugiura, T. & Waku, K. Composition of alkyl ether-linked phospholipids in mammalian tissues. In Snyder, F. (ed). *Platelet-Activating Factor and Related Lipid Mediators* (1987), pp. 55–85. Plenum Press, New York.
72 Tence, M., Jouvin-Marche, E., Bessou, G., Record, M. & Benveniste, J. Etherphospholipids composition in neutrophils and platelets. *Thromb. Res.* (1985), **38**, 207–214.
73 Natarajan, V., Zuzarte-Augstin, M., Schmid, H. H. O. & Graff, G. The alkylacyl and alkenylacyl glycerophospholipids of human platelets. *Thromb. Res.* (1983), **30**, 119–125.
74 Camussi, G., Bussolino, F., Salvidio, G., & Baglioni, C. Tumor necrosis factor/cachectin stimulates peritoneal macrophages, polymorphonuclear neutrophils, and vascular endothelial cells to synthesize and release platelet-activating factor. *J. Exp. Med.* (1987), **166**, 1390–1404.
75 Chilton, F. H., Ellis, J. M., Olson, S. C. & Wykle, R. L. 1-O-alkyl-2-arachidonoyl-*sn*-glycero-3-phosphocholine, a common source of platelet-activating factor and arachidonate in human polymorphonuclear leukocytes. *J. Biol. Chem.* (1984), **259**, 12 014–12 019.
76 Swendsen, C. L., Ellis, J. M., Chilton, F. H., O'Flaherty, J. T. & Wykle, R. L. 1-O-alkyl-2-acyl-*sn*-glycero-3-phosphocholine: a novel source of arachidonic acid in neutrophils stimulated by the calcium ionophore A23187. *Biochem. Biophys. Res. Commun.* (1983), **113(1)**, 72–79.
77 Lin, A. H., Morton, D. R. & Gorman, R. R. Acetyl glyceryl ether phosphorylcholine stimulates leukotriene B_4 synthesis in human polymorphonuclear leukocytes. *J. Clin. Invest.* (1982), **70**, 1058–1065.
78 Chilton, F. H., O'Flaherty, J. T., Walsh, C. E. *et al.* Platelet activating factor—stimulation of the lipoxygenase pathway in polymorphonuclear leukocytes by 1-O-alkyl-2-O-acetyl-*sn*-glycero-3-phosphocholine. *J. Biol. Chem.* (1982), **257**, 5402–5407.
79 Camussi, G., Bussolino, F., Tetta, C., Piacibello, W. & Aglietta, M. Biosynthesis and release of platelet-activating factor from human monocytes. *Int. Arch. Allergy Appl. Immunol.* (1983), **70**, 245–251.
80 Billah, M. M., Eckel, S., Myers, R. F. & Siegel, M. I. Metabolism of platelet-activating factor (1-O-alkyl-acetyl-*sn*-glycero-3-phosphocholine) by human promyelocytic leukemic HL60 cells. *J. Biol. Chem.* (1986), **261**, 5824–5831.
81 Arnoux, B., Duval, D. & Benveniste, J. Release of platelet-activating factor (PAF-acether) from alveolar macrophages by the calcium ionophore A23187 and phagocytosis. *Eur. J. Clin. Invest.* (1980), **10**, 437–441.

82 Alam, I. & Silver, M. J. Metabolism of 1-alkyl-2-acyl-GPC in human platelets in response to stimulation by thrombin. *Thromb. Res.* (1987), **45**, 311–322.
83 Lee, T.-c., Malone, B., Wasserman, S. I., Fitzgerald, V. & Snyder, F. Activities of enzymes that metabolize platelet-activating factor (1-alkyl-2-acetyl-*sn*-glycero-3-phosphocholine) in neutrophils and eosinophils from humans and the effect of a calcium ionophore. *Biochem. Biophys. Res. Commun.* (1982), **105**, 1303–1308.
84 Mencia-Huerta, J.-M., Lewis, R. A., Razin, E. & Austen, K. F. Antigen-initiated release of platelet-activating factor (PAF-acether) from mouse bone marrow-derived mast cells sensitized with monoclonal IgE. *J. Immunol.* (1983), **131**, 2958–2964.
85 Lichtenstein, L. M., Schleimer, R. P., MacGlashan, D. W. *et al. In vitro* and *in vivo* studies of mediator release from human mast cells. In Kay, A. B., Austen, K. F. & Lichtenstein, L. M. (eds) *Asthma: Physiology, Immunopharmacology, and Treatment. Third International Symposium* (1984), pp. 1–18. Academic Press, London.
86 Lewis, R. A., Goetzl, E. J., Wasserman, S. I., Valone, F. H., Rubin, R. H. & Austen, K. F. The release of four mediators of immediate hypersensitivity from human leukemic basophils. *J. Immunol.* (1975), **114**, 87–92.
87 Dulioust, A., Vivier, E., Salem, P., Benveniste, J. & Thomas, Y. Immunoregulatory functions of PAF-acether. I. Effect of PAF-acether on cell proliferation. *J. Immunol.* (1988), **140**, 240–245.
88 Rola-Pleszcynski, M., Pignol, B., Pouliot, C. & Braquet, P. Inhibition of human lymphocyte proliferation and interleukin-2 production by platelet activating factor (PAF-acether): reversal by a specific antagonist, BN 52021. *Biochem. Biophys. Commun.* (1987), **142**, 754–760.
89 Bussolino, F., Foa, R., Malavasi, F., Ferrando, M. L. & Camussi, G. Release of platelet-activating factor (PAF)-like material from human lymphoid cell lines. *Exp. Hematol.* (1984), **12**, 688–693.
90 Foa, R., Bussolino, F., Ferrando, M. L. *et al.* Release of platelet-activating factor in human leukemia. *Cancer Res.* (1985), **45**, 4483–4485.
91 Malavasi, F., Tetta, C., Funaro, A. *et al.* Fc receptor triggering induces expression of surface activation antigens and release of platelet-activating factor in large granular lymphocytes. *Proc. Nat. Acad. Sci. (USA).* (1986), **83**, 2443–2447.
92 Prescott, S. M., Zimmerman, G. A. & McIntyre, T. M. Human endothelial cells in culture produce platelet-activating factor (1-alkyl-2-acetyl-*sn*-glycero-3-phosphocholine) when stimulated with thrombin. *Proc. Nat. Acad. Sci. (USA).* (1984), **81**, 3534–3538.
93 Alam, I., Silver, M. J. Mueller, S. N. & Levine, E. M. Metabolism of 1-O-[^{3}H]alkyl-2-lyso-GPC by adult human iliac vein endothelial cells (HIVE). In *Proceedings of Second International Conference on Platelet-Activating Factor and Structurally Related Alkyl Ether Lipids* (1986). Gatlinburg, Tennessee, p. 58.
94 Bussolino, F., Breviario, F., Aglietta, M., Sanavio, F., Bosia, A. & Dejana, E. Studies on the mechanism of interleukin-1 stimulation of platelet activating factor synthesis in human endothelial cells in culture. *Biochim. Biophys. Acta* (1987), **927**, 43–54.
95 Bussolino, F., Camussi, G. & Baglioni, C. Synthesis and release of platelet-activating factor by human vascular endothelial cells treated with tumor necrosis factor or interleukin-1α. *J. Biol. Chem.* (1988), **263**, 11 856–11 861.
96 Marcus, A. J., Weksler, B. B., Jaffe, E. A., & Broekman, M. J. Synthesis of prostacyclin from platelet-derived endoperoxides by cultured human endothelial cells. *J. Clin. Invest.* (1980), **66**, 979–986.
97 Murphy, R. C., Fitzpatrick, F. A. & Maclouf, J. Transcellular biosynthesis of eicosanoids and inflammation. In Henson, P. M. & Murphy R.C. (eds) *Handbook*

of Inflammation: Mediators of the Inflammatory Process, Vol. 6 (1989), Elsevier, Amsterdam, in press.

98 Maclouf, J. A. & Murphy, R. C. Transcellular metabolism of neutrophil-derived leukotriene A_4 by human platelets. A potential cellular source of leukotriene C_4. *J. Biol. Chem.* (1988), **263**, 174–181.

99 Friedman, B. F., Grandel, K. E. & Farr, R. S. Platelet activating factor-like lipid in the nasal washings of allergic individuals following specific nasal antigen challenge. *Clin. Res.* (1986), **34**, 625A (Abstract).

100 Valone, F., Shalit, M., Atkins, P., Goetzl, E. & Zweiman, B. Platelet activating factor release in allergic skin sites in humans. *J. Allergy Clin. Immunol.* (1987), **79**, 248A (Abstract).

101 Grandel, K. E., Wardlow, M. L. & Farr, R. S. Platelet activating factor in sputum of patients with asthma and COPD. *J. Allergy Clin. Immunol.* (1985), **75**, (Suppl 2), 184 (Abstract).

102 Stenmark, K. R., Eyzaguirre, M., Westcott, J. Y., Henson, P. M., Murphy, R. C. Potential role of eicosanoids and PAF in the pathophysiology of bronchopulmonary dysplasia. *Am. Rev. Resp. Dis.* (1987), **136**, 770–772.

103 Grandel, K. E., Farr, R. S., Wanderer, A. A., Eisenstadt, T. C. & Wasserman, S. I. Association of platelet-activating factor with primary acquired cold urticaria. *New Engl. J. Med.* (1985), **313**, 405–409.

104 Caramelo, C., Fernandez-Gallardo, S, Santos, J. C. *et al.* Increased levels of platelet-activating factor in blood from patients with cirrhosis of the liver. *Eur. J. Clin. Invest.* (1987), **17**, 7–11.

105 Mallet, A. I. & Cunningham, F. M. Structural identification of platelet activating factor in psoriatic scale. *Biochem. Biophys. Res. Commun.* (1985), **126**, 192–198.

106 Cox. C.P., Wardlow, M. L., Jorgensen, R. & Farr, R. S. The presence of platelet-activating factor (PAF) in normal human mixed saliva. *J. Immunol.* (1981), **127**, 46–50.

107 Lianos, E. A. & Zanglis, A. Biosynthesis and metabolism of 1-O-alkyl-2-acetyl-*sn*-glycero-3-phosphocholine in rat glomerular mesangial cells. *J. Biol. Chem.* (1987), **262**, 8990–8993.

108 Neuwirth, R., Singhal, P., Diamond, B. *et al.* Evidence for immunoglobulin Fc receptor-mediated prostaglandin $F_{2\alpha}$ and platelet-activating factor formation by cultured rat mesangial cells. *J. Clin. Invest.* (1988), **82**, 936–944.

109 Hoffman, D. R., and Truong, C. T. & Johnston, J. M. Metabolism and function of platelet-activating factor in fetal rabbit lung development. *Biochim. Biophys. Acta* (1986), **879**, 88–96.

110 Kumar, R., King, R. J., Martin, H. M. & Hanahan, D. J. Metabolism of platelet-activating factor (alkylacetylphosphocholine) by type-II epithelial cells and fibroblasts from rat lungs. *Biochim. Biophys. Acta* (1987), **917**, 33–41.

111 Denizot, Y., Michel, L., Thomas, Y., Benveniste, J. & Dubertret, L. Human epidermal cells produce PAF-acether *in vitro. FASEB J.* (1989), **3**, A609 (Abstract).

112 Chang, J., Musser, J. H. & McGregor, H. Phospholipase A_2: function and pharmacological regulation. *Biochem. Pharmacol.* (1987), **36**, 2429–2436.

113 Alonso, F., Henson, P. M. & Leslie, C. C. A cytosolic phospholipase in human neutrophils that hydrolyzes arachidonoyl-containing phosphatidylcholine. *Biochim. Biophys Acta* (1986), **878**, 273–280.

114 Ribbes, G., Ninio, G., Fontan, P. *et al.* Evidence that biosynthesis of platelet-activating factor (PAF-acether) by human neutrophils occurs in an intracellular membrane. *FEBS Lett.* (1985), **191**, 195–199.

115 Doebber, T. W. & Wu, M. S. Platelet-activating factor (PAF) stimulates the PAF-synthesizing enzyme acetyl-CoA:1-alkyl-*sn*-glycero-3-phosphocholine O-acetyltransferase and PAF synthesis in neutrophils. *Proc. Nat. Acad. Sci. (USA)* (1987), **84**, 7557–7561.

116 Ninio, E., Mencia-Huerta, J. M. & Benveniste, J. Biosynthesis of platelet-activating factor (PAF-acether). V. Enhancement of acetyltransferase in murine peritoneal cells by calcium ionophore A23187. *Biochim. Biophys Acta* (1983), **751**, 298–304.

117 Ninio, E., Joly, F., Hieblot, C., Bessou, G, Mencia-Huerta, J.M & Benveniste, J. Biosynthesis of PAF-acether. IX. Role for a phosphorylation-dependent activation of acetyltransferase in antigen-stimulated mouse mast cells. *J. Immunol.* (1987), **139,** 154–160.

118 Comez-Cambronero, J., Velasco, S., Mato, J. M. & Sanchez Crespo, M. Modulation of lyso-platelet activating factor:acetyl-CoA acetyltransferase from rat splenic microsomes. The role of cyclic AMP-dependent protein kinase. *Biochim. Biophys. Acta* (1985), **845**, 516–519.

119 Lenihan, D. J. & Lee, T-c. Regulation of platelet activating factor synthesis: modulation of 1-alkyl-2-lyso-*sn*-glycero-3-phosphocholine:acetyl-CoA acetyltransferase by phosphorylation and dephosphorylation in rat spleen microsomes. *Biochem. Biophys. Res. Commun.* (1984), **120**, 834–839.

120 Domenech, C., Machado-De Domenech, E. & Soling, H. D. Regulation of acetyl-CoA: 1-alkyl-*sn*-glycero-3-phosphocholine O-acetyltransferase (lyso-PAF-acetyltransferase) in exocrine glands. *J. Biol. Chem.* (1987), **262**, 5671–5676.

121 Whatley, R. E., Lewis, M. S., Zimmerman, G. A. *et al.* The regulation of synthesis of platelet-activating factor by endothelial cells. *Chest* (1988), **93**, 110S–111S.

122 Chignard, M, Le Couedic, J. P., Tence, M., Vargaftig, B. B. & Benveniste, J. The role of platelet-activating factor in platelet aggregation. *Nature* (1979), **279**, 799–800.

123 Arnoux, B., Jouvin-Marche, E, Arnoux, A. & Benveniste, J. Release of PAF-acether from human blood monocytes. *Agents & Actions* (1982), **12**, 713–716.

124 Joly, F., Bessou, G., Benveniste, J. & Ninio, E. Ketotifen inhibits PAF-acether biosynthesis and β-hexosaminidase release in mouse mast cells stimulated with antigen. *Eur. J. Pharmacol.* (1987), **144**, 133–139.

125 Jouvin-Marche, E., Cerrina, J., Coeffier, E., Duroux, P. & Benveniste, J. Effect of the Ca^{2+} antagonist nifedipine on the release of platelet-activating factor (PAF-acether), slow-reacting substance and β-glucuronidase from human neutrophils. *Eur. J. Pharmacol.* (1983), **89**, 19–26.

126 Billah, M. M., Siegel, M. I., Calmodulin antagonists inhibit formation of platelet-activating factor in stimulated human neutrophils. *Biochem. Biophys. Res. Commun.* (1984), **118**, 629–635.

127 Touqui, L., Shaw, A. M., Dumarey, C., Jacquemin, C. & Vargaftig, B. B. The role of Ca^{2+} in regulating the catabolism of PAF-acether (1-O-alkyl-2-acetyl-*sn*-glycero-3-phosphocholine) in rabbit platelets. *Biochem. J.* (1987), **241**, 555–560.

128 Ninio, E., Joly, F. & Bessou, G. Biosynthesis of PAF-acether. XI. Regulation of acetyltransferase by enzyme-substrate imbalance. *Biochim. Biophys. Acta* (1988), **963**, 288–294.

129 Camussi, G., Tetta, C., Bussolino, F. & Baglioni, C. Synthesis and release of platelet-activating factor is inhibited by plasma a_1-proteinase inhibitor or a_1-antichymotrypsin and is stimulated by proteinases. *J. Exp. Med.* (1988), **168**, 1293–1306.

130 Chilton, F. H. & Murphy, R. C. Remodelling of arachidonate-containing phosphoglycerides within the human neutrophil. *J. Biol. Chem.* (1986), **261**, 7771–7777.

131 Triggiani, M. Chilton, F. H. & Lichtenstein, L. M. Metabolism of platelet activating factor (PAF) in human and murine mast cells. *FASEB J.* (1989), **3,** A1277 (Abstract).
132 Swendsen, C. L., Chilton, F. H., O'Flaherty, J. T., *et al.* Human neutrophils incorporate arachidonic acid and saturated fatty acids into separate molecular species of phospholipids. *Biochim. Biophys. Acta* (1987), **919**, 79–89.
133 Strasser, T., Fischer, S. & Weber, P. C. Leukotriene B_5 is formed in human neutrophils after dietary supplementation with icosapentaenoic acid. *Proc. Nat. Acad. Sci. (USA)* (1985), **82**, 1540–1543.
134 Lee, T. H., Hoover, R. L., Williams, J. D. *et al.* Effect of dietary enrichment with eicosapentaenoic and docosahexaenoic acids on *in vitro* neutrophil and monocyte leukotriene generation and neutrophil function. *New Engl. J. Med.* (1985), **312,** 1217–1224.
135 Lee, T. H., Menica-Huerta, J,-M., Shih, C., Corey, E. J., Lewis, R. A. & Austen, K. F. Characterization and biologic properties of 5,12-dihydroxy derivatives of eicosapentaenoic acid, including leukotriene B_5 and the double lipoxygenase product. *J. Biol. Chem.* (1984), **259,** 2383–2389.
136 Prescott, S. M. The effect of eicosapentaenoic acid on leukotriene B production by human neutrophils. *J. Biol. Chem.* (1984), **259**, 7615–7621.
137 Codde, J. P., Vandongen, R., Mori, T. A., Beilin, L. J. & Hill, K. J. Can the synthesis of platelet-activating factor, a potent vasodilator and pro-aggregatory agent, be altered by dietary marine oils? *Clin. Exp. Pharmacol. Physiol.* (1987), **14**, 197–202.
138 Kawasaki, T., Blank, M. L. & Snyder, F. Arachidonic acid regulates platelet activating factor (PAF) synthesis in HL-60 cells. *FASEB J.* (1988), **2,** A1376 (Abstract).
139 Ramesha, C. S. & Pickett, W. C. Platelet-activating factor and leukotriene biosynthesis is inhibited in polymorphonuclear leukocytes depleted of arachidonic acid. *J. Biol. Chem.* (1986), **261**, 7592–7595.
140 Mollinedo, F., Gomez-Cambronero, J, Cano, E. & Sanchez Crespo, M. Intracellular localization of platelet-activating factor synthesis in human neutrophils. *Biochem. Biophys. Res. Commun.* (1988), **154**, 1232–1239.
141 Record, M. & Snyder, F. Biosynthesis of platelet activating factor (PAF) via alternate pathways: Subcellular distribution of products in HL-60 cells. *Fed. Proc.* (1986), **45**, 1529 (Abstract).
142 Eliakim, R., Karmeli, F., Razin, E. & Rachmilewitz, D. Role of platelet-activating factor in ulcerative colitis. *Gastroenterology* (1988), **95**, 1167–1172.
143 Chignard, M., Le-Couedic, J. P., Andersson, P. & Brange, G. Use of steroidal antiinflammatory drug provides further evidence for a potential role of PAF-acether in bronchial anaphylaxis. *Int. Arch. Allergy Appl. Immunol.* (1986), **81,** 184–185.
144 Fradin, A., Rothhut, B., Poincelot-Canton, B., Errasfa, M. & Russo-Marie, F. Inhibition of eicosanoid and PAF formation by dexamethasone in rat inflammatory polymorphonuclear neutrophils may implicate lipocortins. *Biochim. Biophys. Acta* (1988), **963**, 248–257.
145 Parente, L. & Flower, R. J. Hydrocortisone and macrocortin inhibit the zymosan-induced release of lyso-PAF from rat peritoneal leukocytes. *Life Sci.* (1985), **36,** 1225–1231.
146 Chilton, F. H., Schmidt, D. Torphy, T., Goldman, D., & Undem B. cAMP inhibits platelet activating factor (PAF) biosynthesis in the human neutrophil. *FASEB J.* (1989), **3,** A308 (Abstract).
147 Seyama, K. Ishibashi, T. Biochemical characterization of acetyl-CoA:1-alkyl-2-

lyso-*sn*-glycero-3-phosphocholine acetyltransferase in rat spleen microsomes. *Lipids* (1987), **22(3)**, 185–189.
148 Wykle, R. L., Malone, B. & Snyder, F. Enzymatic synthesis of 1-alkyl-2-acetyl-*sn*-glycero-3-phosphocholine, a hypotensive and platelet-aggregating lipid. *J. Biol. Chem.* (1980), **225**, 10 256–10 260.
149 Shen, T. Y., Hwang, S. B., Doebber, T. W. & Robbins, J. C. The chemical and biological properties of PAF agonists, antagonists and biosynthetic inhibitors. In Snyder, F. (ed.) *Platelet-Activating Factor and Related Lipid Mediators* (1987), pp. 153–190. Plenum Press, New York.
150 Walsh, C. E., Dechatelet, L. R., Chilton, F. H., Wykle, R. L. & Waite, M. Mechanism of arachidonic acid release in human polymorphonuclear leukocytes. *Biochim. Biophys. Acta* (1983), **750**, 32–40.
151 Walsh, C. E., Waite, B. M., Thomas, M. J. & DeChatelet, L. R. Release and metabolism of arachidonic acid in human neutrophils. *J. Biol. Chem.* (1981), **256**, 7228–7234.
152 Chilton, F. H. Potential phospholipid source(s) of arachidonate used for the synthesis of leukotrienes by the human neutrophil. *Biochem. J.* (1989), **258**, 327–333.
153 Lotner, G. Z., Lynch, J. M., Betz, S. J. & Henson, P. M. Human neutrophil-derived platelet activating factor. *J. Immunol.* (1980), **124**, 676–684.
154 Nieto, M. L., Velasco, S. & Sanchez Crespo, M. Biosynthesis of platelet-activating factor in human polymorphonuclear leukocytes. *J. Biol. Chem.* (1988), **263**, 2217–2222.
155 Schleimer, R. P., Macglashan, D. W. Jr, Peters, S. P., Pinckard, R. N. Adkinson, N. F. & Lichtenstein, L. M. Characterization of inflammatory mediator release from purified human lung mast cells. *Am. Rev. Resp. Dis.* (1986), **133**, 614–617.
156 Camussi, G., Tetta, C., Coda, R. & Benveniste, J. Release of platelet-activating factor in human pathology. I. Evidence for the occurrence of basophil degranulation and release of platelet-activating factor in systemic lupus erythematosus. *Lab. Invest.* (1981), **44**, 241–251.
157 Bussolino, F., Breviario, F., Tetta, C., Aglietta, M., Mantovani, A. & Dejana, E. Interleukin-1 stimulates platelet-activating factor production in cultured human endothelial cells. *J. Clin. Invest.* (1986), **77**, 2027–2033.
158 Camussi, G., Bussolino, F., Ghezzo, F. & Pegoraro, L. Release of platelet-activating factor from HL-60 human leukemic cells following macrophage-like differentiation. *Blood* (1982), **59**, 16–22.
159 Arnoux, B., Durand, J., Rigaud, M., Vargaftig, B. B. & Benveniste, J. Release of platelet-activating factor (PAF-acether) and arachidonic acid metabolites from alveolar macrophages. *Agents & Actions* (1981), **11**, 555–556.

Chapter 3
PAF receptors

Gordon Dent, Dieter Ukena and Peter J. Barnes

Introduction

The precise structural requirements for PAF activity and the existence of specific antagonists to the actions of PAF indicate the presence of specific receptors for PAF on the surface of target cells (see Chapter 4). Several studies recently have demonstrated the specific binding of radiolabelled PAF and PAF antagonist molecules to intact cells and tissues, as well as to purified cell membranes. Preliminary steps have also been taken towards elucidation of the events following the occupation by PAF of its receptors and, thus, of the mechanisms by which PAF produces its various effects on cell function. The range of cell types in which PAF receptors are evident includes circulating blood elements, namely platelets, and polymorphonuclear and mononuclear leukocytes, as well as eosinophils from both peripheral blood and inflammatory exudates. PAF receptors have also been shown to occur in lung tissues. In this chapter, we shall review the numerous studies characterizing the PAF receptors on these various cell types before examining the putative mechanisms of action of this potent inflammatory mediator.

[^{3}H]PAF binding sites

The characteristics of [^{3}H]PAF binding sites so far identified are summarized in Table 3.1. We shall discuss the binding characteristics for each cell type in turn.

Table 3.1 Characteristics of [^{3}H]PAF binding sites*

Cell type	Temperature (°C)	K_D (nM)	B_{max}	Reference
Human platelets	4	0.25	300 fmol/mg	[5]
	20	37	1400/cell	[1]
	22	0.053	240/cell	[2]
	25	0.016	240/cell	[3]
	37	0.26	245/cell	[4]
	37	9.2	1600/cell	[4]
Human PMNL	4	0.22	1100/cell	[10]
	20	3.5	49600/cell	[12]
	37	0.11	5200000/cell	[9]
Human lung	4	0.49	140 fmol/mg	[15]
Human lymphocytes	4	5.7	11 100/cell	[14]
Rabbit platelets	25	0.5	400/cell	[6]
Dog platelets	25	0.23	911 fmol/mg	[7]

* Binding sites were not found in rat platelets [8].
PMNL = Polymorphonuclear leukocytes.

Platelets

The first investigations of specific PAF receptors were performed in human platelets and demonstrated the binding of the radioligand [^{3}H]PAF (a mixture of C_{16} and C_{18} forms) to washed platelets in a time- and concentration-dependent manner [1]. The binding of the highest concentration of radioligand was >80% complete within 2 min at 20°C, coinciding with the time of initiation of aggregation by PAF, and was complete within 5 min. The specific binding isotherms indicated two distinct binding sites: (i) a saturable high-affinity site with an equilibrium dissociation constant (K_D) of 37 nM and a receptor density—calculated from the maximal capacity (B_{max}), assuming 1:1 stoichiometry—of 1400 sites/platelet; and (ii) a low-affinity site with almost infinite binding capacity, consistent with non-receptor binding or cellular uptake of the radioligand. At saturation, non-specific binding accounted for >60% of total binding, possibly reflecting the lipophilic nature of the ligand, which may readily become incorporated into cell membranes. The binding of [^{3}H]PAF was inhibited by a range of alkylglyceryl ether phosphocholine analogues with a rank order corresponding to their ability to induce platelet aggregation. The structural requirements for high-affinity binding were found to be an ether linkage at position *sn*-1, a short-chain fatty acid at *sn*-2 and a choline moiety at *sn*-3. Incubation of washed platelets with PAF for 5 min at 37°C desensitized the platelets to subsequent PAF stimulation and reduced the specific binding of [^{3}H]PAF; the time course of these reactions showed a 50% reduction in receptor number at the time when the aggregation response to PAF was abolished [1].

The kinetics of the binding reaction were investigated by Kloprogge & Akkerman [2]. Saturation of binding of [^{3}H]PAF to washed human platelets was found between 15 and 90 min at 22°C. The amount and kinetics of binding were identical at 4°C, 22°C and 37°C although non-specific binding increased with increasing temperature within this range, amounting to approximately 33% of total binding at saturating concentrations of radioligand at 22 °C. The lesser extent of non-specific binding found by Kloprogge & Akkerman, compared to that reported by Valone *et al.* [1], could be accounted for by the longer incubation times used by the former (90 min, compared to 5 min); kinetic experiments indicated increasing non-specific binding only during the first 5 min of exposure, whereas specific binding is saturated, at lower PAF concentrations, after about 90 min [2]. Equilibrium binding isotherms indicated the existence of a single class of high-affinity binding sites with a K_D of 53 pM and B_{max} corresponding to 242 sites/platelet; non-equilibrium kinetic experiments gave a K_D of 59 pM [2]. The great disparity between these results and those of Valone *et al.* may arise from the use by the latter group of an unconventional method of conducting saturation binding experiments and a very short incubation time (see above).

In close accordance with the findings of Kloprogge & Akkerman were those of Ukena *et al.* [3] and Tuffin *et al.* [4]. Specific binding of [^{3}H]C_{18}-PAF to gel-filtered human platelets at 25°C was saturable and inhibited by either of two specific PAF receptor antagonists (Fig. 3.1). The K_D for [^{3}H]PAF was 16 pM, only marginally lower than that shown by Kloprogge & Akkerman [2], whilst the receptor density of 240 sites/platelet was identical [3]. Tuffin *et al.* [4] found specific binding of [^{3}H]C_{18}-PAF to two distinct sites on washed human platelets: (i) a high-affinity site with a K_D of 259 pM; and (ii) a low-affinity site with a K_D of 9.2 nM at 37°C; the respective B_{max} values corresponded to receptor densities of 245 and 1616 sites/platelet. Although the affinity of the high-affinity site described by Tuffin *et al.* is markedly lower than the affinities reported by Kloprogge & Akkerman [2] and by Ukena *et al.* [3], the receptor densities calculated from the three separate studies are almost identical.

Specific binding sites for [^{3}H]PAF have also been found on platelets from other species. Hwang *et al.* [5] described a single site on rabbit platelet membranes with a K_D of 1.4 nM at 0 °C and B_{max} of 2.6 pmol/mg protein, which corresponded to approximately 150–300 sites/platelet (depending on vesicle orientation). The kinetics of the binding of [^{3}H]PAF to rabbit platelet membranes were similar to those described for intact human platelets by Kloprogge & Akkerman [2] and by Tuffin *et al.* [4]. A single site was also described on intact washed rabbit platelets with a K_D of 500 pM at 25°C and binding capacity of 400 sites/platelet [6]. [^{3}H]PAF was rapidly internalized by rabbit platelets but no down-

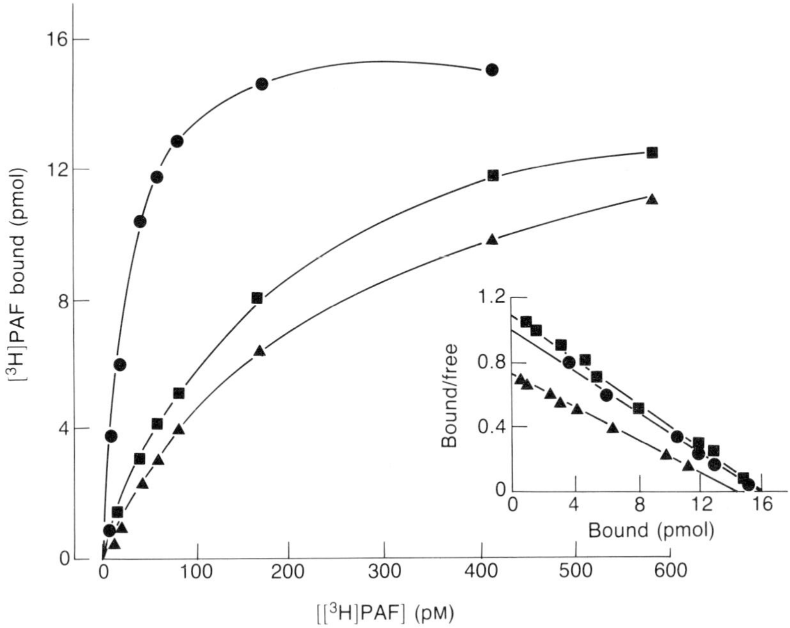

Fig. 3.1 Specific binding of [^{3}H]PAF to gel filtered human platelets (4×10^7 per assay) in the absence of any competing drug (●) and in the presence of 100 nM 52770 RP (■) and 100 nM WEB 2086 (▲). From Ukena *et al.* [3].

regulation of receptor sites was observed in platelets desensitized by previous exposure to PAF [6]. In canine platelet membranes, [^{3}H]PAF labelled a single population of binding sites with a K_D of 230 pM and binding capacity of 911 fmol/mg [7]. The ability of PAF antagonists to displace this binding correlated closely with their potency as inhibitors of PAF-induced aggregation of canine platelets [7].

Rat platelets, which do not respond to PAF, did not exhibit specific binding of [^{3}H]PAF [8].

Polymorphonuclear leukocytes

PAF binding to neutrophils was first studied by Valone & Goetzl [9]. The binding of [^{3}H]C_{16}/C_{18}-PAF to intact human neutrophils was complete within 20–30 min and maximal at 37°C. As in their study with human platelets [1], two types of binding site were found: (i) a high-affinity site, with a K_D of 110 pM at 37°C and binding capacity of 5 200 000 sites/cell; and (ii) a low-affinity, high-capacity site probably corresponding to non-receptor binding and uptake of the radioligand [9]. The large binding capacity of the high-affinity site suggested that PAF may be incorporated into cellular structures or converted to a metabolite with a lower affinity for specific receptors. However, no metabolites could be found associated with the cell pellet [9]. O'Flaherty *et al.* [10] similarly demonstrated the presence of two classes of binding site for [^{3}H]C_{16}-PAF on human neutrophils: (i) a high-affinity site with a K_D at equilibrium of 200 pM at 4°C and binding capacity of 1100 sites/cell; and (ii) a low affinity site with K_D of 200 nM and binding capacity of 200 000 sites/cell. The K_D of the high-affinity site is similar to that reported by Valone & Goetzl but the total receptor number is some 4700-fold lower. The binding sites were strictly associated with cell-surface and membrane markers [10]: there is no evidence that neutrophil granules bear receptors for PAF, although chemotactic peptide receptors have been found on or within specific granules [11]. Membranes prepared from nitrogen cavitated cells were purified so that 90% of the binding sites were recovered as particulate material. [^{3}H]PAF binding to the membrane preparations gave similar results to the experiments with intact cells, fitting a two-site model with K_D values for the high- and low-affinity sites of 200 pM and 500 nM, respectively [10]. Marquis *et al.* [12] demonstrated binding of [^{3}H]PAF to a single class of binding sites on human neutrophils with a K_D of 3.5 nM and binding capacity corresponding to 49 600 sites/cell. The kinetics of this reaction were very similar to those described by Valone & Goetzl [9].

In binding studies using [^{3}H]PAF with leukocytes, the problems of uptake and metabolism of the radioligand are severe. O'Flaherty *et al.* found uptake of [^{3}H]PAF by human neutrophils to be temperature-dependent: 18% of added [^{3}H]PAF was incorporated into cells at 4°C and this incorporation was significantly inhibited in the presence of an excess of unlabelled PAF, whereas at 37°C, 95% of added radioligand was incorporated and this uptake was unaffected by the presence of unlabelled PAF. At 37°C, virtually all cell-associated radioactivity was in the form of 1-O-[hexadecyl-9,10-$^3H_2$]-2-fatty acyl-*sn*-glycero-3-phosphocholine, indicating rapid metabolism of cell-incorporated PAF at physiological temperatures [10]. This extensive uptake and metabolism of the radioligand may account for the very high apparent receptor number described at high temperatures by Valone & Goetzl [9].

Lymphocytes

The observation that phytohaemagglutinin-induced lymphocyte proliferation and interleukin-2 production were inhibited by PAF [13] suggested a possible immunoregulatory function for this mediator. The existence of PAF receptors on human lymphocytes was demonstrated by direct binding studies using peripheral mononuclear cell preparations containing 85–90% lymphocytes. [^{3}H]PAF bound time-dependently, reversibly and saturably to a single class of binding sites with an equilibrium K_D of 5.7 nM at 4°C and binding capacity of 11 100 sites/cell [14]. Binding was displaced competitively by both unlabelled PAF and a range of specific receptor antagonists.

Lung tissues

Specific and saturable binding of [^{3}H]PAF to membrane preparations of human lung tissues was demonstrated by Hwang *et al.* in 1983. A single class of binding sites was found with an equilibrium K_D of 49 pM and B_{max} of 140 fmol/mg [15]. Non-specific binding was very high (60–70% of total binding at a radioligand concentration of 1 nM); however, the binding sites were PAF-specific and [^{3}H]PAF binding was displaced by a series of structural analogues of PAF with the same order of potency as observed for rabbit platelet membranes [5]. However, in human lung membrane preparations, the C_{16}-PAF showed a higher affinity than the octadecyl form, whereas in rabbit platelet membranes the two forms were equipotent in competing for [^{3}H]PAF binding sites [15]. Although PAF receptors were revealed in whole lung homogenates, this gave no indication of the cellular localization of PAF receptors in the lung.

PAF antagonist radioligands

Binding studies with [^{3}H]PAF have often proved difficult because of the high level of non-specific binding and the metabolism and uptake of the radioligand, as described above. It was thought that the development of antagonist radioligands might overcome this problem, particularly if the antagonist molecule were hydrophilic and consequently less prone to receptor-independent incorporation into lipid membranes. Several PAF antagonists had been shown to displace [^{3}H]PAF from its binding sites on target cells but, although the ability of these compounds to displace [^{3}H]PAF binding correlated fairly closely with their potency as inhibitors of PAF-induced platelet aggregation in a variety of species, the correlation between receptor binding and functional antagonism had not been investigated in other cell types. Also, PAF antagonists can be broadly divided into two classes, namely those with PAF-like structures (e.g. CV-3988, ONO-6240) and those whose molecules contain multiple hydrogen-bonding substituents (e.g. kadsurenone, BN 52021); despite some common structural features, there was no certainty that they interacted at a common binding site within the PAF receptor [16]. The development of antagonist radioligands has allowed closer examination of the mechanism by which these particular compounds exert their PAF-antagonistic actions.

As with [^{3}H]PAF binding, we will review the work describing antagonist radioligand binding on each cell type, in turn.

Platelets

The first PAF antagonist to be developed as a radioligand for receptor binding studies was a derivative of the *Piper futokadsurae* extract, kadsurenone. Palladium/charcoal-catalysed hydrogenation of the 5-allyl group of kadsurenone with tritium gas produced [^{3}H]dihydrokadsurenone (Fig. 3.2a) with a specific activity of 57 Ci/mmol [16]. Dihydrokadsurenone was marginally more potent than kadsurenone in displacing [^{3}H]PAF binding to rabbit platelet membranes [16]. [^{3}H]-Dihydrokadsurenone itself bound specifically to rabbit platelet membranes with an equilibrium K_D of 17 nM at 0°C and B_{max} of 2.3 pmol/mg; this receptor number is in very close agreement with the value of 2.6 pmol/mg reported by Hwang *et al.* for [^{3}H]PAF binding to rabbit platelet membranes [5], suggesting that [^{3}H]dihydrokadsurenone and [^{3}H]PAF label a common receptor population [16]. PAF analogues and PAF receptor antagonists which displaced [^{3}H]PAF binding from rabbit platelet membranes also displaced [^{3}H]dihydrokadsurenone binding to a similar extent, whereas selected pharmacological agents which did not affect [^{3}H]PAF binding also exhibited no effect on [^{3}H]dihydrokadsurenone binding. This suggests that PAF and dihydrokadsurenone share a common binding site in a distinct PAF receptor [16]. However, differences in the relative potency were observed for inhibition by PAF antagonists of [^{3}H]PAF and [^{3}H]dihydrokadsurenone binding; also the K_D derived from direct binding studies for [^{3}H]-dihydrokadsurenone (17 nM) was substantially different from the antagonist affinity constant (K_B) calculated from the inhibition of [^{3}H]PAF binding by dihydrokadsurenone (90 nM) [16]. Therefore, it appears that [^{3}H]dihydrokadsurenone may only partially share the binding site for PAF in the PAF receptor.

The pyrrolo[1,2-*c*]thiazole derivative, 52770 RP, in tritiated form, has been used to label PAF binding sites on intact rabbit platelets, as well as crude platelet membranes. 52770 RP was radiolabelled by catalytic tritium exchange of iodine at position 2 of the chlorophenyl ring (Fig. 3.2b) and had a specific activity of 28 Ci/mmol. In both preparations, [^{3}H]52770 RP bound specifically, reversibly and saturably to a single class of binding sites. The [^{3}H]52770 RP binding sites on intact washed rabbit platelets had a K_D of 8.5 nM and numbered 2420 sites/platelet; [^{3}H]52770 RP bound to crude platelet membranes with a K_D of 7.5 nM and B_{max} of 3.66 pmol/mg [17]. In washed rabbit platelets, the inhibition constants (K_i) of a range of 52270 RP analogues for displacement for [^{3}H]PAF binding correlated closely with their K_i versus [^{3}H]52770 RP binding.

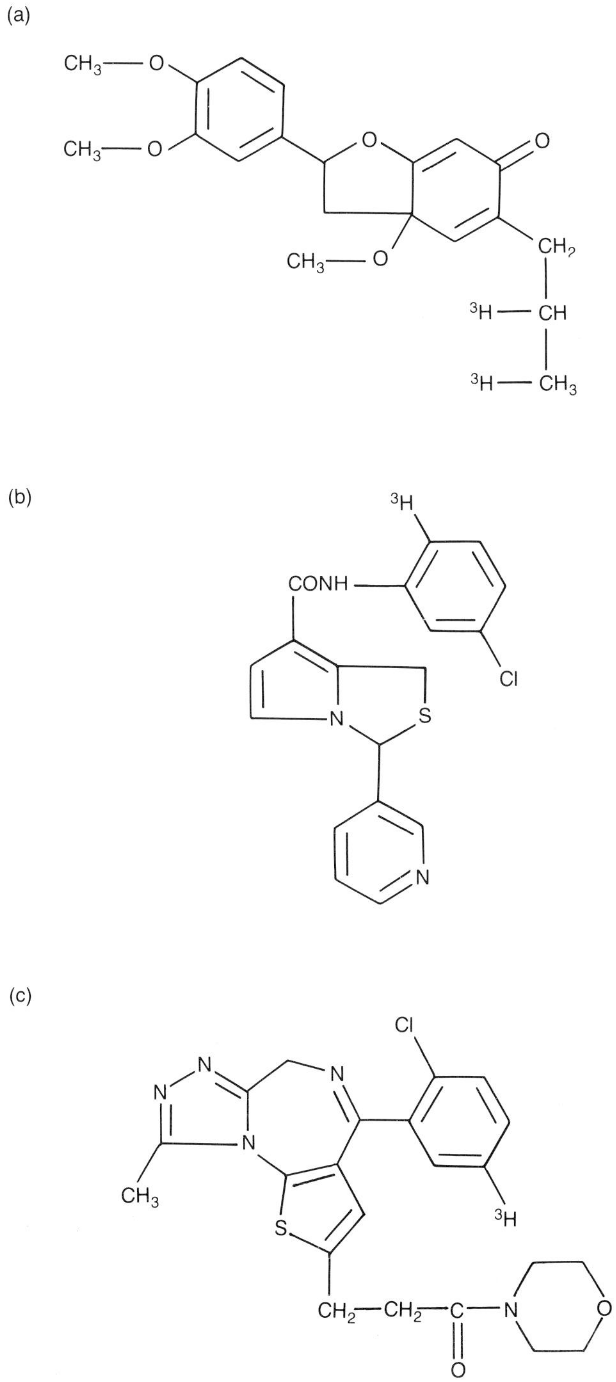

Fig. 3.2 Labelled PAF antagonists. Chemical structures of (a) [^{3}H]dihydrokadsurenone; (b) [^{3}H]52770 RP; and (c) [^{3}H]WEB 2086.

Analysis of the inhibition of [^{3}H]52770 RP binding by PAF showed the PAF inhibition to be of a competitive nature: the K_D for [^{3}H]52770 RP increased with increasing concentrations of PAF but the B_{max} was unaffected [17]. Although the K_i of 52770 RP displacement of [^{3}H]52770 RP binding was 11.2 nM, which is quite close to the K_D for [^{3}H]52770 RP binding, 52770 RP inhibited PAF-induced aggregation of washed rabbit platelets with a K_B of 19.5 nM, which is 2.3-fold higher than the K_D calculated for 52770 RP from direct binding experiments. Also, the K_i for displacement of [^{3}H]52770 RP by PAF was 2.7 nM, three times higher than the K_i of 890 pM found for PAF displacement of [^{3}H]PAF binding [17]. At the same time it was noted that approximately 13% of [^{3}H]52770 RP specific binding was not displaced by PAF at concentrations as high as 10 μM. Thus, although 52770 RP appeared to be a

Table 3.2 Radioligand binding to intact human platelets: characteristics of binding

Radioligand	K_D (nM)	Number of sites per cell
[^{3}H]PAF	0.016	240
[^{3}H]WEB 2086	6.1	260
[^{3}H]52770 RP	14.8	3750

useful antagonist radioligand for labelling PAF receptors, there were certain caveats against its use.

Binding experiments performed with [^{3}H]52770 RP in human platelets seemed to contradict the view of 52770 RP as a specific label of PAF receptors. Gel-filtered human platelets which bound [^{3}H]PAF with a K_D of 16 pM at 25°C and B_{max} corresponding to 240 sites/platelet also bound [^{3}H]52770 RP to a single site. The K_D for this reaction was 15 nM, not dissimilar to that reported for rabbit platelets; however, the binding capacity for [^{3}H]52770 RP was 3750 sites/platelet (Table 3.2), some 15-fold higher than the value calculated from [^{3}H]PAF binding [3]. Also, although 52770 RP displaced [^{3}H]PAF binding (Fig. 3.1) with a K_i of 13.8 nM, very close to the K_D for [^{3}H]52770 RP binding, PAF did not displace specific [^{3}H]52770 RP binding at concentrations up to 10 μM (Table 3.3), indicating that [^{3}H]52770 RP was binding to a site distinct from the PAF receptor in human platelets [3,18]. In the same study, the thienotriazolodiazepine, WEB 2086 was used as a receptor antagonist to [^{3}H]PAF and, in tritiated form, as an antagonist radioligand. WEB 2086 displaced [^{3}H]PAF binding to gel-filtered human platelets (Fig. 3.1) with a K_i of 9.9 nM, suggesting an affinity for the PAF binding site similar to that observed for 52770 RP. Like 52770 RP, WEB 2086 could be labelled with tritium at the 2-position of the chlorophenyl ring (Fig. 3.2c) but with a lower specific activity of 14 Ci/mmol. [^{3}H]WEB 2086 bound specifically and saturably to a single site on gel filtered human platelets (Fig. 3.3) with a K_D of 6.1 nM, in the same range as the K_i of WEB 2086 versus [^{3}H]PAF binding and a higher affinity than 52770 RP, and a binding capacity of 260 sites/platelet, which is in close agreement with the value of 240 sites/platelet obtained for [^{3}H]PAF, in contrast to 52770 RP which bound to 15 times as many sites (Table 3.2). WEB 2086, like PAF, did not inhibit binding of [^{3}H]52770 RP to human platelets at concentrations up to 10 μM (Table 3.3) [3,18]. These results, taken together, demonstrated that, in human platelets, the binding sites for [^{3}H]WEB 2086 are identical

Table 3.3 Radioligand binding to intact human platelets: inhibition of binding

	K_i (nM)		
Compound	[^{3}H]PAF	[^{3}H]WEB 2086	[^{3}H]52770 RP
C_{16}-PAF	0.024	0.019	–
Lyso-PAF	–	–	–
WEB 2086	9.9	5.3	–
52770 RP	13.8	14.5	18.9

-Indicates that binding was not inhibited at a drug concentration of 10 μm [3].

to those of [^{3}H]PAF binding while those for [^{3}H]52770 RP are not. Despite the low specific activity of the available material, WEB 2086 was taken as the most appropriate ligand for labelling of PAF receptors in our subsequent studies in different cell types.

Polymorphonuclear leukocytes

[^{3}H]52770 RP was used again as a radioligand in a study by Marquis *et al.* of PAF receptors on human neutrophils [12]. [^{3}H]PAF was shown to bind to a single class of binding sites with markedly different characteristics to those reported previously [9,10] (Table 3.1). This binding was inhibited by 52770 RP with a K_i of 7 nM. [^{3}H]52770 RP itself bound to a single class of binding sites with a K_D of a 4.2 nM at 20°C and a binding capacity of 43 600 sites/cell; this value was in very close agreement with the binding capacity of 49 600 sites/cell for [^{3}H]PAF, suggesting that, in human neutrophils, unlike human platelets, 52770 RP may bind specifically and selectively to the PAF receptor. The displacement of

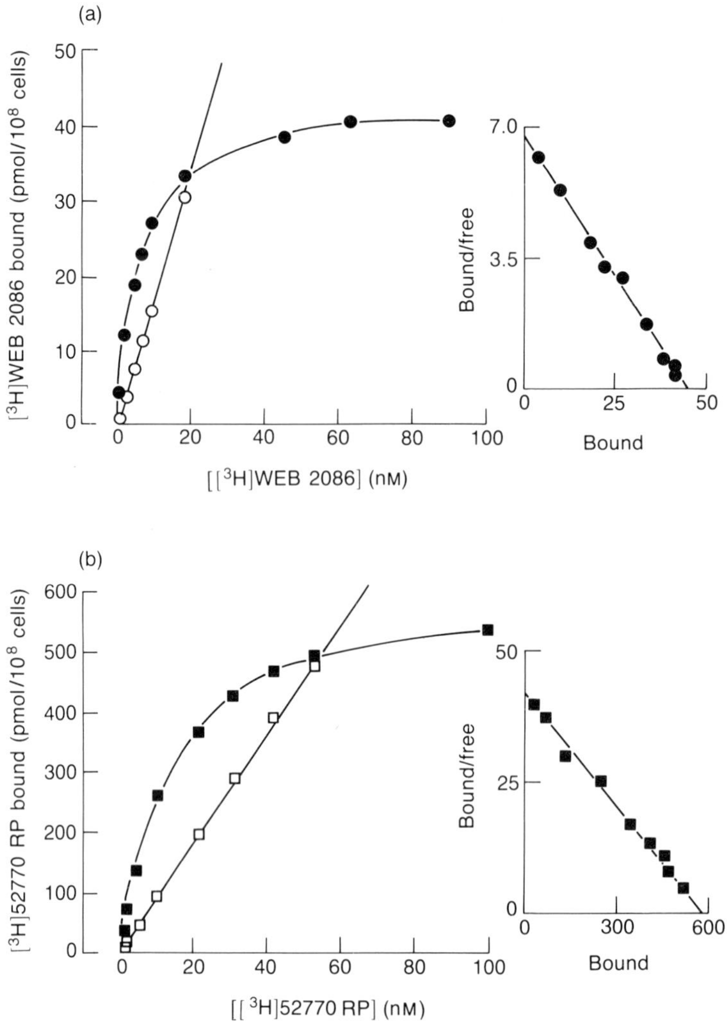

Fig. 3.3 Binding of radiolabelled PAF antagonists to gel filtered human platelets: (a) specific (●) and non-specific binding (○) of [^{3}H]WEB 2086. *Inset*: Scatchard plot of the same data, indicating a single population of binding sites; and (b) specific (■) and non-specific binding (□) of [^{3}H]52770 RP. *Inset*: Scatchard plot of the same data, indicating a single population of binding sites. From Ukena *et al.* [3].

[^{3}H]52770 RP binding to human neutrophils by a series of known PAF antagonists correlated closely [12].

In order to discover whether WEB 2086 exerted its PAF antagonistic actions through direct interaction with the PAF receptor, we investigated the correlation between binding and function in human neutrophils [18–20]. WEB 2086 inhibited PAF-induced lysosomal enzyme release in a competitive manner, with a K_B of 11.9 nM (Fig. 3.4a), while [^{3}H]WEB 2086 bound to a single site with a K_D of 19 nM at 25°C (Fig. 3.4b). The K_i of WEB 2086 versus [^{3}H]WEB 2086 binding was 16.3 nM. Thus, the affinities of WEB 2086 for functional PAF receptors and [^{3}H]WEB 2086 binding sites is similar. The affinity of PAF for [^{3}H]WEB 2086 binding sites was 170 pM, which is in the same range as the K_D values for [^{3}H]PAF binding to human neutrophils reported by

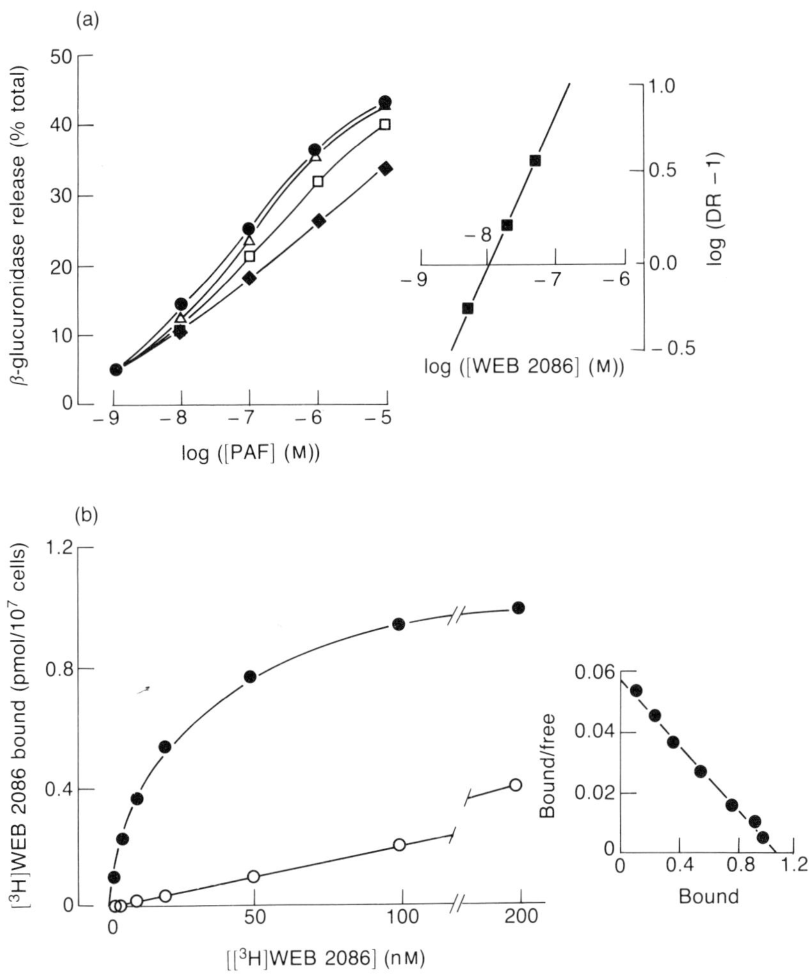

Fig. 3.4 (a) PAF-induced β-glucuronidase release from human neutrophils in the absence of any competing drug (●) and in the presence of 5 nM (△), 20 nM (□) and 50 nM WEB 2086 (◆). *Inset*: Schild plot of the same data, indicating competitive inhibition by WEB 2086, (b) specific (●) and non-specific binding (○) of [^{3}H]WEB 2086 to human neutrophils. *Inset*: Scatchard plot of the same data, indicating a single population of binding sites. From Dent *et al.* [20].

O'Flaherty *et al.* [10] and Valone & Goetzl [9], suggesting that the site of [^{3}H]WEB 2086 binding is, indeed, the PAF receptor. The binding capacity of 40 000 sites/cell for [^{3}H]WEB 2086 is very similar to the values of 49 600 and 43 600 sites/cell reported by Marquis *et al.* for binding of [^{3}H]PAF and [^{3}H]52770 RP, respectively, to human neutrophils [12].

Eosinophils

The studies performed using [^{3}H]WEB 2086 as a radioligand were reproduced in preparations of purified eosinophils obtained from peritoneal exudates of polymyxin B-treated guinea pigs [21] and from peripheral blood of human patients with the hypereosinophilic syndrome (HES) [19]. Guinea-pig eosinophils released the granule enzyme, eosinophil peroxidase (EPO) upon stimulation with PAF [21,22] and this response was inhibited by WEB 2086 with a K_B of 7.3 nM (Fig, 3.5a) while [^{3}H]WEB 2086 bound to guinea-pig eosinophils with a K_D of 17.8 nM at

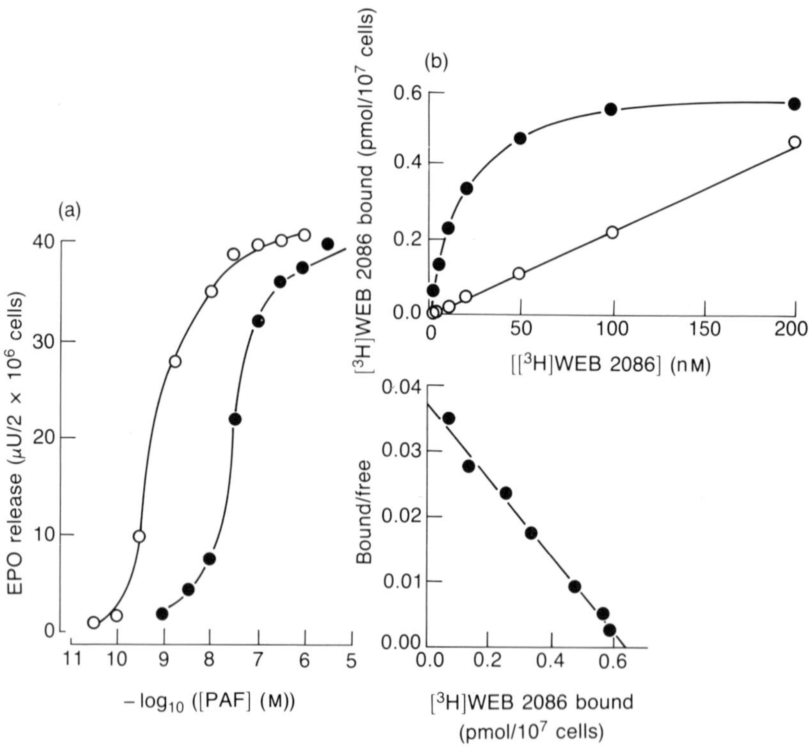

Fig. 3.5 (a) PAF-induced eosinophil peroxidase release from guinea-pig eosinophils in the absence of any competing drug (○) and in the presence of 200 nM WEB 2086 (●); (b) *upper*: specific (●) and non-specific binding (○) of [^{3}H]WEB 2086 to guinea-pig eosinophils. *Lower*: Scatchard plot of the same data, indicating a single population of binding sites. From Ukena *et al.* [21].

25°C (Fig. 3.5b) [21]. Whilst there is a degree of similarity between these affinity constants, it is not so pronounced as that observed in human neutrophils. The K_i of PAF displacement of [^{3}H]WEB 2086 binding (230 pM) and the binding capacity for [^{3}H]WEB 2086 (35 500 sites/cell) were both strikingly similar to the values obtained for human neutrophils [19, 20].

In human eosinophils, PAF-induced lucigenin-enhanced chemiluminescence was inhibited by WEB 2086 with a K_B of 16.4 nM (Fig. 3.6a), while

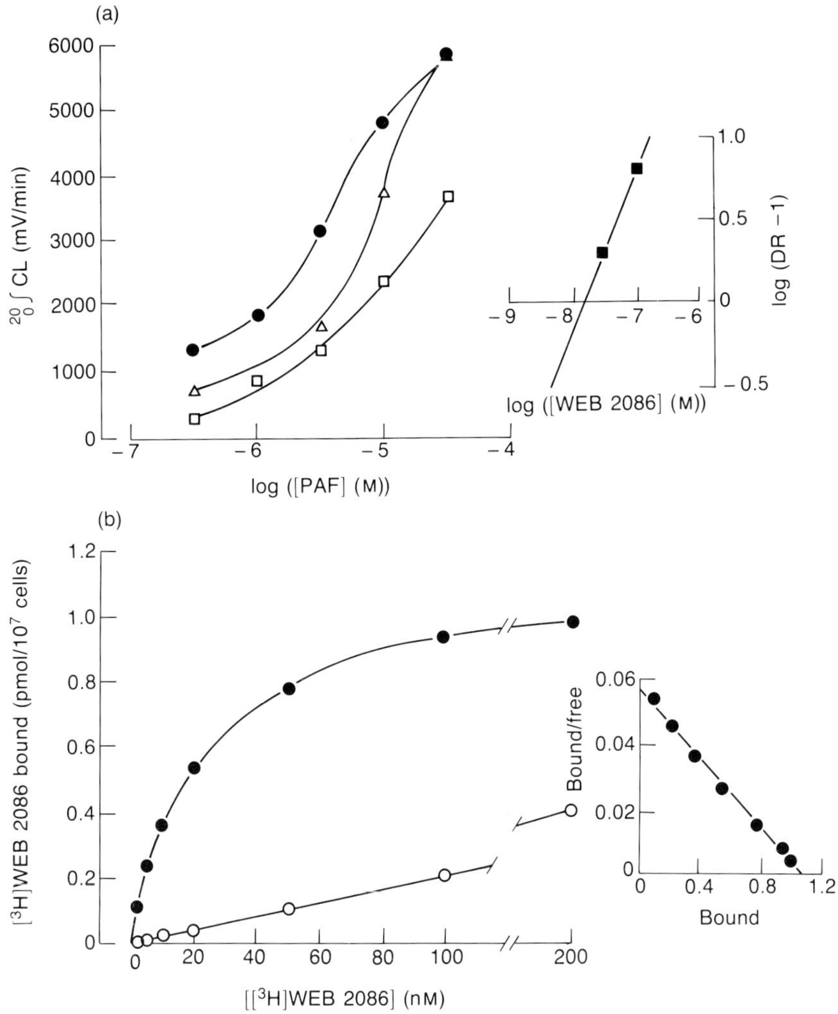

Fig. 3.6 (a) PAF-induced lucigenin-enhanced chemiluminescence of human eosinophils in the absence of any competing drug (●) and in the presence of 32 nM (△) and 100 nM WEB 2086 (□). *Inset*: Schild plot of the same data, indicating competitive inhibition, (b) specific (●) and non-specific binding (○) of [^{3}H]WEB 2086 to human eosinophils. *Inset*: Scatchard plot of the same data, indicating a single population of binding sites.

[^{3}H]WEB 2086 bound to the same cells with a K_D of 18.5 nM (Fig. 3.6b) [19]. These results suggest, again, a common binding site for PAF and WEB 2086. The K_i for PAF displacement of this binding (500 pM) was slightly higher than that observed in human neutrophils [20] and guinea-pig eosinophils [21], as was the binding capacity (64 400 sites/cell).

Lung tissues

A striking characteristic of [^{3}H]PAF binding to human lung membranes was the very high degree of non-specific binding, amounting to as much as 70% of total binding [15]. It was hoped that the use of a lipophobic antagonist radioligand would overcome this difficulty.

We investigated the binding of [^{3}H]WEB 2086 to crude membrane preparations from guinea-pig and human lung homogenates. [^{3}H]WEB 2086 binding was saturable to a single class of binding sites on guinea-pig lung membranes, with a K_D of 17 nM at 25°C and a B_{max} of 203 fmol/mg; binding to human lung membranes followed a similar pattern, giving a K_D of 23 nM and B_{max} of 157 fmol/mg (Fig. 3.7) [23]. In both cases, non-specific binding amounted to <38% of total binding at a radioligand concentration of 20 nM. The identity of the [^{3}H]WEB 2086 binding site was investigated by competition experiments, summarized in Table 3.4. The binding sites identified in lung membranes had the

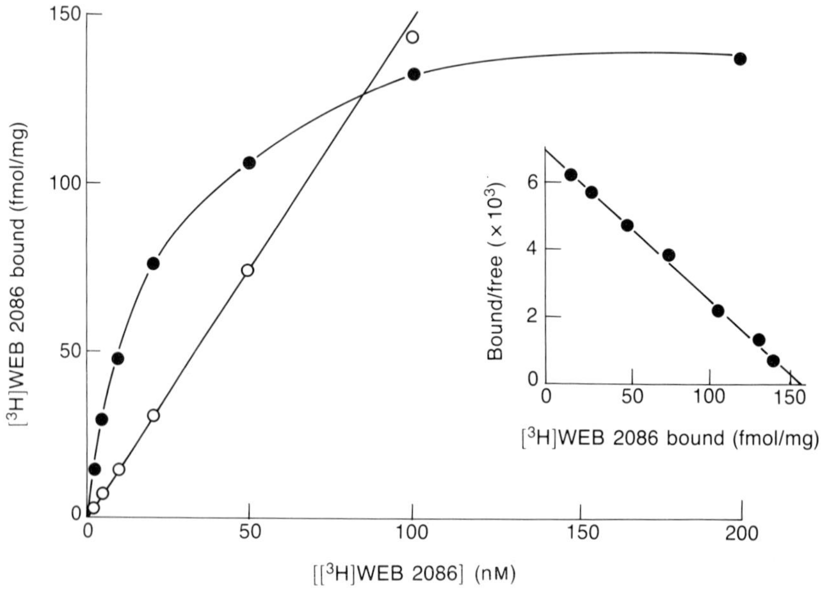

Fig. 3.7 Specific (●) and non-specific binding (○) of [^{3}H]WEB 2086 to human lung membranes. *Inset*: Scatchard plot of the same data, indicating a single population of binding sites.

Table 3.4 Inhibition of [^{3}H]WEB 2086 binding to lung membranes

	K_i (nM)	
Compound	Guinea pig	Human
C_{16}-PAF	7.9	9.8
Lyso-PAF	–	–
WEB 2086	19.4	20.1

-Indicates that binding was not inhibited at a drug concentration of 10 μM [23].

characteristics of PAF receptors and displayed an affinity for the antagonist radioligand, [^{3}H]WEB 2086 similar to that reported for human platelets [3], neutrophils [19,20] and eosinophils [19,21]. The B_{max} for [^{3}H]WEB 2086 was in very close agreement with the value of 140 fmol/mg reported for [^{3}H]PAF to human lung membranes [15]; however, the affinity of PAF for [^{3}H]WEB 2086 binding sites was approximately 50 times lower than the binding affinity reported for [^{3}H]PAF [15].

Coupling to intracellular pathways

It has been observed in several cell types that GTP inhibits binding of PAF to its specific receptors [24–26]. This is generally accepted to indicate the coupling of the receptor to a guanine nucleotide-binding regulatory protein (G-protein). In confirmation of this hypothesis, PAF causes a dose-dependent hydrolysis of [γ-^{32}P]GTP in membranes from rabbit and human platelets [24,27] and human neutrophils [28], a GTPase activity characteristic of the α-subunits of G-proteins. Binding of [^{3}H]PAF to rabbit platelet membranes was inhibited by Na^+ [24], a characteristic previously confined to those receptors related to adenylate cyclase inhibition [29–31], and, indeed, PAF has been shown to inhibit adenylate cyclase in rabbit platelets [25,32]. However, the GTPase activity stimulated by PAF in human platelets is distinct from the well-characterized 'G_i', the adenylate cyclase-inhibiting G-protein coupled to the receptors of agents such as α_2-adrenoceptor agonists and opiates, and also from the G_s adenylate cyclase-stimulatory protein coupled to receptors for, among other agents, β_2-adrenoceptor agonists and E-series prostaglandins [27,33,34].

PAF has been found to increase the intracellular level of free Ca^{2+} and to stimulate the turnover of polyphosphoinositides in a variety of cells (see below). In the rabbit neutrophil, PAF-induced Ca^{2+} mobilization was unaffected by pertussis toxin, which ADP-ribosylates the α-subunit of G_i, whereas polyphosphoinositide turnover and degranulation were potently inhibited [33]. There is a plasma membrane-bound GTPase activity in rabbit and human neutrophils, linked to the receptors for formylmethionyl chemotactic peptides, the complement fraction C5a, and leukotriene B_4 (LTB_4), which has been likened to G_i in view of its sensitivity to pertussis and insensitivity to cholera toxin [35,36]. Hwang [28] has demonstrated inhibition by both pertussis and cholera toxins of the PAF-stimulated GTPase activity in human neutrophil membranes but an absence of inhibition by either toxin of the activity in human platelet membranes. This may indicate a distinction between platelet and neutrophil PAF receptors (see below), but further obscures the identity of the PAF receptor-linked G-protein in both cell types.

Intracellular mechanisms

Turnover of inositol phosphates

PAF has been shown to stimulate an early degradation of phosphatidylinositol-4, 5-bisphosphate (PIP_2) in horse and rabbit platelets [37,38]. In both species, the major phospholipid changes observed were an increase in cellular levels of phosphatidic acid (PA) and of phosphatidylinositol (PI)—reflecting activation of the PI cycle via PI-specific phospholipase (phospholipase C) [39,40], and a later increase in levels of phosphatidylinositol-4-phosphate (PIP) and PIP_2. In rabbit platelets, a maximal aggregation response was measured within 30–60 s of addition of PAF [38]. The kinetics of the phospholipid changes were: decreased PIP_2 and increased PA within 10 s followed by an increase in PI at 30 s, with increases in PIP and PIP_2 becoming significant at 60 s [38]. The initial hydrolysis of PIP_2 in horse platelets was accompanied by a loss of PIP and PI, as well as an accumulation of PA and lyso-PI. These early events (5–10 s) were followed by re-synthesis of PIP_2, PIP and PI, which was proportional to the concentration of PAF [37]. Prostacyclin, which elevates cellular cyclic-3′, 5′-adenosine monophosphate (cAMP) levels via G_s-dependent activation of adenylate cyclase, inhibited the formation of PA and lyso-PI, as well as the subsequent re-synthesis of polyphosphoinositides, without affecting the initial degradation of PIP_2 [37]. The findings that agents which raise intracellular cAMP levels inhibit PAF-induced cell responses in human platelets [41] and guinea-pig alveolar macrophages [42] may suggest that the latter events in the inositol phosphate pathway may be of equal importance in the activation of cellular functions to the initial loss of PIP_4, which has been linked to the initiation of cellular activation by mobilization of membrane-bound Ca^{2+} stores [43].

Modulation of intracellular Ca^{2+} concentrations

PAF was shown to increase intracellular calcium ion concentrations ($[Ca^{2+}]_i$) in human platelets [44] and endothelial cells [45] in a dose-dependent manner. An increase in $[Ca^{2+}]_i$ of approximately 50% of the maximal increase achievable with PAF was associated with a 100% aggregation response in platelets and pre-incubation with low concentrations of PAF abolished the $[Ca^{2+}]_i$ increases, as well as the aggregation, induced by subsequent addition of PAF [44]. Increases in $[Ca^{2+}]_i$ induced by PAF in platelets were largely dependent upon extracellular Ca^{2+}, the response in platelets incubated in Ca^{2+}-free buffer being approximately 25% of that obtained in platelets incubated at physiological extracellular Ca^{2+} concentrations [44]. PAF induced an efflux of Ca^{2+} from pre-loaded vascular endothelial and smooth-muscle cells [45, 46], suggesting that there is a mobilization of intracellular stores of Ca^{2+}. These observations were repeated in murine peritoneal macrophages, where $[Ca^{2+}]_i$ increases stimulated by PAF were 19 times higher in the presence of 1 mM extracellular Ca^{2+} than in its absence [47]. In guinea-pig peritoneal eosinophils, PAF-stimulated increases in $[Ca^{2+}]_i$ were almost completely inhibited by the Ca^{2+} chelator, ethylene glycol tetra-acetic acid (EGTA), and the Ca^{2+} translocation blocker, Ni^{2+}, but not by dihydropyridines, indicating that Ca^{2+} entry via receptor-operated Ca^{2+} channels may be involved in PAF activation of eosinophils (Fig. 3.8) [48]. This view was reinforced by the use with human neutrophils of high extracellular concentrations of Mn^{2+}—a divalent cation which does not block Ca^{2+} channels—which showed a stimulated influx of Mn^{2+} after discharge of intracellular Ca^{2+} stores, indicating that PAF stimulates divalent cation entry by a mechanism independent of changes in $[Ca^{2+}]_i$ [49]. In addition, depolarization by high extracellular K^+ concentrations or antagonism of L-type Ca^{2+} channels did not affect either $[Ca^{2+}]_i$ or Mn^{2+} entry, showing that voltage-dependent Ca^{2+} channels are not involved in PAF-stimulated Ca^{2+} entry into human neutrophils [49].

The relationship of Ca^{2+} mobilization to functional PAF responses of cells has not been demonstrated conclusively. Hartiala *et al.* [50] demonstrated that low concentrations of formyl-methionyl peptide, C5a, LTB_4 and PAF all induced a rapid rise in $[Ca^{2+}]_i$ in rabbit neutrophils but the agents differed greatly in their ability to induce the respiratory burst. The peptides induced strong single chemiluminescence responses while the lipids produced weaker, two-peaked responses [50]. Also the peptide-induced responses were dependent on extracellular Ca^{2+}, whereas the lipids required both Ca^{2+} and Mg^{2+}, although this could be due to a requirement of Mg^+ for receptor binding of the lipid mediators. Thus, the intracellular pathways leading to activation appear to depend upon the nature of the stimulus [50].

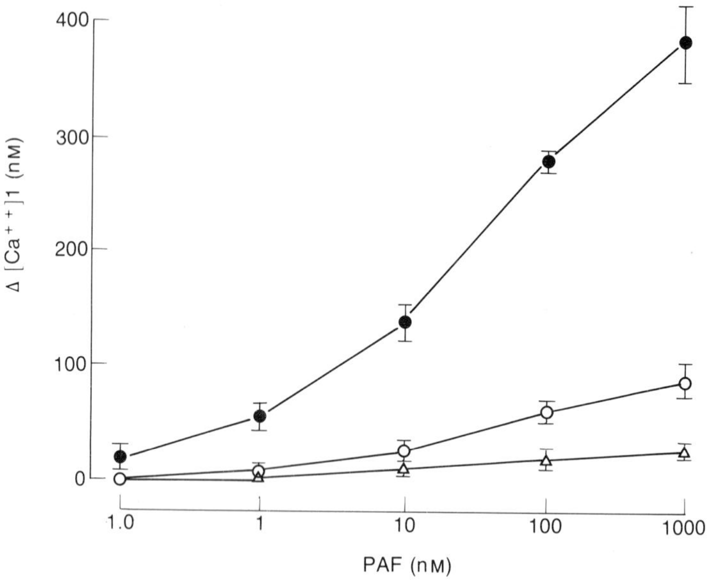

Fig. 3.8 PAF-induced increase in cytoplasmic $[Ca^{2+}]$ of guinea-pig eosinophils in the presence of: 1 mM Ca^{2+} (●); in the absence of extracellular Ca^{2+} and the presence of 5 mM EGTA (○); and in the presence of 1 mM Ni^{2+} (△). From Kroegel *et al.* [48].

PAF-receptor sub-types

Multiple molecular species of PAF have been reported [51–55]. However, it has not been clearly demonstrated whether they act upon the same receptor or on different sub-types of PAF receptor. Lambrecht & Parnham [56] proposed the existence of PAF-receptor sub-types based on the different potency of kadsurenone in inhibiting PAF-induced chemiluminescence of guinea-pig peritoneal macrophages and aggregation of pig peripheral leukocytes. It has been argued that the difference in potency of the antagonists may be due to a species difference of the PAF receptor, as demonstrated for the human and rabbit platelet [28], rather than to a difference in sub-types of PAF receptor between macrophages and circulating leukocytes [28]. No significant difference was observed between the potencies with which a number of PAF analogues and antagonists inhibited $[^3H]$PAF binding to human platelet membranes and human lung membranes [15]. However, when the relative potencies were compared in human platelets and human neutrophils, it was found that one antagonist, ONO-6240, was about 8-fold less potent in neutrophils than in platelets in both binding and functional assays [28]. There were differences, also, in ionic effects on the binding of $[^3H]$PAF to the two cell types: although Mg^{2+}, Ca^{2+} and K^+ potentiated the specific binding in both systems, Na^+ and Li^+ inhibited the specific binding to platelets but not to leukocytes. Finally, the sensitivity to pertussis and cholera toxins of the G-protein activated by the occupation by PAF of its receptors was different in the two cell types: the GTPase activity stimulated by PAF in human luekocytes could be abolished by both pertussis toxin and cholera toxin, whereas these toxins had no effect on the platelet GTPasè activity. It was suggested, on the basis of this evidence, that the PAF receptor on human polymorphonuclear leukocytes is structually different from the receptor characterized in human platelets, and that the G-proteins coupled to the PAF receptors in the two cell types also differ from one another [28].

Future directions

Much progress has been made in the identification and characterization of PAF receptors in a variety of cell types. However, much work remains to be done to develop our current knowledge into an understanding of the function of PAF in cellular regulation and thus of the role of PAF in health and disease and the potential of PAF antagonists in therapeutics.

Although we can demonstrate the presence of PAF receptors in tissues and on purified cells, the low specific activity of currently available ligands restricts the ability to identify lower affinity states of receptors. The development of better ligands may turn up important details about the regulation of PAF receptors, in terms of both affinity and receptor numbers. The demonstration of PAF receptor sub-types will depend upon the identification or development of drugs which are selective for each type. The existence of one antagonist with a greater affinity for the PAF receptor on one cell type than on another cannot be taken as strong evidence for the existence of PAF receptor sub-classes unless drugs are found which show the opposite selectivity.

The isolation and purification of the PAF receptor, allowing cloning of the receptor protein, will allow precise study of the regulation of receptor affinity. The separation of a lipid-binding protein presents major technical problems but the development of high-affinity, hydrophilic antagonist affinity ligands may surmount these problems. The purification of the receptor would also allow the development of radioreceptor assays for PAF which would be many times more sensitive than existing bioassays and more reproducible and specific than the highly complicated measurement by gas chromatography/mass spectroscopy.

Finally, investigation of the potential role of PAF in lung disease, such as bronchial asthma, requires precise localization of PAF receptors among the conglomeration of cells within the lung. Autoradiographic localization also requires the development of better ligands: highly specific activity radiolabels with high affinity for PAF receptors. Tritiated ligands are unsuitable for such work and the introduction of PAF antagonists labelled with high-energy β- or γ-emitting radioisotopes is awaited.

References

1 Valone, F. H., Coles, E., Reinhold, V. R. & Goetzl, E. J. Specific binding of phospholipid platelet-activating factor by human platelets. *J. Immunol.* (1982), **129**, 1637–1641.

2 Kloprogge, E. & Akkerman, J. W. N. Binding kinetics of PAF-acether (1-O-alkyl-2-acetyl-*sn*-glycero-3-phosphocholine) to intact human platelets. *Biochem. J.* (1984), **223**, 901–909.

3 Ukena, D., Dent, G., Birke, F. W., Robaut, C., Sybrecht, G. W. & Barnes, P. J. Radioligand binding of antagonists of platelet-activating factor to intact human platelets. *FEBS Lett.* (1988), **228**, 285–289.

4 Tuffin, D. P., Davey, P., Dyer, R. L., Lunt, D. O. & Wade, P. J. Binding of [3H]-1-O-octadecyl PAF-acether to washed human platelets. In Westwick, J., Scully, M. F., MacIntyre, D. E. & Kakkar, V. J. (eds) *Mechanisms of Stimulus–Response Coupling in Human Platelets.* (1985), Plenum Press, New York.

5 Hwang, S-B., Lee, C-S.C., Cheah, M. J. & Shen, T. Y. Specific receptor sites for 1-O-alkyl-2-O-acetyl-*sn*-glycero-3-phosphocholine (platelet activating factor) on rabbit platelet and guinea pig smooth muscle membranes. *Biochemistry* (1983), **22**, 4756–4763.

6 Homma, H., Tokumura, A. & Hanahan, D. J. Binding and internalization of platelet-activating factor 1-O-alkyl-2-acetyl-3-*sn*-glycero-3-phosphocholine in washed rabbit platelets. *J. Biol. Chem.* (1987), **262**, 10 582–10 587.

7 Tarahoui, L., Floch, A., Mondot, S. & Cavero, I. High affinity specific binding sites for tritiated platelet-activating factor in canine platelet membranes: counterparts of platelet-activating factor receptors mediating platelet aggregation. *Mol. Pharmacol.* (1988), **34**, 145–151.

8 Inarrea, P., Gomez-Cambronero, J., Nieto, M. & Crespo, M. S. Characteristics of the binding of platelet-activating factor to platelets of different animal species. *Eur. J. Pharmacol.* (1984), **105**, 309–315.

9 Valone, F. H. & Goetzl, E. J. Specific binding by human polymorphonuclear leukocytes of the immunological mediator 1-O-hexadecyl/octadecyl-2-acetyl-*sn*-glycero-3-phosphorylcholine. *Immunology* (1983), **48**, 141–149.

10 O'Flaherty, J. T., Surles, J. R., Redman, J., Jacobson, D., Piantadosi, C. & Wykle, R. L. Binding and metabolism of platelet-activating factor by human neutrophils. *J. Clin. Invest.* (1986), **78**, 381–388.

11 Gallin, J. I., Gallin, E. K. & Schiffmann, E. Mechanism of leukocyte chemotaxis. *Adv. Inflammatory Res.* (1979), **1**, 123–130.

12 Marquis, O., Robaut, C. & Cavero, I. [^{3}H]52770 RP, a platelet-activating factor receptor antagonist, and tritiated platelet-activating factor label a common specific binding site in human polymorphonuclear leukocytes. *J. Pharmacol. Exp. Ther.* (1988), **244**, 709–715.

13 Rola-Pleszcynski, M., Pignol, B., Pouliot, C. & Braquet, P. Inhibition of human lymphocyte proliferation and interleukin-2 production by platelet activating factor (PAF-acether): reversal by a specific antagonist, BN 52021. *Biochem. Biophys. Res. Commun.* (1987), **142**, 754–760;

14 Ng, D. S. & Wong, K. Specific binding of platelet-activating factor (PAF) by human peripheral blood mononuclear leukocytes. *Biochem. Biophys. Res. Commun.* (1988), **155**, 311–316.

15 Hwang, S-B., Lam, M-H. & Shen, T. Y. Specific binding sites for platelet activating factor in human lung tissues. *Biochem. Biophys. Res. Commun.* (1985), **128**, 972–979.

16 Hwang, S-B., Lam, M-H, & Chang, M. N. Specific binding of [^{3}H]dihydrokadsurenone to rabbit platelet membranes and its inhibition by the receptor agonists and antagonists of platelet-activating factor. *J. Biol. Chem.* (1986), **261**, 13 720–13 726.

17 Robaut, C., Durand, G., James, C., *et al.* PAF binding sites: characterization by [^{3}H]52770 RP, a pyrrolo[1,2,*c*]thiazole derivative, in rabbit platelets. *Biochem. Pharmacol.* (1987), **36**, 3221–3229.

18 Ukena, D., Dent, G., Sybrecht, G. W. & Barnes, P. J. Radioligand binding of antagonists of platelet-activating factor to human platelets and polymorphonuclear leukocytes. *FASEB J.* (1988), **2**, A1575.

19 Dent, G., Ukena, D., Chanez, P., Sybrecht, G. W. & Barnes, P. J. Characterization of platelet-activating factor (PAF) receptors in human neutrophils and eosinophils using the new competitive PAF antagonist, WEB 2086. *Am. Rev. Resp. Dis.* (1988), **137**, A236 (Abstract).

20 Dent, G., Ukena, D., Chanez, P., Sybrecht, G. W. & Barnes, P. J. Characterization of PAF receptors on human neutrophils using the specific antagonist, WEB 2086: correlation between receptor binding and function. *FEBS Lett.* (1989), **244**, 365–368.

21 Ukena, D., Kroegel, C., Dent, G., Yukawa, T., Sybrecht, G. W. & Barnes, P. J. PAF receptors on eosinophils: identification with a novel ligand, [^{3}H]WEB 2086. *Biochem. Pharmacol.* (1989), **38**, 1702–1704.

22 Kroegel, C., Yukawa, T., Dent, G., Chanez, P., Chung, K. F. & Barnes, P. J. Platelet-activating factor induces eosinophil peroxidase release from purified human eosinophils. *Immunology* (1988), **64**, 559–562.

23 Dent, G., Ukena, D., Mak, J. C. W., Sybrecht, G. W. & Barnes, P. J. Platelet-activating factor receptors in human and guinea pig lung: demonstration using the novel antagonist ligand [^{3}H]WEB 2086. *Am. Rev. Resp. Dis.* (1989), **139**, A94 (Abstract).

24 Hwang, S-B., Lam, M-H. & Pong, S-S. Ionic and GTP regulation of binding of platelet-activating factor to receptors and platelet-activating factor-induced activation of GTPase in rabbit platelet membranes. *J. Biol. Chem.* (1986), **261**, 532–537.

25 Williams, K. A. & Haslam, R. J. Effects of NaCl and GTP on the inhibition of platelet adenylate cyclase by 1-O-octadecyl-2-O-acetyl-*sn*-glyceryl-3-phosphorylcholine (synthetic platelet-activating factor). *Biochim. Biophys. Acta* (1984), **770**, 216–223.

26 Ng, D. A. & Wong, K. GTP regulation of platelet-activating factor binding to human neutrophil membranes. *Biochem. Biophys. Res. Commun.* (1986), **141**, 353–359.

27 Houslay, M. D., Bojanic, D. & Wilson, A. Platelet activating factor and U44069 stimulate a GTPase activity in human platelets which is distinct from the guanine nucleotide regulatory proteins, N_s and N_i. *Biochem. J.* (1986), **234**, 737–740.

28 Hwang, S-B. Indentification of a second putative receptor of platelet-activating factor from human polymorphonuclear leukocytes. *J. Biol. Chem,* (1988), **263**, 3225–3233.

29 Motulsky, H. J. & Insel, P. A. [^{3}H]Dihydroergocryptine binding to alpha-adrenergic receptors of human platelets. A reassessment using the selective radioligands [^{3}H]prazosin, [^{3}H]yohimbine, and [^{3}H]rauwolscine. *J. Biol. Chem.* (1983), **258**, 3913–3919.

30 Pong, S-S. & DeHaven, R. N. Characterization of a leukotriene D_4 receptor in guinea pig lung. *Proc. Nat. Acad. Sci. (USA)* (1983), **80**, 7415–7419.

31 Koski, G., Streaty, R. A. & Klee, W. A. Modulation of sodium-sensitive GTPase by partial opiate agonists. An explanation for the dual requirement for Na^+ and GTP in inhibitory regulation of adenylate cyclase. *J. Biol. Chem.* (1982), **257**, 14 035–14 040.

32 Haslam, R. J. & Vanderwel, M. Inhibition of platelet adenylate cyclase by 1-O-alkyl-2-O-acetyl-*sn*-glyceryl-3-phosphorylcholine (platelet-activating factor). *J. Biol. Chem.* (1982), **257**, 6879–6885.

33 Naccache, P. H., Molski, M. M., Volpi, M., Becker, E. M. & Sha'afi, R. I. Unique inhibitory profile of platelet activating factor induced calcium mobilization, polyphosphoinositide turnover and granule enzyme secretion in rabbit neutrophils towards pertussis toxin and phorbol ester. *Biochem. Biophys. Res. Commun.* (1985), **130**, 677–684.

34 Lad, P. M., Olson, C. V., Grewal, I. S. & Scott, S. J. A pertussis toxin-sensitive GTP-binding protein in the human neutrophil regulates multiple receptors, calcium mobilization and lectin-induced capping. *Proc. Nat. Acad. Sci. (USA)* (1985), **82**, 8643–8647.

35 O'Flaherty, J. T. & Nishihira, J. Arachidonate metabolites, platelet-activating factor, and the mobilization of protein kinase C in human polymorphonuclear neutrophils. *J. Immunol.* (1987), **138**, 1889–1895.

36 Feltner, D. E., Smith, R. H. & Marasco, W. A. Characterization of the plasma membrane bound GTPase from rabbit neutrophils. I. Evidence for an N_i-like protein coupled to the formyl peptide, C5a, and leukotriene B_4 chemotaxis receptors. *J. Immunol.* (1986), **137**, 1961–1970.

37 Billah, M. M. & Lapetina, E. G. Platelet-activating factor stimulates metabolism of phosphoinositides in horse platelets: possible relationship to Ca^{2+} mobilization during stimulation. *Proc. Nat. Acad. Sci. (USA)* (1983) **80**, 965–968.

38 Mauco, G., Chap, H. & Douste-Blazy, L. Platelet activating factor (PAF-acether) promotes an early degradation of phosphatidylinositol-4, 5-bisphosphate in rabbit platelets. *FEBS Lett.* (1983), **153**, 361–365.

39 Rittenhouse-Simmons, S. Production of diglyceride from phosphatidylinositol in activated human platelets. *J. Clin. Invest.* (1979), **63**, 580–587.

40 Mauco, G., Chap, H. & Douste-Blazy, L. Characterization and properties of a phosphatidylinositol phosphodiesterase (phospholipase C) from platelet cytosol. *FEBS Lett.* (1979), **100**, 367–370.

41 Gorman, R. R., Morton, D. R., Hopkins, N. K. & Lin, A. H. Acetyl glyceryl ether phosphorylcholine stimulates leukotriene B_4 synthesis and cyclic AMP accumulation in human polymorphonuclear leukocytes. *Adv. Prost. Thromb. Leuk. Res.* (1983), **12**, 57–63.

42 Bachelet, M., Adolfs, M. J. P., Masliah, J., Bereziat, G., Vargaftig, B. B. & Bonta, I. L. Interaction between PAF-acether and drugs that stimulate cyclic AMP in guinea-pig alveolar macrophages. *Eur. J. Pharmacol.* (1988), **149**, 73–78.

43 Billah, M. M. & Lapetina, E. G. Formation of lysophosphatidylinositol in platelet stimulated with thrombin or ionophore A23187. *J. Biol. Chem.* (1982), **257**, 12 707–12 708.

44 Valone, F. H. & Johnson, B. Modulation of cytoplasmic calcium in human platelets by the phospholipid platelet-activating factor 1-O-alkyl-2-acetyl-*sn*-glycero-3-phosphorylcholine. *J. Immunol.* (1985), **134**, 1120–1124.

45 Bussolino, F., Aglietta, M., Sanavio, F., Stacchini, A., Lauri, D. & Camussi, G. Alkyl-ether phosphoglycerides influence calcium fluxes into human endothelial cells. *J. Immunol.* (1985), **135**, 2748–2753.

46 Doyle, V. M., Creba, J. A. & Ruegg, U. T. Platelet-activating factor mobilises intracellular calcium in vascular smooth muscle stores. *FEBS Lett.* (1986), **197**, 13–16.

47 Conrad, G. W. & Rink, T. J. Platelet-activating factor raises intracellular calcium ion concentration in macrophages. *J. Cell. Biol.* (1986), **103**, 439–450.
48 Kroegel, C., Pleass, R., Yukawa, T., Chung, K. F., Westwick, J. & Barnes, P. J. Characterization of platelet-activating factor-induced elevation of cytosolic free calcium concentration in eosinophils. *FEBS Lett.* (1989), **243**, 41–46.
49 Merrit, J. E., Jacob, R. & Hallam, T. J. Use of manganese to discriminate between calcium influx and mobilization from internal stores in stimulated human neutrophils. *J. Biol. Chem.* (1989), **264**, 1522–1527.
50 Hartiala, K. T., Scott, I. G., Viljanen, M. K. & Akerman, K. E. O. Lack of correlation between calcium mobilization and respiratory burst activation induced by chemotactic factors in rabbit polymorphonuclear leukocytes. *Biochem. Biophys. Res. Commun.* (1987), **144**, 794–800.
51 Clay, K. L., Murphy, R. C., Andres, J. L., Lynch, J. & Henson, P. M. Structure elucidation of platelet activating factor derived from human neutrophils. *Biochem. Biophys. Res. Commun.* (1984), **121**, 815–825.
52 Mueller, H. W., O'Flaherty, J. T. & Wykle, R. L. The molecular species distribution of platelet-activating factor synthesized by rabbit and human neutrophils. *J. Biol. Chem.* (1984), **259**, 14 554–14 559.
53 Pinckard, R. N., Jackson, E. M., Hoppens, C., Weintraub, S. T., Ludwig, J. C., McManus, L. M. & Mott, G. E. Molecular heterogeneity of platelet-activating factor produced by stimulated human polymorphonuclear leukocytes. *Biochem. Biophys. Res. Commun.* (1984), **122**, 325–332.
54 Oda, M., Satouchi, K., Yasunaga, K. & Saito, K. Molecular species of platelet-activating factor generated by human neutrophils challenged with ionophore A23187. *J. Immunol.* (1985), **134**, 1090–1093.
55 Weintraub, S. T., Ludwig, J. C., Mott, G. E., McManus, L. M., Lear, C. & Pinckard, R. N. Fast atom bombardment–mass spectrometric identification of molecular species of platelet-activating factor produced by stimulated human polymorphonuclear leukocytes. *Biochem. Biophys. Res. Commun.* (1985), **129**, 868–876.
56 Lambrecht, G. & Parnham, M. J. Kadsurenone distinguishes between different platelet activating factor receptor subtypes on macrophages and polymorphonuclear leucocytes. *Br. J. Pharmacol.* (1986), **87**, 287–289.

Chapter 4
PAF-receptor antagonists

David Hosford, Clive P. Page, Peter J. Barnes and Pierre Braquet

Introduction

The importance of the patho-physiological role of PAF has only been more fully elucidated since the discovery in the early 1980s of compounds capable of specifically antagonizing the various biological activities of PAF bioactions. These compounds are specific and displace the PAF molecule from its receptor-binding sites, in most cases without themselves initiating any response. Their action is therefore a receptor-mediated process, competitive and generally reversible. Indeed, binding studies using [^{3}H]PAF have revealed high-affinity receptors for the mediator in human [1–4] and rabbit platelets [2,5], human neutrophils [6], human lung membranes [7], gerbil brain [8], rat retinal tissue [9] and pigmented rabbit iris and ciliary body [10].

PAF antagonists have allowed a more detailed investigation of these binding sites and also revealed PAF binding sites in guinea pig platelets, macrophages and polymorphonuclear leukocytes (PMNL) [11], rat PMNL [12], and rabbit and guinea pig smooth muscle membranes [5]. Interestingly, rat platelets do not aggregate, secrete or demonstrate Ca^{2+} uptake in response to PAF or posses high-affinity binding sites for the mediator [2].

The fact that PAF has such a diverse range of biological activities means that PAF antagonists may be of considerable medicinal value as therapeutic agents. In this review we will consider the pharmacology of the various specific PAF receptor antagonists. These compounds can generally be classed as: (i) synthetic antagonists, which may or may not be related to the structure of PAF; and (ii) natural antagonists and their derivatives. In addition to the present article, PAF antagonists have been the subject of several reviews, most recently by Braquet [13], Braquet & Godfroid [14] and Braquet *et al.* [15].

Specific PAF antagonists of synthetic origin

The majority of PAF antagonists of synthetic origin are modified derivatives of the PAF molecule (compound **1**), the glycerol backbone (or modified glycerol backbone) either being non-constrained as is the case with CV-3988 [16], Ro 19-3704 [17], SRI 63-119 [18] and RU 45-703 [19] or constrained as in SRI 63-072 [20] and SRI 63-675 [21]. There are relatively few antagonists of synthetic origin unrelated to the PAF structure, although 48740 RP and 52770 RP [22] derived from a (3-pyridyl)-1H,3H-pyrrolo[1,2*c*]thiazole framework and the diazepam-related agents, alprazolam, triazolam [23], brotizolam, WEB 2086 and WEB 2170 [24] show potent PAF-antagonistic properties.

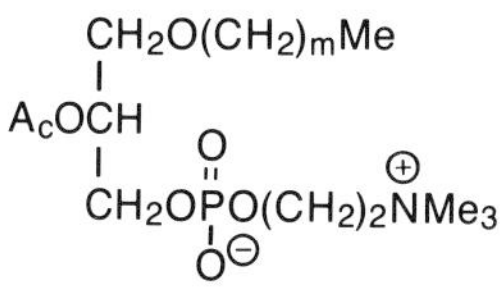

(**1**) PAF
(*n* is usually 15 or 17)

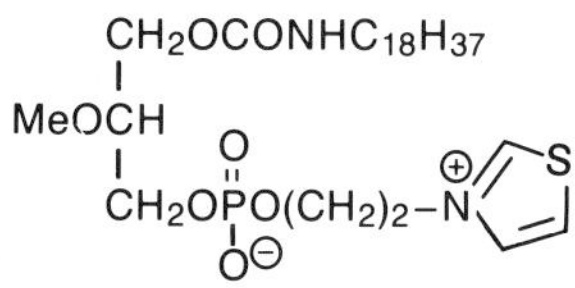

(**2**) CV-3988

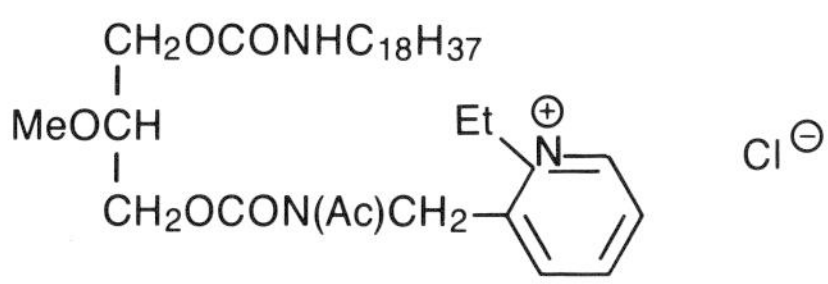

(**3**) CV-6209

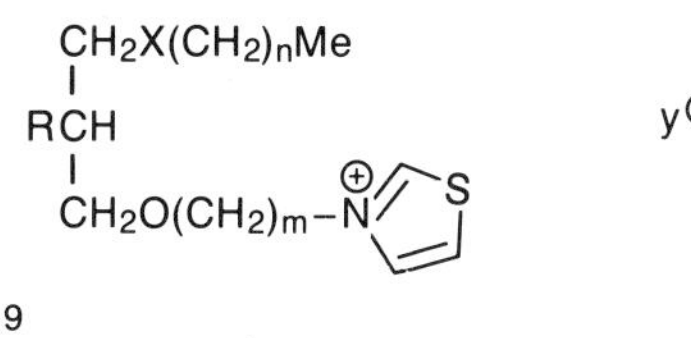

(**4a**) SRI 63-119
n = 17, X = OCONH, R = OMe, m = 4, y = I

(**4b**) ONO-6240
n = 15, X = O, R = OEt, m = 7, y = $MeSO_3$

(**4c**) Ro 19-3704
n = 17, X = OCONH, R = OCO_2Me, m = 4, y = I
n = 17, X = OCONi-Pr, R = OCONHMe, m = 4

Fig. 4.1 PAF antagonists (compounds **1**–**4**).

Non-constrained PAF framework-related antagonists

These antagonists derive directly from the PAF structure and are open-chain analogues of the mediator CV-3988 (compound **2**; Takeda), the first product described in this series. Incorporating an octadecyl carbamate in position 1, a methylether in position 2 and a thiazolium ethyl phosphate in position 3, this compound was discovered during an investigation of carbamate analogues of lysophospholipids as potential anti-fungal and cytotoxic agents [16]. The K_i values of CV-3988 for the specific binding of $[^3H]$PAF to human, rabbit and guinea pig platelets are, respectively 0.16, 0.12 and 0.18 μM [16], showing it to be a potent antagonist. A weak agonistic activity has also been described, but only at high doses. The first report by Terashita *et al.* [16] claimed that CV-3988 specifically inhibited PAF-induced platelet aggregation, however more recent studies have shown that at higher concentrations, the compound also displays antagonistic properties against arachidonic acid, ADP and collagen [25].

CV-3988 effectively antagonizes endotoxin-induced shock in the rat [26], the related gastrointestinal damage [27] and disseminated intravascular coagulation [28]. This compound also counteracts the decrease in blood pressure induced by unclipping of the renal artery in the one-kidney, one-clip hypertensive rat [29] and evokes a dose-dependent inhibition of the vascular permeability increase induced by PAF in rat skin [30]. CV-3988 also prevents the alteration of mucus secretion, respiratory and circulatory changes caused by the administration of PAF in the ferret [31] and the airway hyper-responsiveness observed in beagles subjected to ozone inhalation [32]. Furthermore, CV-3988 has recently entered phase-1 clinical trials [33]. Human volunteers who received an i.v. infusion of CV-3988 (750–2000 μg/kg) in a double-blind, placebo-controlled study, showed reduced *ex vivo* platelet sensitivity to PAF. However, blood pressure, pulse, and respiratory rate were unaffected, although, there was a small but clinically insignificant change in plasma haemoglobin and serum haptoglobin [33].

CV-6209 (compound **3**), is an analogue of CV-3988 where the phosphate group has been replaced by an acetylcarbamate group. This modification produces a marked increase in PAF inhibitory activity and the compound is some 80-fold more active than CV-3988. CV-6209 specifically inhibits PAF-induced aggregation of rabbit and human platelets (IC_{50} = 75 nM and 0.17 μM, respectively) and abolishes PAF-induced hypotension in rats [34].

SRI 63-119 (compound **4a**), a compound recently described by Sandoz, is a non-phosphorus containing thiazolium PAF-receptor antagonist that inhibits PAF-induced human platelet aggregation with an IC_{50} of 3.8×10^{-6} M [35]. It also antagonizes PAF-induced hypotension in the rat

[36], haemoconcentration, bronchoconstriction [37] and microvascular leakage in the guinea pig [38], and haemoconcentration in the primate [39]. In addition, studies in the rat have demonstrated that the compound effectively inhibits effects produced by endotoxin and PAF-induced bowel necrosis [40]. The *d* and *l*-forms of the SRI 63-119 are equipotent against PAF-induced bronchoconstriction and haemoconcentration in the guinea pig, indicating a lack of enantiomeric selectivity [41]. It is interesting to note however, that SRI 63-119 only partially inhibits dermal extravasation in the reverse arthus reaction suggesting the involvement of vasoactive mediators other than PAF in this type of pathology [42].

Replacement of the phosphoryl moiety of CV-3988 with a heptamethylene thiazolium, yields another series of antagonists among which ONO-6240 (compound **4b**) is the most potent [43]. This compound protects against PAF-induced guinea pig platelet aggregation ($IC_{50} = 0.2$ μM), and at 0.1–1 mg/kg i.v. prevents hypotension and bronchoconstriction in rats and guinea pigs [43]. ONO-6240 also partially prevents the decrease in cardiac output and systemic arterial pressure induced by *E. coli*-derived endotoxin in the sheep [44].

Other modifications of the non-constrained PAF framework, have led Hoffmann–La Roche to develop a further series of antagonistic compounds. The two closely-related tetramethylene derivatives, both designated Ro 19-3704 (compounds **4c**), are the most efficient and inhibit PAF-induced rabbit platelet aggregation with an IC_{50} of 3.0 and 0.4 μM respectively [19]. These compounds inhibit PAF-induced aggregation of rabbit, human and guinea pig platelets, as well as bronchoconstriction, hypotension, thrombocytopenia, leukopenia and increased vascular permeability in the guinea pig [45]. In addition, they prevent PAF-induced activation of alveolar macrophages, and the formation of thromboxane by isolated and perfused PAF-stimulated guinea pig lungs. Although this antagonist fails to counteract bronchoconstriction of homologous passive systemic anaphylaxis, it does inhibit bronchospasm due to aerosolized antigen [45].

Replacement of the phosphate group in CV-3988 with $-COCH_3$ and alteration of the $-OCH_2$ moiety leads to the structures Ro 18-8736, Ro 19-1400 and Ro 18-7953 (compounds **5a**, **b**, **c**) [17]. These antagonists have an IC_{50} against PAF-induced human platelet aggregation of 0.5, 0.4 and 0.7 μM, respectively [46]. The closely-related Hoechst-Roussel compound, RU 45703 (compound **5d**), is obtained by substitution of the phosphoryl group by an ester linkage. This antagonist is a potent inhibitor of PAF-induced aggregation of rabbit platelet-rich plasma (PRP) with an IC_{50} of 8 μM and also protects against PAF-induced bronchoconstriction and hypotension *in vivo*.

Very recently two further series of non-constrained PAF-related antagonists have been reported. The Sankyo product, designated 137-224

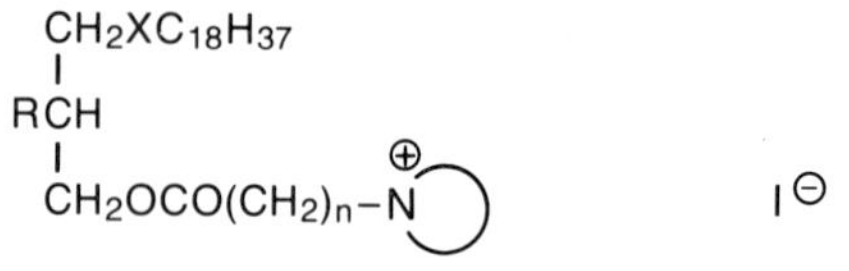

(**5a**) Ro 18-7953
X = OCONH, R = OMe, *n* = 3

(**5b**) Ro 19-1400
X = OCONH, R = OCO_2Me, *n* = 3

(**5c**) Ro 18-8736
X = OCONH, R = $NHCO_2Me$, *n* = 3

(**5d**) RU 45,703
X = O, R = OEt, *n* = 4

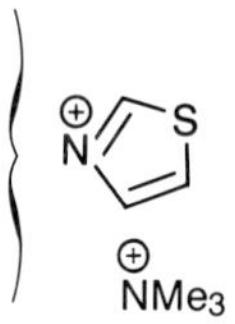

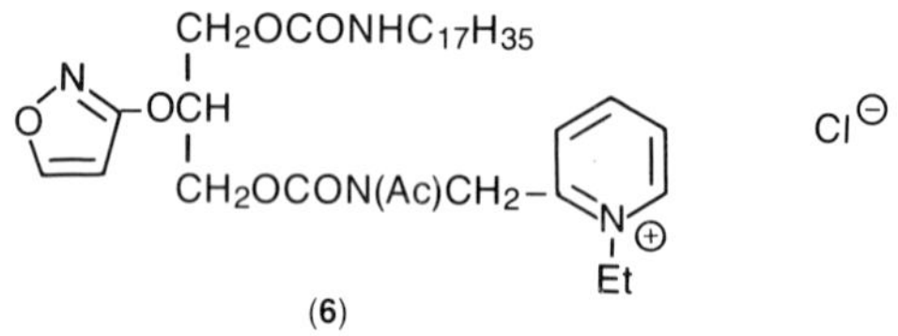

(**6**)

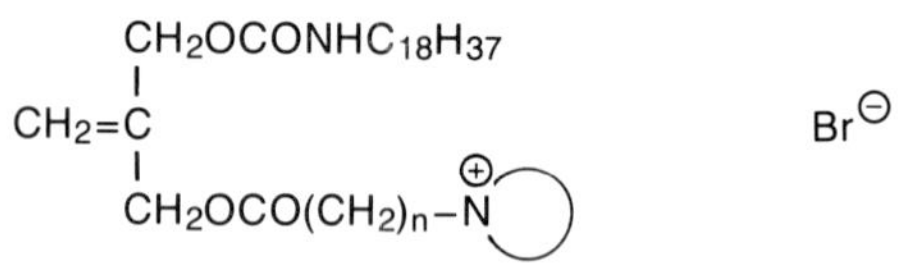

(**7a**) GS 1065-180, n = 5

(**7b**) GS 1160-180, n = 6

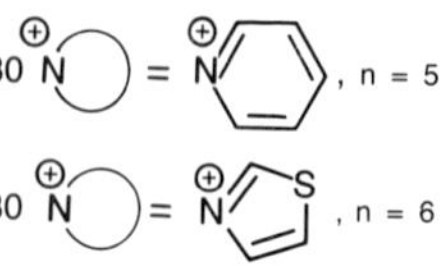

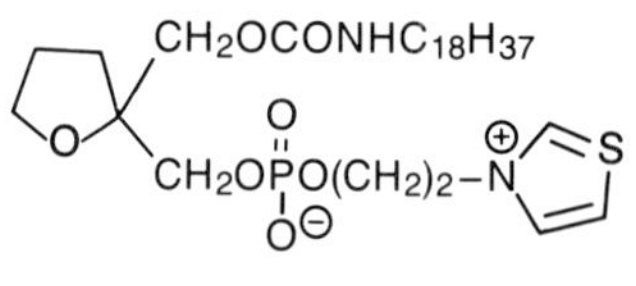

(**8**)

Fig. 4.2 PAF antagonists (compounds **5**–**8**).

(compound **6**) and structurally defined as 2-[*N*-acetyl-*N*-[3-(*N*-heptadecylcarbamoyloxy)-2-(3-isoxazolyloxy)propoxycarbonyl]-1-ethyl-pyridinium chloride [47] is a potent PAF antagonist which inhibits PAF-induced hypotension in rats ($ID_{50} = 0.004$ mg/kg i.v.) and PAF-induced rabbit platelet aggregation *in vitro* ($IC_{50} = 0.081$ μM). The compound displays good duration of action and bioavailability, and a variety of glycerol derivatives of the parent structure have been synthesized to establish structure–activity relationships in this series.

Finally, researchers from Leo Pharmaceuticals have reported the synthesis of two new achiral PAF antagonists, GS 1065–180 (compound **7a**) and GS 1160–180 (compound **7b**) from 2-methyleneproane-1, 3-diol [48]. *In vitro* platelet aggregation experiments with PRP from rabbits revealed GS 1160–180 as the most effective PAF antagonist (EC_{50} = 0.25 μM) twice active as GS 1065–180 and 80 times more active than CV-3988. Neither GS 1065–180 nor GS 1160–180 induced platelet aggregation at concentrations $\leqslant 10^{-4}$ M, or exhibited any inhibitory effect on platelet aggregation induced by collagen or adenosine diphosphate (ADP).

In vivo experiments with PAF-induced bronchoconstriction in guinea pigs demonstrated that GS 1160–180 (ED_{50} = 0.1 mg/kg i.v.) was twice as active as GS 1065–180 and 35 times more active than CV-3988 as PAF antagonists. In this system the difference in activity was less marked with the PAF-induced hypotension in rats, the two antagonists being equipotent (ED_{50} = 0.5 mg/kg i.v.) and only twice as active as CV-3988 [48].

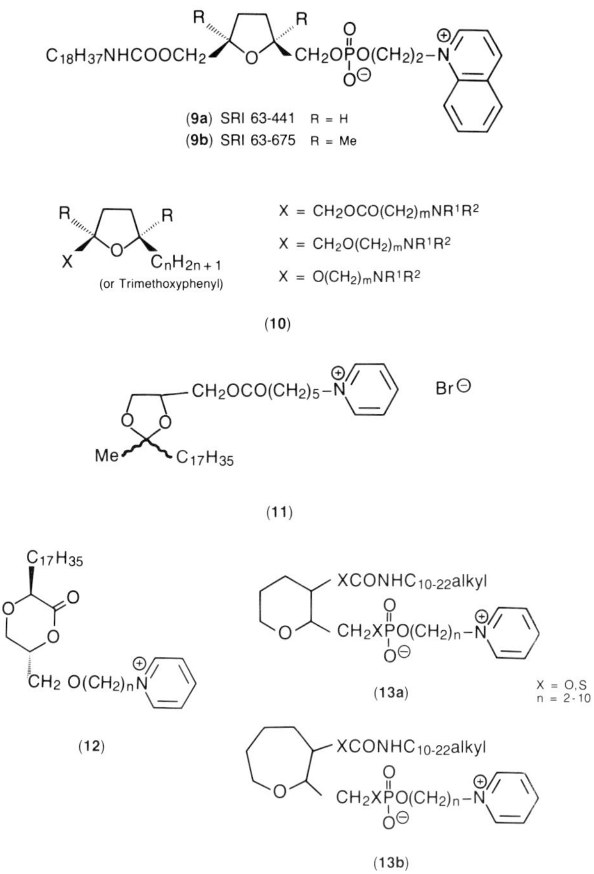

Fig. 4.3 PAF antagonists (compounds **9**–**13**).

Constrained PAF framework-related antagonists

Cyclization of parts of the PAF molecular backbone produces the second family of PAF-related antagonists, with a constrained framework. For example, insertion of a tetrahydrofuran ring has led to derivatives such as SRI 63-072 (compound **8**), SRI 63-441 (compound **9a**), SRI 63-675 (compound **9b**) and BN 55009 (compound **10**). The inclusion of a 1,3-dioxolane has given rise to BN 52111 (compound **11**) and analogues, while Roche have synthesized a series of 1,4-dioxane antagonists, exemplified by compound **12**. Other constrained framework inhibitors contain a tetrahydropyran ring (compounds **13a** and **13b**), while inclusion of a piperidine produces the inhibitor, SRI 63-073 (compound **14**). Incorporation of a 2-

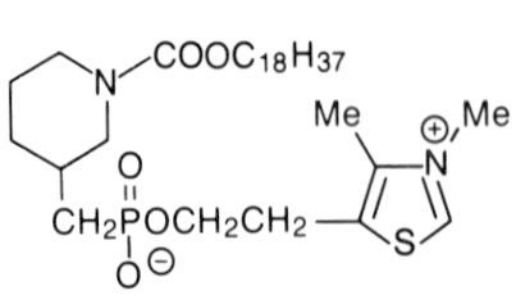

(**14**) SRI 63-073

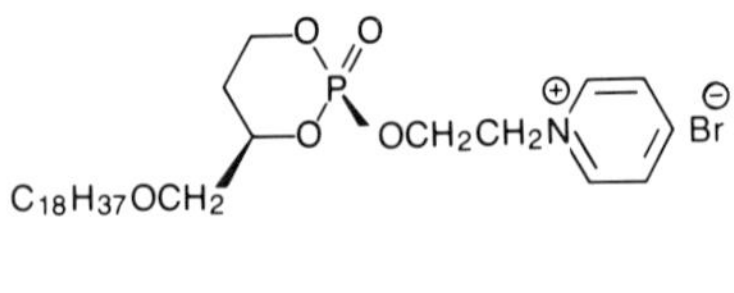

(**15**) Ro 18-6977

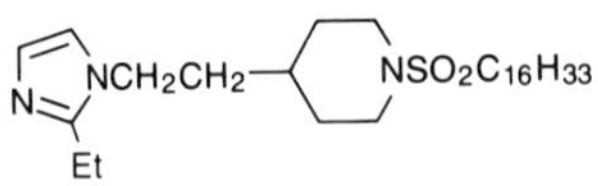

(**16**) SRI 62-586

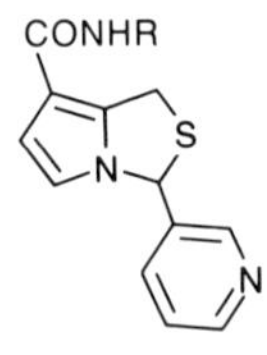

(**17a**) 48740 RP R = H
(**17b**) 52770 RP R = $_m$Cl-C_6H_4

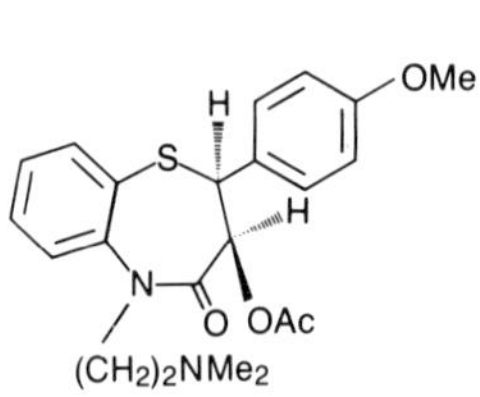

(**18**) Diltiazem

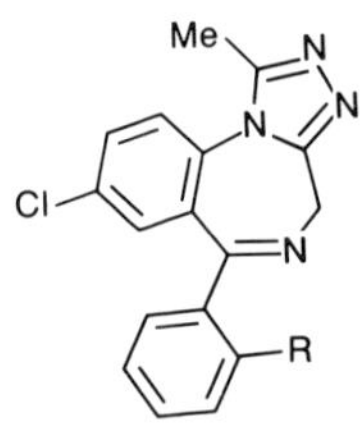

(**19a**) Alprazolam R = H
(**19b**) Triazolam R = Cl

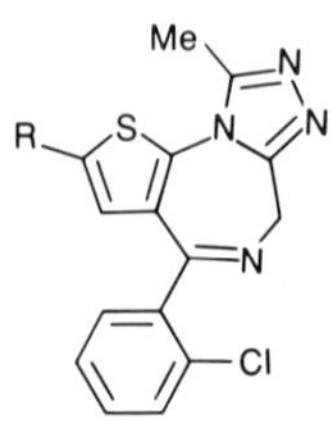

(**20a**) Brotizolam R = Br
(**20b**) Etizolam R = Et

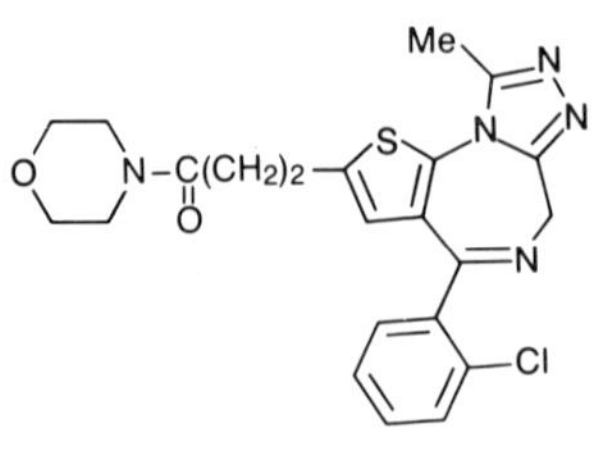

(**21**) WEB 2086

Fig. 4.4 PAF antagonists (compounds **14**–**21**).

oxo-1,3,2-dioxaphosphorinane gives compound **15** and related antagonists. Finally, Sandoz have also synthesized an antagonist containing a piperidine, designated SRI 62-586 (compound **16**).

SRI 63-072 (compound **8**) [20] is an inhibitor of PAF-induced human, guinea pig, rabbit, dog and baboon platelet aggregation with $IC_{50} = 22.3$, 1.4, 4.7, <100, and 19.0 μM, respectively [49]. The antagonist also prevents PAF-induced bronchoconstriction and haemoconcentration in the guinea pig [41] and haemoconcentration in a primate *(Cebus appella)* [39]. In the rat, SRI 63-072 not only abolishes PAF-induced ischaemic bowel necrosis [50], but also PAF-, endotoxin-, and human IgG-induced hypotension [51]. In the primate this antagonist also protects against PAF-induced bronchoconstriction [52]. Further studies have shown that SRI 63-072 partially inhibits dermal extravasation in the reverse, passive Arthus reaction in guinea pigs [53] and rats [54], and also in this latter species diminishes glomerulonephritis induced by immune complexes [54]. SRI 63-072, similar to SRI 63-119, does not exhibit enantiospecificity either *in vitro* or *in vivo* [41].

The closely-related *cis*-2,5-disubstituted tetrahydrofuran analogue, SRI 63-441 (compound **9a**), is a more potent PAF antagonist. It inhibits PAF binding to human platelets with an IC_{50} of 0.35 μM [55] and PAF-induced aggregation of guinea pig, rabbit, dog, baboon and human platelets aggregation with IC_{50} values of 0.3, 0.8, 10.2, 0.3 and 3.3 μM, respectively. *In vivo* SRI 63-441 effectively inhibits many of the PAF responses in the guinea pig, rat, dog and primate (reviewed by Handley [56]). However, the antagonist does not block the acute IgE-mediated airways response to *Ascaris suum* [57] and has no effect on the allergic reaction in awake dogs with natural asthma [58]. It also fails to prolong renal xenograft survival and function in a model of pig-to-dog heterotransplantation [59].

SRI 63-675 (compound **9b**), the *cis*-2,5-dimethyl analogue of SRI 63-441, shows a similar profile of activity against PAF-induced effects both *in vitro* and *in vivo* [21]. For example, at doses of 0.1 mg/kg i.v. SRI 63-675 prevents PAF-induced airway microvascular leakage of colloidal carbon tracer in guinea pigs [60]. We have also recently developed a series of tetrahydrofuran-containing antagonists as exemplified by BN 55006 (compound **10**) and thc pharmacological activity is currently being investigated.

BN 52111 (compound **11**) and related analogues which contain a 1,3-dioxolane ring are another series of PAF inhibitors developed by Institut Henri Beaufour (Braquet, P. & Broquet, C., unpublished). BN 52111 inhibits [^{3}H]PAF binding to rabbit platelets and PAF-induced platelet aggregation, with IC_{50} values of 35 nM and 0.4 μM, respectively. The antagonist also blocks PAF-induced aggregation of rat neutrophils *in vitro* ($IC_{50} = 0.5$ μM), the PAF-induced calcium mobilization in washed rabbit platelets and enhanced benzodiazepine binding in the rat cortex. When administered i.v., BN 52111 and analogues prevent PAF-induced thrombus formation in the rat mesenteric artery and counteract PAF-induced bronchoconstriction and hypotension in the guinea pig (Braquet, P. & Broquet, C., unpublished). However, the antagonists in this interesting series are inactive when administered orally and also show a high degree of toxicity, and thus are not likely to constitute future pharmacological agents. Interestingly, moderate PAF antagonism has also been reported for a series of 1,4-dioxanes of which compound **12** is representative [17].

Developed by Sankyo, the tetrahydropyran-based constrained-framework antagonist (compound **13a**) inhibits hypotension induced by PAF ($ED_{50} = 0.8$ mg/kg i.v.) or endotoxin ($ED_{50} = 0.058$ mg/kg i.v.) in the rat [61]. The related oxethane derivative (compound **13b**) also displays similar PAF antagonistic activity.

The novel piperidine derivative SRI 63-073 (compound **14**) was designed by including a polar head of thiamine phosphate in the modified PAF framework [62]. This compound has a relatively low potency, inhibiting PAF-induced aggregation of human and guinea-pig platelets with IC_{50} values of 37 and 15 μM, respectively. Although five-membered cyclic phosphorodiamidic derivatives of this compound are devoid of any PAF-antagonistic activity, six-membered cyclic phosphates, especially the equatorial isomer (compound **15**) has an IC_{50} of 2.1 μM of 2.1 μM against PAF-induced aggregation of rabbit platelets [63].

Finally, with respect to the family of constrained antagonists, the Sandoz piperidine derivative SRI 62-586 (compound **16**) shows moderate inhibition of PAF-induced human platelet aggregation ($IC_{50} = 32.6$ μM) and [^{3}H]PAF receptor binding ($IC_{50} = 22.7$ μM) [18]. Administered to guinea pigs at 2.45 mg/kg i.v. it inhibits PAF-induced haemoconcentration by 70% and increase of pulmonary inflation pressure by 85% [18].

Synthetic antagonists unrelated to the PAF framework

There are relatively few PAF inhibitors which are not structurally related to the mediator itself or to the various naturally-occurring antagonistic compounds. However, although small, this significant group contains antagonists including 48740 RP, which derives from a (3-pyridyl)-1H,3H-pyrrolo[1,2*c*]thiazole framework, the calcium channel blocker, diltiazem, and various triazolobenzodiazepine-derived pharmacological agents such as WEB 2086, which exhibits highly potent PAF antagonistic properties.

48740 RP (compound **17a**) inhibits PAF-induced human ($IC_{50} =$ 69 μM) and rabbit ($IC_{50} = 16$ μM) platelet aggregation, [^{3}H]PAF binding to rabbit platelets ($K_i = 2.3$ μM [64] and PAF-elicited elastase release by human neutrophils [65]. At 10 mg/kg i.v. the antagonist suppresses PAF-induced bronchoconstriction in the guinea pig [64] and thrombocytopenia in the rabbit [22]. A 7 day clinical study of four human volunteers administered 48740 RP at 1000 mg/day orally gave >60% inhibition of PAF-induced platelet aggregation and a slight inhibition of TXB_2 production in *ex vivo* studies [66]. Recently a more potent analogue has been reported: 52770 RP (compound **17b**) inhibits [^{3}H]PAF binding in human leukocytes with a K_i of 7 nM[67]. The (+)-52770 RP isomer is *ca.* 300 times more potent than the (−)-isomer at displacing [^{3}H]52770 RP from intact rabbit platelets[68].

Diltiazem (compound **18**), a drug used clinically as a Ca^{2+} antagonist, shows selective and competitive inhibition of PAF-induced aggregation of human (IC_{50} = 28 μM) and rabbit (IC_{50} = 13 μM) platelets and inhibits [^{3}H]PAF binding to human platelets (IC_{50} = 47 μM) [69]. The PAF antagonistic properties of diltiazem and other Ca^{2+}-channel blockers suggest that the PAF receptor and membrane Ca^{2+} channels may be linked in some way in the platelet.

The triazolobenzodiazepines alprazolam (compound **19a**) and triazolam (compound **19b**) are widely used psychotropic drugs. These compounds are also specific inhibitors of PAF-induced human platelet aggregation with respective IC_{50} values of *ca.* 5 and 3 μM [23], rabbit platelet aggregation with IC_{50} values of 2.5 and 0.6 μM [70], and [^{3}H]PAF receptor binding on human platelets (IC_{50} = *ca.* 5 μM and 1 μM [23]. The inhibitory activity of triazolam against PAF-induced platelet aggregation is not blocked by the benzodiazepine receptor antagonist Ro 15-1788 indicating that the PAF and CNS properties can be separated [71]. Pretreatment with triazolam (20–100 mg/kg p.o.) inhibited the intra-thoracic accumulation and aggregation of [^{111}In]-labelled platelets in the guinea pig after a PAF challenge [72]. However triazolam, at doses which cause sedation, has no effect on PAF-induced skin responses in normal volunteers (Roberts, N. & Barnes, P., unpublished).

Brotizolam (compound **20a**) is a *s*-triazolo[3,4*c*]thieno[2,3*e*]-[1,4] diazepine which is clinically useful as a hypnotic agent. It inhibits PAF-induced human platelet (IC_{50} = 0.54 μM) and neutrophil (IC_{50} = 0.21 μM) aggregation [72], and [^{3}H]PAF receptor binding (IC_{50} = 0.5 μM) [71]. Administered at 0.05–1.0 mg/kg i.v. or 1.0–10.0 mg/kg p.o., brotizolam dose-dependently inhibits PAF-induced bronchoconstriction in the guinea pig, hypotension in the rat, and intra-thoracic accumulation of [^{111}In]-labelled platelets in the guinea-pig. Interestingly, the PAF-inhibiting activity of brotizolam is not blocked when co-administered with the benzodiazepine receptor antagonist Ro 15-1788 [71]. Etizolam (compound **20b**, another clinically-useful drug administered for relief of anxiety, inhibits PAF-induced rabbit platelet aggregation (IC_{50} = 1.3 μg/ml) and at doses of 0.01–1 mg/kg i.v. or 1–10 mg/kg p.o. prevents PAF-induced bronchoconstriction in the guinea pig, hypotension in the rat, and lethal shock in the mouse [73].

A separation of the CNS and PAF antagonistic properties in the triazolothienodiazepine series has been achieved with the synthesis of the hetrazopine compounds WEB 2086 (compound **21**). This compound selectively inhibits PAF-induced human platelet ($IC_{50} = 0.17$ μM) and neutrophil aggregation ($IC_{50} = 0.36$ μM) and [^{3}H]PAF receptor binding ($K_D = 0.15$ μM) [24]. WEB 2086 inhibits PAF-induced bronchoconstriction ($IC_{50} = 0.07$ mg/kg p.o. and 0.017 mg/kg i.v.), hypotension ($IC_{50} = 0.66$ mg/kg p.o. and 0.015 mg/kg i.v.), thrombocytopenia and neutropenia in the guinea pig [24,74] and hypotension ($ED_{50} =$ 0.052 mg/kg i.v.) in the rat. It also protects against PAF-induced gastric lesions in the rat, mortality in the mouse and intra-thoracic accumulation of [^{111}In]-labelled platelets in the guinea pig. In addition, the antagonist protects against *E. coli*-derived endotoxin-induced hypotension in the rat [75], decreases bronchoconstriction and leukopenia induced by antigen in mepyramine-treated passively-sensitized guinea pigs, and decreases the ovalbumin-induced anaphylactic effects in the mouse and guinea pig. [^{3}H]WEB 2086 shows a high affinity of binding to PAF receptors in human platelets, neutrophils and eosinophils [76,77]. In rat isolated lungs, WEB 2086 dose-dependently inhibits the increase in PAF-induced pulmonary artery perfusion and bronchial inflation pressure [78].

Restricting the rotation of the alkylene side chain in WEB 2086 by forming a cyclopentane ring between the α-carbon and C7 produces WEB 2170 (compound **22a**) and the CH_2 analogue STY 2108 (compound **22b**. Both WEB 2170 and STY 2108 inhibit PAF-induced human platelet aggregation ($IC_{50} = 0.30$ and 0.04 μM, respectively) with no significant effect on that induced by ADP, adrenaline, collagen, 5-HT or arachidonic acid. *In vivo*, WEB 2170 ($ED_{50} = 0.008$ mg/kg i.v., 0.16 mg/kg p.o.) and STY 2108 ($ED_{50} = 0.007$ mg/kg i.v., 0.033 mg/kg p.o.) inhibit PAF-induced bronchoconstriction in the guinea pig and hypotension ($ED_{50} =$ 0.011 mg/kg i.v. and 0.013 mg/kg i.v., respectively) in the rat. Hypotension induced by endotoxin derived from *E. coli* in the rat was also blocked in a dose-dependent manner by both compounds [78].

Recently, Tilley *et al.* (79) have synthesized a series of *N*-[(hetero-aryl)alkyl]pyrido[2,1*b*]quinazolines and evalulated them for PAF antagonism. The most potent compounds in this series were found to be pyrido-[2,1*b*]quinazoline-8-carboxamides possessing a 4 or 6 carbon chain between the carboxamide *N* and a 3-pyridinyl or 5-pyrimidinyl moiety [79]. The most potent antagonists were found to be the racemic compound 2-(1-methyl-ethyl)-*N*-[1-methyl-4-(3-pyridinyl)butyl]-11-oxo-11H-pyrido-[2,1*b*]-quinazoline-8-carboxamide (compound **23**) and the corresponding (*R*)-enantiomer. These compounds inhibited the binding of [^{3}H]PAF to its receptor on dog platelets with IC_{50} values of 0.4 and 0.25 μM

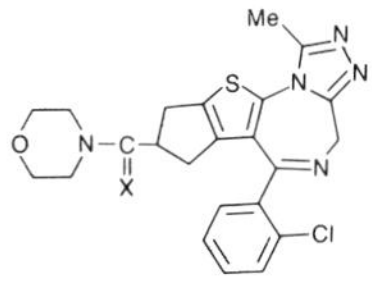

(**22a**) WEB 2170 X = O
(**22b**) STY 2108 X = H_2

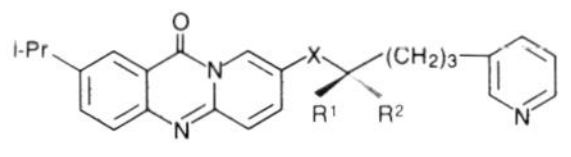

X = CONH R^1 = Me R^2 = H

(**23**)

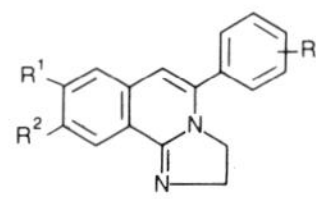

R = H, Cl, alkyl, alkoxy, alkylthio
R^1 = R^2 = H, Cl, F, alkyl (C_1-C_3)

(**24**)

Compound n°	Ginkgolide	IHB nomenclature	R^1	R^2	R^3
a	A	BN 52020	OH	H	H
b	B	BN 52021	OH	OH	H
c	C	BN 52022	OH	OH	OH
d	J	BN 52024	OH	H	OH
e	M	BN 52023	H	OH	OH
f	Synthetic	BN 50580	OH	OMe	H
g	Synthetic	BN 50585	OH	OEt	H

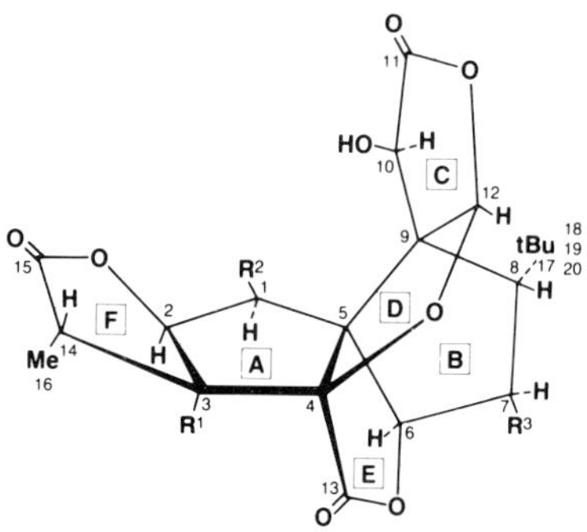

(**25**) Ginkgolides A, B, C, J, M, and the 1-methoxy and 1-ethoxy derivates of ginkgolide B

Fig. 4.5 PAF antagonists (compounds **22**–**25**).

respectively. Compound **23** also inhibited transient PAF-induced thrombocytopenia and decreased blood pressure in guinea pigs after i.v. or p.o. administration and has a duration of action of >5 h after a p.o. dose of 200 mg/kg. Thus, these compounds represent prototypes of a new class of orally-active PAF antagonists.

Finally, with regard to synthetic structurally-unrelated PAF antagonists, Houlihan *et al.* [80] have reported that a series of 5-aryl-2,3-dihydroimidazo[2,1*a*]isoquinolines, as represented by structure **24**, display PAF-antagonistic properties. However, the effectiveness of these compounds in inhibiting the binding of [^{3}H]PAF to its various receptors remains to be reported.

Naturally-occuring PAF antagonists and their derivatives

The second class of PAF antagonists comprises natural products and their synthetic derivatives. Indeed, it appears that 'PAF antagonists' may have been amongst the first indigenous natural drugs utilized by man. The Chinese in particular, have always placed great importance on herbal medicines and still use a considerable number of plants for their medicinal properties. One of the oldest of these natural therapeutic agents is a leaf-extract of the 'fossil tree', *Ginkgo biloba.* This tree has apparently always been part of the traditional Chinese pharmacopoeia, being referred to in the medicinal book *Chen Noung Pen T'sao,* published in 2800 BC. In the modern Chinese pharmacopoeia, Ginkgo is still recommended as 'beneficial for the heart and lungs' and inhalation of a decoction of the leaves is used to alleviate asthma. Another plant of therapeutic value is *Piper futokadsurae,* which is widely used in southern China for its anti-rheumatic and anti-allergic properties.

These plants are of particular importance to the present review; *Ginkgo biloba* leaves provide the only natural source of the unique C_{20} cage molecules, the ginkgolides, while kadsurenone and other lignans with interesting pharmacological properties have been isolated from *Piper futokadsurae.* These two groups of chemicals, together with some gliotoxin-related compounds produced by various fungi and bacteria, constitute the three groups of naturally-occurring PAF antagonists. Indeed, the traditional medicinal properties of the plant extracts can be largely explained by modern pharmacology in terms of their inhibition of PAF-induced effects.

Ginkgolides

Ginkgolides (compounds **25a–g**) are unique C_{20} cage molecules, incorporating a *t*-butyl group and six 5-membered rings A to F including a spiro[4.4]nonane, a tetrahydrofuran cycle and three lactone rings. The *cis*-fused cyclopentanoid rings F, A, D and C are folded in such a way that a semi-spherical cavity of significant size is formed (*c.* 4 Å wide × 5 Å deep). In relative molecular terms the cavity is sufficiently large to receive most atoms (e.g. Fe^{2+}, Ca^{2+}) or organic moieties (e.g. the trimethylammonium group). The two parallel sides of the cavity are defined by the C_{11} and C_{15} lactone carbonyls included in the F and C rings, respectively. The head or the cap of the cavity is defined by rings A and D. The tetrahydrofuran ring (D) occupies a central position in the cage; its etheral oxygen, along with F and C ring ester oxygens and the C_{10} hydroxyl oxygen consitute a polydentate system similar to that observed in the 'crown' ether series. This electron-rich cavity is ideally suited to the charged binding of cationic or positively polarized molecules. It is important to note that the *t*-butyl group is very prominent outside the main framework. Due to the shape of the cavity, if binding does occur, it may well be stereospecific.

These compounds were first isolated in 1932 by Furukawa [81] from the bitter principles of *Ginkgo biloba* but their structures have only been resolved recently. In 1967, Nakanishi's group reported their structures and called them 'ginkgolides A, B, C and M' (compounds **25a**, **b**, **c**, **e**) [82]. These are termed BN 52020, BN 52021, BN 52022 and BN 52023 respectively in Institut Henri Beaufour (IHB) nomenclature. A new ginkgolide, J (BN 52024; compound **25d**) has been recently identified [83]. All these compounds differ only by the number and the position of hydroxyl groups which may be present on C_1, C_3 or C_7 of the spirononane framework.

The ginkgolide structures initially deduced by chemical methods, have been confirmed by NMR and X-ray crystallography [84]. Recently, Roumestand *et al.* [85] have employed very high-field proton and [^{13}C] NMR experiments to determine an unequivocal structural assignment. These high-field studies confirmed the structures already reported, but showed that the stereochemistry of the H/R2 arrangement at the 1 position of the A ring is the reverse of that previously described. This feature may be important as OH–OH interactions of the C_1 and C_{10} positions may influence conformational changes during binding. The structures of compounds **25a–e** presented diagrammatically are those unequivocally determined by high-field [^{13}C]-NMR.

Ginkgolide structure–activity relationships

Ginkgolides inhibit the binding of [^{3}H]PAF to its membrane platelet receptor [86, 87]. This inhibition is competitive, ginkgolides displacing [^{3}H]PAF in an excess of cold PAF. The IC_{50} values obtained are 0.25 μM, 0.74 μM, 7.1 μM and 54.0 μM for BN 52021, BN 52020, BN 52022 and BN 52024, respectively [86]. Characterized by the presence of two hydroxyl groups on C_1 and C_3, ginkgolide B is the most powerful antagonist. Conversely, BN 52022 and BN 52024 which have a hydroxyl group on C_7, in the α-position of the lipophilic *t*-butyl moiety, are less active. As for BN 52024, the loss of the hydroxyl group on C_1 further decreases the activity in comparison with BN 52022. The 1-methoxy (BN 50580; compound **25f**) and 1-ethoxy (BN 50585; compound **25g**) derivatives of BN 52021 have also been prepared and show similar activity to the natural product (Braquet, P., unpublished).

A substantial loss of antagonism is also apparent after opening of the ginkgolide lactone rings. Relative to the natural product, the inhibitory activity of BN 52021 (10 μM) with opened lactone rings on PAF-induced rabbit platelet aggregation is decreased by 64% and the IC_{50} is shifted to 0.2–0.8 mM (Domingo, M. T., personal communication).

It is interesting to note that the ginkgolide structure bears a close resemblance to that of bilobalide, another sesquiterpene found in *Ginkgo biloba* which contains three γ-lactone rings and a *t*-butyl group but which is devoid of the spiro[4.4]nonane nucleus and tetrahydrofuran cycle [88]. Interestingly, bilobalide does not inhibit PAF-induced platelet aggregation suggesting the importance of the two latter moieties for activity (Braquet, P., unpublished).

The fact that BN 52021 displaces the [^{3}H]PAF from its receptor-like unlabelled PAF in both human [25] and rabbit [86] platelets further demonstrates its high specificity as an antagonist. The potent binding capacity of BN 52021 to PAF receptors is also evidenced by the fact that platelets pretreated with the antagonist and then washed, do not respond to further stimulation by PAF [25, 86].

These binding data are further corroborated by the results on the inhibition of PAF-induced aggregation of washed human [25] and rabbit [86] platelets. BN 52021 is the most efficient compound with an IC_{50} of 1.8 μM and 0.18 μM for human and rabbit platelets, respectively. BN 52022 is the least effective with IC_{50} values of 21.1 μM and 1.53 μM, respectively, for inhibition of aggregation of the above cell types. The antagonism induced by ginkgolides is specific for PAF; they do not inhibit other pro-aggregating agents such as ADP, collagen, arachidonic acid, thrombin or A23187.

Pharmacological properties

BN 52021 and related ginkgolides are the most advanced PAF antagonists in terms of clinical investigation. A complete description of their pharmacology is beyond the scope of the present review and thus their effects on airway hyper-reactivity, shock and cellular immunity are considered. For a more extensive review of the effects of BN 52021 as diverse as cardiac anaphylaxis, kidney physiology, ocular diseases, the central nervous system and cerebral ischaemia, the interested reader is referred to a review by Braquet [89].

The importance of PAF in airway hypersensitivity has been confirmed by the protective effect exerted by BN 52021 and related ginkgolides, mainly BN 52020 [90] in: (i) PAF-induced bronchoconstriction and airway hyper-reactivity in both humans and animals; (ii) various models of immune anaphylaxis and airway hyper-reactivity in animals; and (iii) antigen-induced bronchial provocation tests in asthmatic patients.

BN 52021 given i.v. (0.5–2 mg/kg) or p.o. (5–15 mg/kg) dose-dependently antagonizes both the cardiovascular impairments and the bronchoconstriction induced by PAF [91]. For example, BN 52021 administered at a dose of 2 mg/kg i.v. almost completely prevents the lowering of blood pressure, alterations in heart rate and the bronchoconstrictive effect of

PAF. Furthermore, BN 52021 significantly inhibits the PAF-induced airway vascular permeability [92,93] and hypertension and oedema in isolated perfused lungs [94]. The effect of BN 52021 results from its high binding capacity to the PAF lung receptor. Interestingly, synthetic products which are better inhibitors of the binding of [^{3}H]PAF to platelets such as L-652731, L-653150, SRI 63-441 and Ro 19-3704 have a lower affinity for pulmonary PAF receptors, suggesting the existence of a receptor sub-type in the lungs different to that detected in platelets. This may explain why BN 52021 is more effective in immune lung anaphylaxis in comparison with other antagonists [95].

BN 52021 also antagonizes PAF-induced airway hyper-responsiveness in guinea pigs [96], its effect again being greater than those of other PAF antagonists like L-653731, kadsurenone, 48740 RP (Touvay, C., unpublished). BN 52021 also dose-dependently prevents thrombocytopenia, leukopenia and the increase in circulating thromboxane induced by PAF [97]. The antagonistic activity of BN 52021 seems to be long-lasting since bronchoconstriction is still markedly inhibited after 40 min [98]. In these studies, the order of antagonist activity observed is: BN 52021 > BN 52020 > BN 52022 > BN 52024.

Ginkgolides also inhibit antigen-induced pulmonary dysfunction. BN 52021 given i.v. (0.1–2 mg/kg) or p.o. (10–15 mg/kg) significantly antagonizes both homologous [99,100] and heterologous [89] passive anaphylaxis in guinea pigs. This antagonist (2–4 mg/kg i.v.) also prevents mortality and counteracts the sustained bronchoconstriction observed in actively-sensitized guinea pigs [89].

Interestingly, in passive anaphylaxis, BN 52021 moderately antagonizes the antigen-induced thrombocytopenia but the accompanying leukopenia is unaffected [91,100]. BN 52021 also antagonizes immune bronchoconstriction when antigen is given by aerosol in passively-sensitized guinea pigs [45].

In addition to antigen-induced airway responses, ginkgolides also protect against endotoxin and IgG-induced shock. In endotoxic shock, BN 52021 provides significant protection both preventively and curatively. In rats treated preventively (5–15 mg/kg s.c.; 10–30 mg/kg p.o.) 30 min before injection of *Salmonella enteritidis* endotoxin (16 mg/kg p.o.), a significant dose-dependent inhibition of the lethality is observed, complete protection being provided by the highest dose of the antagonists [101,102]. The other ginkgolides, BN 52020 and BN 52022 do not afford any protection at 20 mg/kg (p.o., 30 min before endotoxin). However, they do act synergistically with BN 52021 (Etienne, A., unpublished), an effect also observed with a combination of BN 52021 and indomethacin. In guinea pigs injected with *Salmonella typhimurium* endotoxin, protection by BN 52021 is also observed [103,104], this being accompanied by a partial inhibition of the associated thrombocytopenia and leukopenia. In platelet-depleted animals, BN 52021 affords total protection against the drop in arterial pressure, suggesting that platelets contribute to hypotension by the release of an unknown factor, not inhibited by gingkolide B [103,104].

In the late phase of shock, BN 52021 (6 mg/kg i.v.) restores arterial pressure, which returns to basal levels immediately after injection of the antagonists [103,104]. A similar effect is observed if BN 52021 is administered after injection of PAF or aggregates of human IgG [105]. In the dog kidney, BN 52021 significantly restores the functional alterations induced by a local injection of endotoxin in the renal artery *in vivo* (Etienne, A., unpublished), while in the guinea pig, the antagonist dose-dependently inhibits platelet accumulation after endotoxin aerosol [106]. BN 52021 (5 mg/kg i.v., 5 min before challenge) also inhibits the haemodynamic changes induced by i.v. injection of 40 mg/kg of human IgG aggregates in rats [105]. This protection is accompanied by significant inhibition of plasma extravasation and mortality.

Recent studies with BN 52021 have demonstrated that PAF can modulate various immune processes. BN 52021 can inhibit the suppressive effects of PAF on T-lymphocyte proliferation and cytokine production. When PAF is added to human peripheral blood lymphocyte cultures (containing 5–10% monocytes) stimulated with phytohaemagglutinin (PHA) or concanavalin A (Con A), a non-toxic concentration-dependent inhibition of lymphocyte proliferation is observed [107]. This effect is prevented by BN 52021. The antagonist also reverses the PAF-induced suppression of IL-2 production by human lymphocytes [107]. PAF inhibition of lymphocyte proliferation and IL-2 production appears to be due to the activation of T-suppressor cells [108]. Indeed, BN 52021 itself generates some suppressor cell activity, although to a lesser extent than the mediator [108]. BN 52021 also counteracts the effects of PAF on IL-1 production by lipopolysaccharide (LPS)-stimulated human monocytes, inhibiting both its enhancing effect on IL-1 production at low concentrations (1.0 pM to 0.1 nM) and its suppressive action at high concentrations (0.1 nM to 1.0 μM) [109].

Cell-mediated graft rejection is another area in which BN 52021 has been studied. Foegh *et al.* [110] demonstrated that the antagonist increases cardiac allograft survival in rats, acting synergistically with azathioprine and cyclosporin A (CSA). Pirotzky *et al.* [111] have also shown that BN 52021 prevents CSA-induced nephrotoxicity without altering the immunosuppressive effect of the drug. In addition, Pignol *et al.* [112] noted that concomitant treatment with CSA and the ginkgolide mixture BN 52063 produced greater immunosuppression than that induced by CSA alone. Both of these results suggest that PAF may be generated in response to CSA treatment. Although the precise mechanism of ginkgolide protection in graft rejection remains to be defined, it is apparent that these compounds may offer considerable therapeutic potential for treatment of this condition.

Studies with BN 52021 are also leading to an improved understanding of the role of PAF in the generation of cytotoxic lymphocytes. The ginkgolide potentiates allo-antigen recognition in primary and secondary mixed-lymphocyte cultures and enhances the generation of cytotoxic lymphocytes *in vitro* [113], its presence throughout the duration of the culture period having the greatest enhancing effect on cell proliferation. Similar effects are observed in mixed cultures employed to generate cytotoxic T-lymphocytes. Again, the presence of BN 52021 throughout the entire culture period produces an enhanced level of cell-mediated cytotoxicity. This potentiating effect of BN 52021 on allo-antigen recognition is not due to an enhanced production of IL-2 in the antagonist-treated cultures [113]. Recently, Farkas *et al.* [114], have examined the effect of BN 52021, on *in vitro* rat splenic lymphocyte-induced cytotoxicity of Langerhans islets. When these latter cells are pretreated with BN 52021, almost total inhibition of cellular destruction relative to the control is observed, representing a direct effect of BN 52021 on the target cells. When splenic lymphocytes are pretreated with BN 52021, the inhibition of islet destruction is significant with respect to the control cytotoxicity, but slightly lower than that in the above circumstances. As cytotoxic and/or suppressor T-lymphoblasts have been shown to accumulate around Langerhans islets and thus may participate in development of diabetes, the results of Farkas *et al.* [114] provide further support for the use of PAF antagonists in the prevention of the autoimmune form of this disease.

Lignans

Natural lignans and neolignans are a chemical family formed by the oxidative dimerization of various C_6C_3 phenols. These compounds have attracted interest over the years because of their widespread occurrence in nature and broad range of biological effects. Several lignans and neolignans are known to exhibit anti-tumour activity [115] and inhibit fungal growth.

Benzofuranoid lignans

A neolignan isolated from the plant *Piper futokadsurae* was the first natural product discovered as a potent inhibitor of the binding of [^{3}H]PAF to rabbit platelet membrane preparation with an IC_{50} close to 0.1 μM [116]. Named kadsurenone (compound **26**) it was also shown to be a specific and potent inhibitor of PAF-induced rabbit platelet aggregation with an IC_{50} of 0.99 μM.

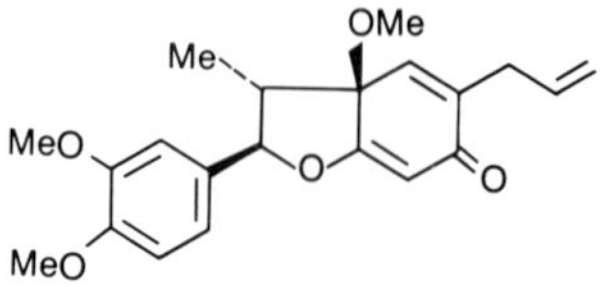

(**26**) Kadsurenone (mirandin series)

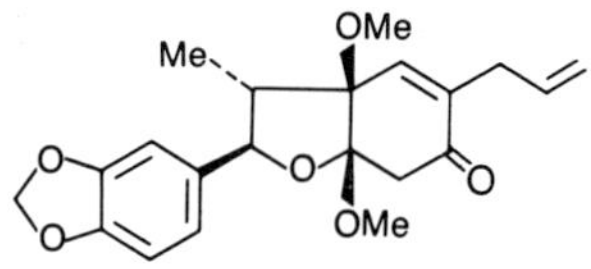

(**27**) Kadsurin A

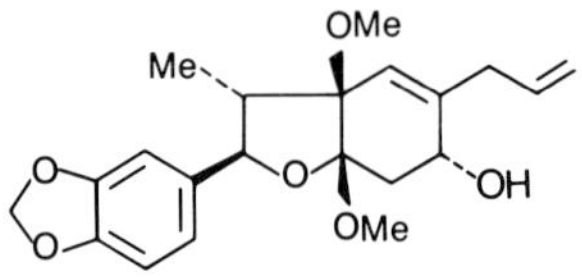

(**28**) Kadsurin B

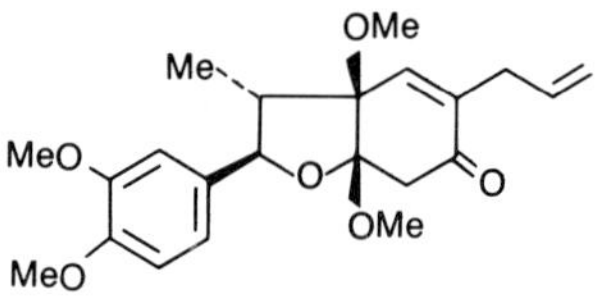

(**29**) Piperenone

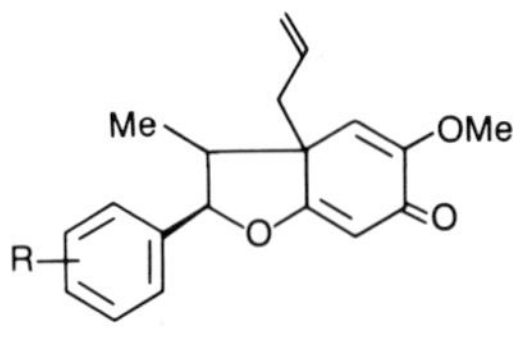

(**30**) Burchellin series

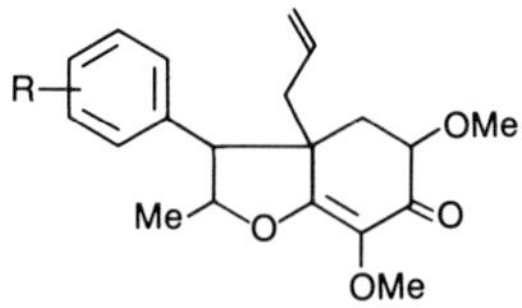

(**31**) Chrysophyllin series

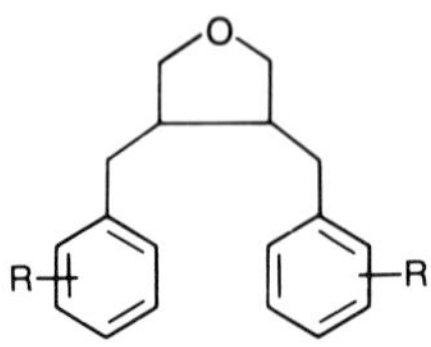

(**32**)

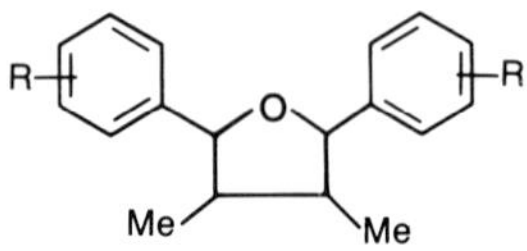

(**33**)

Fig. 4.6 PAF antagonists (compounds **26**–**33**).

This result reflects the potent effect of kadsurenone in inhibiting the binding of [^{3}H]PAF to both its platelet and lung-receptors [117]. The weak activity of several related compounds isolated from the same plant (e.g. kadsurin A, kadsurin B, and piperenone; compounds **27**, **28** and **29**, respectively) and several synthetic analogues with altered stereochemistry or ring substituents, demonstrate the chemical specificity of kadsurenone. Only the dihydro derivative, obtained by hydrogenation of the allyl side chain, retains full activity [118]. The inversion of the configuration at either the 2- or 3a-position results in a significant decrease of activity. Furthermore, the 6-oxo group appears fundamental for antagonism since the related methoxyamino or alcohol analogue are only weak inhibitors.

Interestingly, desallylkadsurenone is relatively inactive, indicating the contribution of a lipophilic allyl or propyl side chain at the 5-position. Kadsurenone inhibits PAF-induced aggregation and degranulation of human neutrophils [116]. In a Langendorff preparation of isolated guinea pig heart perfused at constant pressure, kadsurenone (1 μM) effectively antagonizes the PAF-induced decrease in contractility and coronary flow [119]. The neolignan is also active in antagonizing various PAF-induced phenomena such as increases in cutaneous permeability in the guinea pig [120] and elevated hematocrit and circulating *N*-acetylglucosaminidase levels in the rat. Kadsurenone also partially antagonizes endotoxic shock in this species [121]. However, the compound has a relatively short duration of action, with half-life from 30 min to 2 h in animals. In a study on rhesus monkeys, metabolism has been observed by alkyl side-chain oxidation and glucoronide formation [122].

Substituted furanoid lignans

Several structures in this ligan series are also potent PAF-antagonists such as some tetrahydrofuran compounds belonging to types A (compound **32**) and C (compound **33**) lignans in Haworth's classification. Isolated from *Bursera microphylla* A (Burseraceae), burseran (compound **34**) is a moderate specific inhibitor of PAF-induced rabbit platelet aggregation. Similar results are obtained with 2,3,4,5-tetra-substituted furanoid lignans such as some furoguaiacidin derivatives isolated from *Guaiacum officinale* L. or *Guaiacum sanctum* L. (Zygophyllaceae) or nectandrin A (BN 52010) and nectandrin B (BN 52011) isolated from the Brazilian *Nectandra rigida*. Magnosalicin (BN 52004), a 2,3,4-trisubstituted furanoid lignan isolated from *Magnolia salicifolia* and used for treating nasal allergy in China, also has specific PAF antagonizing properties.

A series of dinor type C tetrahydrofuran lignans has been synthesized (see structure **35** and related compounds). *Trans*-2,5-bis(3,4,5-trimethoxyphenyl)tetrahydrofuran (L-652731; compound **35a**) is orally active and several times more potent tha kadsurenone *in vitro* and *in vivo* [123]. With an IC_{50} of 19 nM, it inhibits [^{3}H]PAF binding and is a very potent inhibitor of PAF-induced rabbit and human platelet aggregation. The *trans*-isomers are generally 10-fold more potent than the corresponding *cis*-isomers in this series. The IC_{50} for inhibition of [^{3}H]PAF to its platelet receptor is increased by three orders of magnitude with the *cis* analog of L-652731 (22 μM).

Aromatic ring substitutions are also relatively specific, with a decrease in methoxy substitution generally leading to reduced activity [123] (e.g. compounds **35b** and **35c**). With a different methoxy substitution of the phenyl rings (e.g., positions 2,3,4), the bistrimethoxyphenyl isomer of L-652731 (compound **35g**) is three orders of magnitude less efficient than the

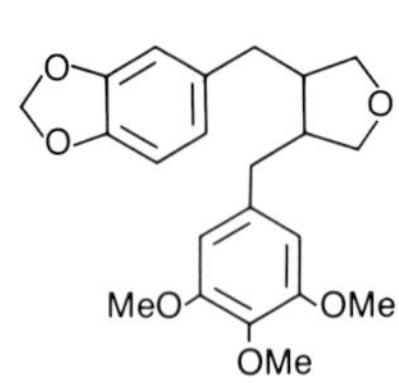

(**34**) Burseran

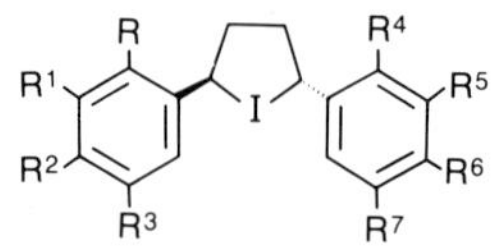

Compound	I	R	R¹	R²	R³	R⁴	R⁵	R⁶	R⁷	ED_{50}*
a	O	H	OMe	OMe	OMe	H	OMe	OH	OMe	2×10^{-8} M
b	O	H	H	OMe	OMe	H	H	OEt	OMe	2×10^{-7} M
c	O	H	OMe	OMe	OMe	H	OMe	H	OMe	8×10^{-7} M
d	O	H	OMe	OEt	OMe	H	OMe	H	OMe	4×10^{-7} M
e	O	H	OMe	Oi-Pr	OMe	H	OMe	Oi-Pr	OMe	3×10^{-5} M
f	O	H	OMe	OMe	OMe	OMe	H	OMe	OMe	$< 30 \mu$M
g	O	OMe	OMe	OMe	H	OMe	OMe	OMe	H	1×10^{-3} M
h	O	H	OMe	OMe	OMe	H	SO_2Me	OPr	OMe	3×10^{-9} M
i	S	H	OMe	OMe	OMe	H	OMe	OH	OMe	2×10^{-8} M
j	CH_2	H	OMe	OMe	OMe	H	OMe	OH	OMe	2×10^{-8} M

* ED_{50} values for inhibition of [3] PAF binding to rabbit platelet membranes

(**35**) and related compounds

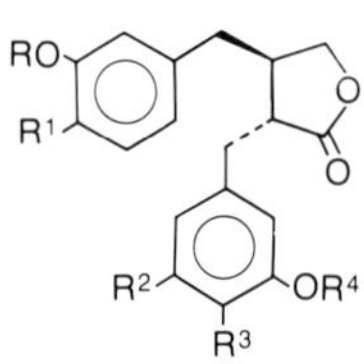

Enterolactone and other mammalian lignans

R	R¹	R²	R³	R⁴	PRODUCT	ORIGIN
H	H	H	H	H	Enterolactone	Mammalian urines
Me	H	H	H	H	3-O-methylenterolactone	Mammalian urines
Me	H	H	H	Me	Di-O-methylenterolactone	Mammalian urines
Me	OMe	H	OMe	H	Prestegane A	Mammalian urines and *Steganotaenia araliacea*
H	OMe	H	OMe	H	Prestegane B	
Me	OMe	H	OMe	Me	Di-O-methylmatairesinol	
Me	OMe	OMe	OMe	Me	5'-methoxymatairesinol	Synthetic

(**36**) and related compounds

Fig. 4.7 PAF antagonists (compounds **34**–**36**).

corresponding bis-3,4,5-trimethoxyphenyl analogue. Similarly, the substitution of methoxy groups by isopropyloxy moieties significantly reduces activity (compound **35e**).

The most potent member of this series synthesized to date is *trans*-2-(3-methoxy-5-methylsulfonyl-4-propoxyphenyl)-5-(3,4,5-trimethoxyphenyl)tetrahydrofuran (L-659989; compound **35h**). This inhibits [^{3}H] binding to rabbit platelet membranes with an ED_{50} of 3 nM and prevents PAF-induced extravasation and lysosomal enzyme release in rats when the antagonist is infused i.v. 1 min before PAF administration [124]. L-659989 is also orally active in female (ED_{50} = 0.2 mg/kg), but not male rats, with an oral duration of action of 12–16 h when given p.o. at a dose of 1 mg/kg. The origin of this gender difference is presently unknown.

Recently, the thioisoster of compound **20a**, *trans*-2,5-bis(3,4,5-trimethoxyphenyl)tetrahydrothiophene, was synthesized [125]. Denoted L-653150 (compound **35i**), it was found to inhibit the binding of 1 nM [^{3}H]PAF to isolated rabbit platelet membranes with an IC_{50} of 19 nM. In addition, it inhibited the rat basophilic leukaemia cell 5-lipoxygenase catalysed transformation of [^{14}C]-arachidonic acid to 5-HETE with an IC_{50} of 5 μM [125]. The superior efficacy and longer duration of action of L-653150 as compared to L-652731, was demonstrated in a variety of *in vitro* (PAF-induced human neutrophil degranulation and aggregation of rabbit platelets, human PMNL and guinea pig PMNL) and *in vivo* (PAF-induced enzyme release, vascular permeability and hypotension) assays. In addition to the thioisoster of **35a**, Chaing *et al.* [126] have reported that the cyclopentane isoster (compound **35j**) and derivatives are also specific PAF antagonists. The substitution of H borne by $-CH_2$ in position 1 with various groups posessing a heteroatom (N or O) can reinforce the inhibitory activity providing the steric hinderance is relatively small and lipophilic. In contrast to this data, we have recently observed that other lignan series such as tetralines, dibenzo[4,5,6,7]cyclooctadienes, (stegane-derived compounds), and furo[3,4*c*]furanoids do not have any significant effect on PAF-induced rabbit-platelet aggregation (Braquet, P., unpublished).

Diabenzylbutyrolactone (butanolide)-derived lignans

Most lignans originate from higher plants; recently however, these compounds have also been identified in human and animal urines [127,128]. These lignans (see structure **36** and related compounds) are characterized by the presence of a dibenzyl-γ-butyrolactone framework and one *m*-OH group in each aryl ring [129]. The main lignan identified in mammalian urine is enterolactone [127,128]. Methyl derivatives have also been detected in minor quantities [128]. These lignans are weak inhibitors of PAF-induced rabbit platelet aggregation with an IC_{50} of 1 μM to 0.1 mM [130].

The biological role of mammalian lignans has never been clearly evaluated, however, their renal excretion increases during the luteal phase of the menstrual cycle and pregnancy in the vervet monkey [127,128]. In contrast, decreased levels are observed in post-menopausal women and during breast cancer [131]. As the level of mammalian lignans is high during early pregnancy [127,128], it has been postulated that these compounds may produce a negative feedback against PAF and plasminogen released during pregnancy [132]. However, at present, their physiological role and possible relationship with PAF is still unknown.

Gliotoxin-related products

Gliotoxin (compound **37**) and other epipolythiodioxopiperazines (ETPS) are toxins produced by a wide range of fungi. This group of chemicals has received considerable attention due to their widespread biological activities. Indeed, the inhibitory effects of gliotoxin on fungal growth were first reported in 1932. The biological effects of ETPs include inhibition of proliferation of some viruses, bacteria, fungi and mammalian cells. The structural feature common to this group of toxins is the ETP nucleus, and

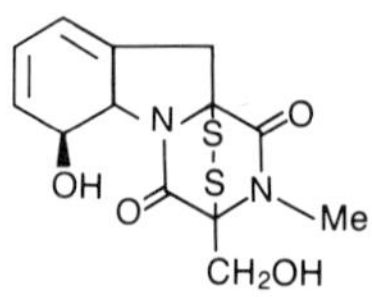

(**37**) Gliotoxin

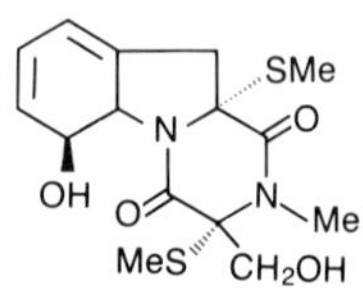

(**38**) FR 49175

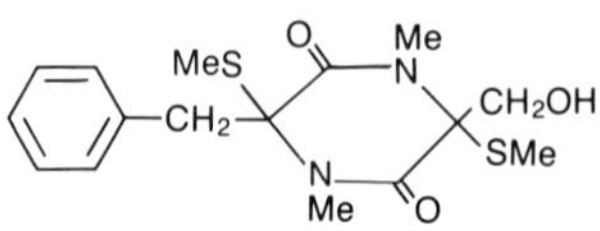

(**39**) FR 106969

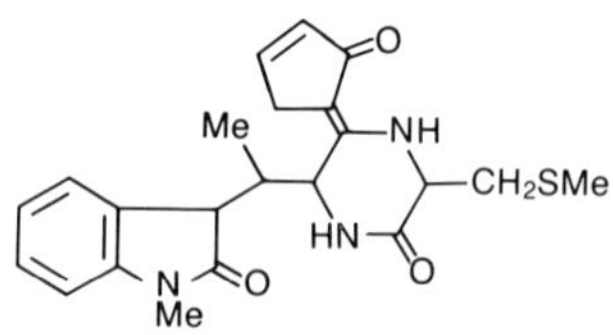

(**40**) FR 900452

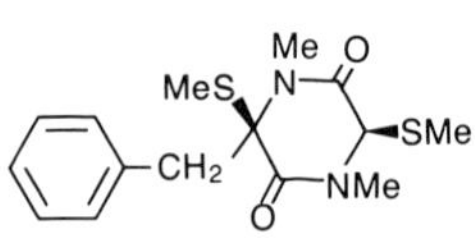

(**41**)

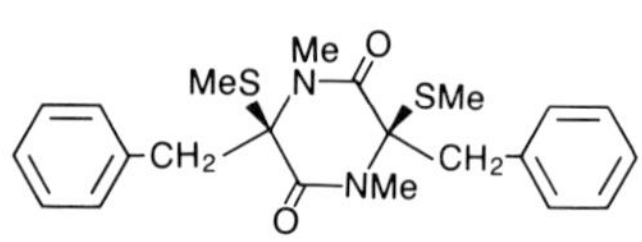

(**42**)

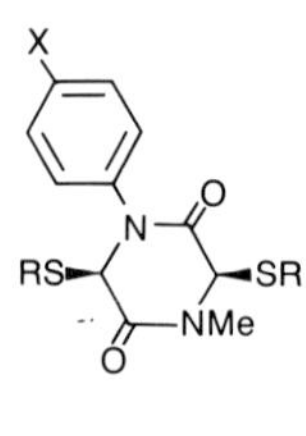

(**43a**) X = H, R = Me (**44a**) X = H, R = Ph
(**43b**) X = Cl, R = Me (**44b**) X = Cl, R = Ph
(**43c**) X = OMe R = Me (**44c**) X = OMe, R = Ph

Fig. 4.8 PAF antagonists (compounds **37**–**44**).

the critical role of the sulfur bridge in the biological activity has been demonstrated by chemical modifications (methylation or elimination of sulfur) which diminish the effects of the toxins on virus, bacteria and eukaryotic cell growth [133].

It is of particular interest to note that researchers of the Fusijawa Pharmaceutical Company recently isolated some PAF antagonists, structurally related to the ETPs, from the fermentation products of certain fungi and actinomycetes [134–137]. Most of these products possess a dialkylthiopiperazinedione skeleton and derive from bisdithiobis(methylthio)gliotoxin (FR 49175; compound **38**).

The three most potent antagonists have been designated FR 49175 (compound **38**; [134,135]), FR 106969 (compound **39**; [138]) and FR 900452 (compound **40**; [136,137]). Isolated from the culture filtrate of *Penicillium terlikowskii, Penicillium citrinum* and *Streptomyces phaeofaciens*, FR 49175, FR 106969 and FR 900452 inhibit PAF-induced rabbit platelet aggregation with an IC_{50} of 4.9, 16.9 and 0.26 μM, respectively. FR 40175 and FR 900452 slightly inhibit collagen-induced aggregation but are inactive against aggregation induced by ADP or arachidonic acid. Interestingly, these compounds do not possess a closed bridge across the ETP nucleus as the sulfur groups are methylated. Thus, while the sulfur bridge is critical for the toxic properties of the ETPs, its absence is desirable for PAF antagonistic activity. Indeed FR 49175 is a far more potent PAF antagonist than gliotoxin, which is relatively inactive.

Structure–activity relationships

Various structure–activity relationships have been deduced from studies using synthetic analogues in PAF-induced *in vitro* platelet aggregation (reviewed by Yoshida *et al.* [138]). Cleavage of the C–N bond of FR 49175 leads to compounds of the FR 106969 type such as compounds **41** and **42**. The IC_{50} values of these compounds are 12.3 and 9.7 μM, respectively, similar to that shown by FR 106969. Alterations of the *p*-position of the phenyl ring produce compounds **43a,b,c**. The IC_{50} values of these decline from 16.9 to 5.2 μM indicating that hydrophobic, electron-donating substituents in this position are desirable for activity. Replacing the methylthio groups of compound **43a** with phenylthio groups (compound **44a**) doubles the activity. When the phenyl ring *p*-position of this compound is substituted as shown (compounds **44a,b,c**), a similar effect on the resulting IC_{50} values is observed, which decline from 5.2 (compound **44a**) to 0.69 μM (compound **44c**).

Compound **45** is also inhibitory with an IC_{50} of 14.5μM, only 2.8 times less potent than compound **44c**. This latter compound (FR 65049) is 6-fold more potent than the natural product, FR 49175, and thus, is the most active compound in this series. In addition, it is a specific PAF inhibitor as

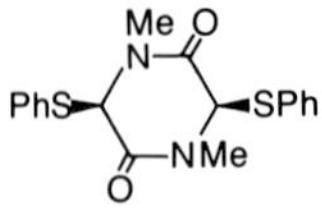

(45)

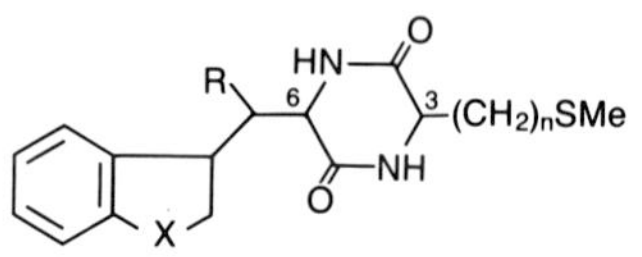

Compound	X	R	n	Configuration C-3	Configuration C-6	IC_{50} μM *
a	NMe	H	1	S	R	7.9
b	NMe	H	1	R	R	36.0
c	NMe	H	1	R	S	>250
d	NMe	H	1	S	S	142
e	NMe	H	2	R	R	2.1
f	$(CH_2)_2$	H	2	R	R	1.4
g	$(CH_2)_2$	(R)-Me	2	R	R	0.18
h	$(CH_2)_2$	(S)-Me	2	R	R	1.9

* IC_{50} values for inhibition of PAF-induced rabbit platelet aggregation

(**46**) and related compounds

Fig. 4.9 PAF antagonists (compounds **45**–**46**).

it has no effect on rabbit platelet aggregation induced by other trigger factors. From a comparison of the structure of FR 900452 with that of compounds **39** and **44c**, Yoshida *et al.* [138] deduced that the oxocylopentyl residue could be removed in favour of the simpler diketopiperazine itself and further, that the oxyindole moiety could be replaced by other similar aromatic nuclei such as N-methylindole and 1-naphthalene without loss of activity. These findings indicate the importance of the *R* configuration at the C_6 position and the irrelevance of the substitution on the diketopiperazine nitrogens group for the biological activity.

The length of the alkylsulfide chain on the piperazine skeleton also modulates the activity. Thus, the methionine derivative, compound **46e**, shows an activity superior to compound **46a**, while the compound without the alkylsulfide is inactive. Antagonistic activity towards PAF is also conferred by the stereochemistry of the tertiary carbon bonded to the aromatic nucleus. Hence, compound **46g** (*R* configuration) possesses an IC_{50} of 0.18 μM and is 10 times more active than the corresponding (*S*) configuration (compound **46h**) and compound **46f** which has no methyl group at this carbon. Compound **46g** (FR 72112) is the most potent derivative in this series being a specific antagonist of PAF-induced platelet aggregation and 1.5 times more active than the natural product,

FR 900452. From their studies on the structure–activity relationship of chemically-synthesized derivatives, Yoshida *et al.* [138] concluded that the stereochemistry of the diketopiperazine moiety is the most important structural requirement for PAF inhibitory activity.

Pharmacological properties

Okamoto *et al.* have evaluated the therapeutic potential of these compounds and examined their pharmacology in various animal models of inflammation and allergy. FR 49175 significantly inhibits PAF-induced bronchoconstriction in guinea pigs (ED_{50} = 0.26 mg/kg i.v.) but fails to prevent PAF-induced hypotension in rats, vascular permeability increase in mice and immune anaphylaxis in guinea pigs [136,137]. FR 90042 is also inactive on antigen-induced increase of airway resistance or hypotension[138]. The effect of FR 900452 was also evaluated on carrageenan oedema, passive cutaneous anaphylaxis (IgE-mediated) and the Arthus reaction in rats, where at 10 mg/kg i.v., it does not show any significant activity in these models. However, antigen-induced hypotension in passively-sensitized adrenalectomized rats is inhibited by 40% after pretreatment by FR 900452 (10 mg/kg i.v.). Thus, although this compound appears to be a specific inhibitor of PAF-induced hypotension, it does not suppress that evoked by acetylcholine, histamine, bradykinin or isoproterenol [135,136].

The antagonistic properties of FR 900542 have also been examined in a model of endotoxin shock, the haemodynamic and haematological manifestations of this condition closely resembling the changes induced by PAF. FR 900452 (10 mg/kg i.v.) almost completely prevents PAF (1 μg/kg i.v.)-induced thrombocytopenia and leukocytopenia in rabbits. It also significantly inhibits *E. coli* LPS endotoxin (30 μg/kg i.v.)-induced thrombocytopenia but not leukocytopenia. The same dose of FR 900452 also causes the decreased arterial blood pressure to return to normal in the endotoxin-induced rat hypotension model, an effect also reported for other PAF inhibitors [26,121]. Finally, FR 900452 has been tested for its therapeutic effect on rat nephrosis induced by aminonucleoside (puromycin, 100 mg/kg i.p). At 100 mg/kg p.o. twice daily for 6 days, the agent significantly reduces urinary protein loss in nephrotic rats [139].

Yoshida *et al.* [138] examined the pharmacology of the two most potent synthetic derivatives. FR 72112 (compound **46g**) showed significant effects on both rat hypotension and mouse vascular permeability tests. This compound inhibited PAF-induced hypotension by 51% (3 mg/kg i.v.) and the increased vasuclar permeability by 40% (10 mg/kg i.v.). However, FR 65049 (compound **44c**; 10 mg/kg i.v.) failed to inhibit PAF-induced hypotension in rats, suggesting the existence of at least two types of PAF receptor *in vivo*, i. e. a platelet type and vascular type.

Conclusions

From the evidence reviewed here it is apparent that a diverse range of both synthetic and natural compounds possess potent PAF antagonistic properties. The emergence of PAF as a mediator having diverse biological activities emphasizes the importance of developing compounds which can attenuate the actions of this molecule. The therapeutic potential of these PAF antagonists remains unknown but the outcome of future clinical trials is eagerly awaited.

References

1 Valone, F. H., Coles, E., Reinhold, V. R. & Goetzl, E. J. Specific binding of phospholipid platelet-activating factor by human platelets. *J. Immunol.* (1982), **129**, 1637–1641.

2 Inarrea, P., Gomez-Cambronero, J., Nieto, M. & Sanchez Crespo, M. Characteristics of the binding of platelet-activating factor to platelets of different animal species. *Eur. J. Pharmacol.* (1984), **105**, 309–315.

3 Kloprogge, E. & Akkerman, J. W. N. Binding kinetics of PAF-acether (1-O-alkyl-2-acetyl-*sn*-glycero-3-phosphocholine) to intact human platelets. *Biochem. J.* (1984), **223**, 901–909.

4 Wade, P. J., Lunt, D. O., Lad, N., Tuffin, D. P. & McCullagh, K. G. Effect of calcium and calcium antagonists on [^{3}H]-PAF-acether binding to washed human platelets. *Thromb. Res.* (1986), **41**, 251–262.

5 Hwang, S. B., Lee, C.S.C., Cheah, M. J. & Shen, T. Y. Specific receptor sites for 1-O-acetyl-*sn*-glycero-3-phosphocholine (platelet activating factor) on rabbit platelet and guinea pig smooth muscle membranes. *Biochemistry* (1983), **22**, 4756–4763.

6 Valone, F. H. & Goetzl, E. J. Specific binding by human polymorphonuclear leukocytes of the immunological mediator 1-O-hexadecyl/octadecyl-2-acetyl-*sn*-glycero-3-phosphorylcholine. *Immunology* (1983), **48**, 141–149.

7 Hwang, S. B., Lam, M. H. & Shen, T. Y. Specific binding sites for platelet activating factor in human lung tissues. *Biochem. Biophys. Res. Commun.* (1985), **128**, 972–979.

8 Domingo, M. T., Spinnewyn, B., Chabrier, P. E. & Braquet, P. (1988), Presence of specific binding sites for platelet-activating factor (PAF) in gerbil brain. *Biochem. Biophys. Res. Comm.* (1988), **151**, 730–736.

9 Doly, M., Braquet, P., Bonhomme, B. & Meyniel, G. Presence of specific PAF-acether receptors inside the retina and their electrophysiological involvement (abstract). *Clin. Exp. Physiol. Pharmacol.* (1988), Suppl. **13**, 15.

10 Domingo, M. T., van Delst, G. L., Nerbey, M. L. G., van Haerinjen, N. G., Chabrier, P. E. & Braquet, P. Specific binding of PAF in iris and ciliary body in pigmented rabbit eye. In *Proceedings of the British Pharmacological Society*, 6–8 January 1988, C106.

11 Lambrecht, G. & Parnham, M. J. Kadsurenone distinguishes between different platelet-activating factor receptor subtypes on macrophages and polymorphonuclear leukocytes. *Br. J. Pharmacol.* (1986), **87**, 287–289.

12 Voelkel, N. F., Worthen, S., Reeves, J. T., Henson, P. M. & Murphy, R. C. Nonimmunological production of leukotrienes induced by platelet-activating factor. *Science* (1982), **218**, 286–288.

13 Braquet, P. The ginkgolides: potent platelet-activating factor antagonists isolated from *Ginkgo Biloba* L. *Drugs of the Future* (1987), **12**, 643–699.
14 Braquet, P. & Godfroid, J. J. PAF-acether specific binding sites: 2. Design of specific antagonists. *Trends Pharmacol. Sci.* (1986), **7**, 397–403.
15 Braquet, P., Chabrier, P. E. & Mencia-Huerta, J. M. The promise of PAF-acether antagonists. In. *Advances in Inflammation Research* (1987), Vol. 12, pp. 135–157. Raven Press, New York.
16 Terashita, Z., Tsushima, S., Yhoshioka, Y., Nomura, H., Inada, Y. & Nishikawa, K. CV 3988—a specific antagonist of platelet activating factor (PAF). *Life Sci.* (1983), **32**, 1975–1982.
17 Burri, K., Barner, R., Cassal, J. M., Hadvary, P., Hirth, G. & Muller, K. PAF from agonists to antagonists by synthesis. *Prostaglandins* (1985), **30**, 691.
18 Winslow, C. M., Vallespir, S. R., Frisch, G. E. *et al.* A novel platelet-activating factor receptor antagonists. *Prostaglandins* (1985), **30**, 697.
19 Wichrowski, B., Jouquey, S., Heymans, F. *et al.* Platelet activating factor analogs from agonists to antagonists by synthesis of carboxylate isosters. In *6th International Conference on Prostaglandins and Related Compounds*, Florence (Italy) June 6 1986, p. 309.
20 Saunders, R., Anderson, R., Handley, D. *et al.* The biological activity of SRI 63-072. In *Second International Conference on Platelet-Activating Factor and Structurally Related Alkyl Ether Lipids* (1986), Gatlingburg, Tennessee, October 26–29, p. 33.
21 Handley, D. A., van Valen, R. G., Winslow, C. M., Tomesch, J. C. & Saunders, R. N. *In vitro* and *in vivo* pharmacological profiles of the PAF receptor antagonist SRI 63-675. *Thromb. Haemost.* (1987), **57**, 187–190.
22 Sedivy, P., Caillard, C. G., Floch, A. *et al.* 48740 RP: a specific PAF-acether antagonist, *Prostaglandins* (1985), **30**, 688.
23 Kornecki, E., Ehrlich, Y. H. & Lenox, R. H. Platelet-activating factor-induced aggregation of human platelets specifically inhibited by triazolobenziodiazepines. *Science* (1985), **226**, 1454–1456.
24 Casals-Stenzel, J., Muacevin, G & Weber, K. H. Pharmacological actions of WEB 2086, a new specific antagonist of platelet activating factor. *J. Pharmacol. Exp. Ther.* (1987), **241**, 974–981.
25 Nunez, D., Chignard, M., Korth, R. *et al.* Specific inhibition of PAF-acether-induced platelet activation by BN 52021 and comparison with the PAF-acether inhibitors kadsurenone and CV-3988. *Eur. J. Pharmacol.* (1986), **123**, 197–205.
26 Terashita, Z., Imura, Y., Nishikawa, K. & Sumida, S. Is platelet activating factor (PAF) a mediator of endotoxin shock? *Eur. J. Pharmacol.* (1985), **109**, 257–261.
27 Wallace, J. L. & Whittle, B. J. R. Prevention of endotoxin-induced gastrointestinal damage by CV-3988, an antagonist of platelet-activating factor. *Eur. J. Pharmacol.* (1986), **124**, 209–210.
28 Imura, Y., Terashita, Z. & Nishikawa, K. Possible role of platelet-activating factor (PAF) in disseminated intravascular coagulation (DIC), evidenced by use of a PAF antagonist, CV-3988. *Life Sci.* (1986), **39**, 111–117.
29 Masugi, F., Ogihara, T., Otsuka, A., Saeki, S. & Kumajara, Y. Effect of 1-alkyl-2-acetyl-*sn*-glycero-3-phosphorylcholine inhibitor on the reduction of one-kidney, one-clip hypertension after unclipping in the rat. *Life Sci.* (1984), **34**, 197–201.
30 Wallace, J. L., Steel, G. & Whittle, B. J. Gastrointestinal leakage in endotoxic shock. Inhibition by prostaglandin E_2 and by a platelet-activating factor antagonist. *Can. J. Physiol. Pharmacol.* (1987), **65**, 1428–1432.
31 Lang, M., Hansen, D. & Hahn, H. L. Effects of the PAF-antagonist CV-3988 on PAF-induced changes in mucous secretions and in the respiratory and circulatory variables in ferrets. *Agents Actions* (1987), (Suppl), **21**, 245–252.

32 Satoh, H. M., Adachi, T., Imai, T., *et al.* The effects of a specific antagonist of PAF (CV-3988) on airway hyperresponsiveness induced by ozone exposure in beagles. *Arerugi* (1987), **36**, 306–312.
33 Arnout, J., van Hecken, A., Delepeleire, I. *et al.* Effectiveness and tolerability of CV-3988, a selective PAF-antagonist, after intravenous administration to man. *Thromb. Haemost.* (1987), **58**, 20.
34 Terashita, Z., Imura, Y., Takatani, M., Tsushima, S. & Nishikawa, K. CV-6209, a highly potent antagonist of platelet-activating factor *in vitro* and *in vivo, J. Pharmacol. Exp. Ther.* (1987), **242**, 263–268.
35 Lee, M. L., Winslow, C. M., Frisch, G. E. *et al.* Enantioselectivity in the binding of analogs and inhibitors of platelet-activating factor to the human platelet receptor. In Lee, M. L. Winslow, C. M. (eds) *New Horizons in Platelet Activating Factor Research* (1987), pp.263–279. John Wiley, Chichester.
36 Melden, M. K., Flury, S., Saunders, R. N. & Handley, D. A. Inhibition and reversal by SRI 63–072 and SRI 63–119 of PAF-induced hypotention in the rat. *Fed. Proc.* (1986), **45**, 856.
37 Farley, C., Melden, M. K., van Valen, R. G. *et al. In vivo* inhibition by SRI 63–072 and SRI 63–119 in PAF-induced hemoconcentration and bronchoconstriction in the guinea pig. *Fed. Proc.* (1986), **45**, 855.
38 O'Donnell, S. R. & Barnett, C. J. K. Microvascular leakage to platelet activating factor in guinea pig trachea and bronchi. *Eur. J. Pharmacol.* (1987), **138**, 385–396.
39 Handley, D. A., van Valen, R. G. & Saunders, R. N. Vascular responses of platelet-activating factor in the *Cebus apella* primate and inhibitory profiles of antagonists SRI 63-072 and SRI 63-119. *Immunopharmacology* (1986), **11**, 175–182.
40 Hseuh, W., Gonzalez-Crussi, F., Arroyana, J. L. *et al.* Platelet-activating factor-induced ischemic bowel necrosis: its prevention by PAF antagonists. In Winslow, C. M. & Lee, M. L. (eds) *New Horizons in Platelet-Activating Factor Research* (1987), pp. 347–355. John Wiley, Chichester.
41 Handley, D. A., Anderson, R. C. & Saunders, R. N. Inhibition by SRI 63-072 and SRI 63-119 of PAF-acether and immune complex effects in the guinea pig. *Eur. J. Pharmacol.* (1987), **141**, 409–416.
42 Handley, D. A., Deacon, R. W., Lee, M. L. & Saunders, R. N. Effect of PAF antagonist SRI 63-072 on dermal extravasation in the reverse passive arthus reaction. In *New Horisons in Platelet-Activating Factor Research. October 15–18 1985, Hilton Head Island* (1987) p. 82.
43 Miyamoto, T., Ohno, H., Yano, T., Okada, T., Hamanaka, N. & Kawasaki, A. Ono-6240: a new potent antagonist of platelet-activating factor. In *Advances in Prostaglandins, Thromboxane and Leukotriene Research*, Hayaisi, O. & Yamamoto, S. (eds) Vol. 15, pp. 719–720. Raven Press, New York.
44 Toyofuku, T., Keishi, K., Kobayashi, T. & Kusama, S. Effects of Ono-6240, a platelet-activating factor antagonist, on endotoxin shock in unanesthetized sheep. *Prostaglandins* (1986), **31**, 271–281.
45 Cirino, M., Lagente, V., Lefort, J. & Vargaftig, B. B. A study with BN 52021 demonstrates the involvement of PAF-acether in IgE-dependent anaphylactic bronchoconstriction. *Prostaglandins* (1986), **32**, 121–126.
46 Hadvary, P. & Baumgartner, H. R. Interference of PAF-acether antagonists with platelet aggregation and with formation of platelet thrombi. *Prostaglandins* (1985), **30**, 694.
47 Nakamura, N., Ookawa, N., Koke, H., Sada, T., Oshima, T. & Iizuka, Y. European Patent No. 238–202 (1988).
48 Grue-Sorensen, G., Nielsen, I. M. & Nielsen, C. K. Derivatives of 2-methylenepropane-1, 3-diol as new antagonists of platelet activating factor. *J. Med. Chem.* (1989), **31**, 1174–1178.

49 Winslow, C. M., Anderson, R. C., D'Aries, F. J., *et al.* Toward understanding the mechanism of action of platelet-activating factor receptor antagonists. In Winslow, C. M. & Lee, M. L. (eds), *New Horizons in Platelet-Activating Factor Research* (1987), pp. 153–164. John Wiley, Chichester.
50 Hseuh, W., Gonzalez-Crussi, F., Arroyave, J. L., Anderson, R. C., Lee, M. L. & Houlihan, W. J. Platelet-activating factor-induced ischemic bowel necrosis. The effect of PAF antagonists. *Eur. J. Pharmacol.* (1986), **123**, 79–83.
51 Handley, D. A., van Valen, R. G., Melden, M. K., Flury, S., Lee, M. L. & Saunders, R. N. Inhibition and reversal of endotoxin-, aggregated IgG and PAF-induced hypotension in the rat by SRI 63-072, a PAF receptor antagonist. *Immunopharmacology* (1986), **12**, 11–17.
52 Patterson, R., Harris, K. E., Lee, M. L. & Houlihan, W. J. Inhibition of rhesus monkey airway and cutaneous responses to platelet-activating factor (PAF) (AGEPC) with the anti-PAF agent SRI 63-072. *Int. Arch. Allergy Appl. Immunol.* (1986), **81**, 168–265.
53 Deacon, R. W., Melden, M. K., Saunders, R. N. & Handley, D. A. PAF involvement in dermal extravasation in reverse passive arthus reaction. *Fed Proc.* (1986), **45**, Abstract 995.
54 Camussi, G., Pawlowski, I., Saunders, R., Brentjens, J. & Andres, G. Receptor antagonist of platelet activating factor inhibits inflammatory injury induced by *in situ* formation of immune complexes in renal glomeruli and in the skin. *J. Lab. Clin. Med.* (1987), **110**, 196–206.
55 Winslow, C. M., Gubler, H. U., DeLillo, A. K., D'Aries, F. J., Tomesch, J. C. & Saunders, R. N. Inhibition of PAF-induced ulcer formation by the specific PAF receptor antagonist, SRI 63-441 (abstract). In *Second International Conference on Platelet-Activating Factor and Structurally Related Alkyl Ether Lipids* (1986), Gatlinburg, Tennessee, October 26–29, p. 33.
56 Handley, D. A. Development and therapeutic indications for PAF receptor antagonists. *Drugs of the Future* (1988), **13**, 137–152.
57 Patterson, R., Harris, K. E., Handley, D. A. & and Saunders, R. N. Evaluation of the effect of a platelet antagonist on platelet-activating factor and *Ascaris* antigen-induced airway responses in rhesus monkeys, *J. Lab. Clin. Med.* (1987), **110**, 606–611.
58 Stenzel, H., Hummer, B. & Han, H. L. Effect of the PAF-antagonist SRI 63-441 on the allergic reaction in awake dogs with natural asthma. *Agents & Actions* (1987), **21**, (Supplement), 253–260.
59 Makowka, L., Miller, C., Chapchap, P. *et al.* Prolongation of pig-to-dog renal xenograft survival by modification of the inflammatory mediator response. *Ann. Surg.* (1987), **206**, 482–495.
60 Jones, S. L., O'Donnell, S. R. & Barnet, C. J. K. A new potent and specific PAF-antagonist drug, SRI 63-675. *Clin. Exp. Physiol. Pharmacol.* (1988), Suppl. **13**, 6.
61 Nakamura, N., Ookawa, N., Koke, H., Sada, T., Oshima, T. & Iizuka, Y. Phosphate ester derivatives, their penetration and their therapeutic use. European Patent 210804-A1 (February 4, 1987).
62 Lee, M. L., Winslow, C. M., Jaeggi, Ch., D'Aries, F., Frisch, G. & Farley, C. Inhibition of platelet-activating factor: synthesis and biological activity of SRI 63-073, a new phospholipid PAF-acether antagonist. *Prostaglandins* (1985), **30**, 690.
63 Hadvary, P. & Weller, T. Conformationally restricted analogs of platelet-activating factor (PAF). *Helv. Chim. Acta* (1986), **69**, 1862–1871.
64 Floch, A., Sedivy, P. & Caillard, C. G. Specific inhibition of PAF-acether-induced bronchoconstriction by 48740RP. *J. Pharmacol.* (1986), **17**, 177.
65 Dewald, B. & Baggiolini, M. Evaluation of PAF-antagonists using human neutrophils in a microliter plate assay. *Biochem. Pharmacol.* (1987), **36**, 2505–2510.

66 Sedivy, P., Weber, S., Gergoire, J. *et al.* 4874HRP inhibits PAF-induced platelet aggregation and thromboxane B_2 generation *ex vivo* in volunteers. *Clin. Exp. Physiol. Pharmacol.* (1988), Suppl. **13**, 13.
67 Marquis, O., Robaut, C. & Carero, I. Influence of mono- and divalent ions on the specific binding of [^{3}H]PAF and [^{3}H]52770RP in human polymorphonuclear leukocytes. *Clin. Exp. Physiol. Pharmacol.* (1988), Suppl. **13**, 13.
68 Robaut, C., Durand, G., James, C., *et al.* PAF binding sites. Characterization by [^{3}H]52770RP, a pyrrolo[1,2*c*]thiazole derivative, in rabbit platelets. *Biochem. Pharmacol.* (1987), **36**, 3221–3229.
69 Valone, F. H. Inhibition of platelet-activating factor binding to human platelets by calcium channel blockers. *Thromb. Res.* (1987), **45**, 427–435.
70 Cox, C. P. & Wood, K. L. Selective antagonism of platelet-activating factor (PAF)-induced aggregation and secretion in washed rabbit platelets by CV-3988, L-652,731, triazolam and alprazolam. *Thromb. Res.* (1987), **47**, 249–257.
71 Casals-Stenzel, J. & Weber, K. H. Triazolobenzodiazepines: dissociation of their PAF (platelet-activating factor) antagonistic and CNS activity. *Br. J. Pharmacol.* (1987), **90**, 139–146.
72 Casals-Stenzel, J. Triazolodiazepines are potent antagonists of platelet-activating factor (PAF) *in vitro* and *in vivo*. *Naunyn-Schmiedeberg's Arch. Pharmacol.* (1987), **335**, 351–355.
73 Tahara, T., Mikashima, H., Terasawa, M. & Maruyama, Y. PAF antagonistic activity of some thieno[3,2*f*][1,2,4]triazolo[4,3*A*]-[1,4]diazepines. *Chem. Pharm. Bull. Japan* (1987), **35**, 2119–2121.
74 Evans, T. W., Dent, G., Rogers, D. F., Aursudkuj, B., Chung, K. F. & Barnes, P. J. Effect of a PAF antagonist, WEB 2086, on airway microvascular leakage in the guinea pig and platelet aggregation in man. *Br. J. Pharmacol.* (1988), **94**, 164–168.
75 Casals-Stenzel, J. Protective effect of WEB 2086, a novel antagonist of platelet-activating factor in endotoxin shock. *Eur. J. Pharmacol.* (1987), **135**, 117–122.
76 Ukena, D., Dent, G., Birke, F. W., Robaut, C., Sybrecht, G. W. & Barnes, P. J. Radioligand binding of antagonists of platelet activating factor to intact human platelets. *FEBS Lett* (1988), **2**, 285–289.
77 Dent, G., Ukena, D., Chanez, P., Sybrecht, G. W. & Barnes, P. J. Characterization of platelet-activating factor receptors in human neutrophils and eosinophils using the new competitive PAF antagonist WEB 2086. *Ann. Rev. Resp. Dis.* (1988), **137**, 236.
78 Heuer, H., Casals-Stenzel, J., Muacevic, G., Stransky, W. & Weber, K. H. Effect of WEB 2170 and STY 2108, two hetrazepines with PAF-antagonistic activity on PAF-induced changes *in vitro* and *in vivo*. *Clin. Exp. Physiol. Pharmacol.* (1988), Suppl. **13**, 7.
79 Tilley, J. W., Burghardt, B., Burghardt, C. *et al.* Pyrido[2,1*b*]quinazolinecarboxamide derivatives as platelet-activating factor antagonists. *J. Med. Chem.* (1988), **31**, 466–472.
80 Houlihan, W. J., Cheon, S. H., Handley, D. A. *et al.* 5-Aryl-2,3-dihydroimidazo[21*a*]isoquinolines. A novel class of platelet-activating factor (PAF) receptor antagonists structurally derived from the PAF molecule. *Prostaglandins* (1988), **35**, 848.
81 Furukawa, S. Constituents of *Ginkgo biloba* L. leaves. *Sci. Papers Inst. Phys. Chem. Res. Tokyo* (1932), **19**, 27–38.
82 Nakanishi, K. The ginkgolides. *Pure Appl. Chem.* (1967), **14**, 89–113.
83 Weinges, K., Hepp, M. & Jaggy, H. Isolierung and Strukturaufklärung eines neuen Ginkgolides. *Liebigs Ann. Chem.* (1987), **6**, 521–526.
84 Dupont, L., Germain, G. & Dideberg, O. Crystal and molecular structure of BN

52021, a PAF-acether antagonist. Comparison with the conformation of kadsurenone and related compounds. *Pharmacol. Res. Comm.* (1986), **18**, 25–42.
85 Roumestand, C., Perly, B., Hosford D. & Braquet, P. Carbon-13 and proton 500 MHz NMR of ginkgolides. *Tetrahedron Lett.* (1989), in press.
86 Braquet, P., Spinnewyn, B., Braquet, M., *et al.* BN 52021 and related compounds: a new series of highly specific PAF-acether receptor antagonists isolated from *Ginkgo biloba. Blood Vessels* (1985), **16**, 559–572.
87 Braquet, P. Involvement of PAF-acether in various immune disorders using BN 52021 (ginkgolide B): a powerful PAF-acether antagonist isolated from *Ginkgo biloba* L. In *Advances in Prostaglandin, Thromboxane and Leukotriene Research* (1986), Vol. 16, pp. 179–198. Raven Press, New York.
88 Nakanishi, K., Habaguchi, K., Nakadaira, Y. *et al.* Structure of bilobalide, a rare *t*-butyl containing sequiterpenoid related to the C_{20} ginkgolides. *J. Am. Chem. Soc.* (1971), **93**, 3544–3546.
89 Braquet, P. *Ginkgolides: Chemistry, Biology, Pharmacology and Clinical Perspectives* (1988), Braquet, P. (ed.). J.R. Prous Science Publishers, Barcelona.
90 Braquet, P., Guinot, P. & Touvay, C. The role of PAF-acether in anaphylaxis demonstrated with the use of the antagonist BN 52021. *Agents & Actions* (1987), **21**, 97–117.
91 Touvay, C., Villain, B., Taylor, J. E., Etienne, A. & Braquet, P. Proof of the involvement of platelet-activating factor (PAF-acether) in pulmonary complex immune systems using a specific PAF-acether receptor antagonist: BN 52021. *Prog. Lipid Res.* (1985), **25**, 277–288.
92 Barnes, P. J., Chung, K. S., Evans, T. W. & Rogers, D. S. Increased airway vascular permeability induced by platelet-activating factor: effect of specific antagonism and platelet depletion. *Br. J. Pharmacol.* (1986), **89**, 764p.
93 Evans, T. W., Chung, K. F., Rogers, D. F. & Barnes, P. J. Effect of platelet-activating factor on airway vascular permeability: possible mechanisms. *J. Appl. Physiol.* (1987), **63**, 479–484.
94 Berti, F. & Rossoni, G. PAF, ginkgolides and active anaphylactic shock in lung and heart. In *The Ginkgolides: Chemistry, Biology, Pharmacology and Clinical Perspectives* (1988), Braquet, P. (ed.). pp. 399–410. J.R. Prous Science Publishers, Barcelona.
95 Braquet, P. & Godfroid, J. J. Conformational properties of the PAF-acether receptor in platelets based on structure–activity studies. In *Platelet-Activating Factor and Related Lipid Mediators* (1987), Synder, F. (ed.). pp. 191–235. Plenum Press, New York.
96 Coyle, A. J., Unwin, S., Touvay, C., Villain, B., Page, C. P. & Braquet, P. The effect of the selective PAF antagonist BN 52021 on antigen-induced eosinophil infiltration and bronchial hyperreactivity. *Eur. J. Pharmacol.* (1988), **148**, 51–58.
97 Desquand, S., Touvay, C., Randon, J. *et al.* Interference of ginkgolide B (BN 52021) with the broncho-pulmonary effects of PAF-acether in the guinea-pig. *Eur. J. Pharmacol.* (1986), **127**, 83–95.
98 Berti, F., Omini, C., Rossoni, G. & Braquet, P. Protection by two ginkgolides, BN 52020 and BN 52021, against guinea-pig lung anaphylaxis. *Pharmacol. Res. Comm.* **18**, 775–793.
99 Vilain, B., Lagente, V., Touvay, C. *et al.* Pharmacological control of the *in vivo* passive anaphylactic shock by the PAF-acether antagonist compound BN 52021. *Pharmacol. Res. Commun.* (1986), **18**, 119–126.
100 Lagente, V., Touvay, C., Randon, J. *et al.* Interference of the PAF-acether antagonist BN 52021 with passive anaphylaxis in the guinea-pig. *Prostaglandins* (1987), **33**, 264–274.

101 Etienne, A., Hecquet, F., Soulard, C., Spinnewyn, B., Clostre, F. & Braquet, P. *In vivo* inhibition of plasma protein leakage and *Salmonella enteritidis*-induced mortality in the rat by a specific PAF-acether antagonist: BN 52021. *Agent & Actions (1985)*, **17**, 368–370.
102 Etienne, A., Guilmard, C., Soulard, C., Clostre, F. & Braquet, P. Hematological changes induced by endotoxin and PAF in the rat: inhibition by BN 52021. *Circul. Shock* (1987), **21**, 368.
103 Adnot, S., Lefort, J., Braquet, P. & Vargaftig, B. B. Interference of the PAF-acether antagonist BN 52021 with endoxtoxin-induced hypotension in the guinea-pig. *Prostaglandins* (1986), **32**, 791–802.
104 Adnot, S., Lefort, J., Lagente, V., Braquet, P. & Vargaftig, B. B. Interference of BN 52021, a PAF-acether antagonist, with endotoxin-induced hypotension in the guinea-pig. *Pharmacol. Res. Comm.* (1986), **18**, 197–200.
105 Sanchez Crespo, M., Fernandez-Gallardo, S., Nieto, M. L., Baranès, J. & Braquet, P. Inhibition of the vascular actions of IgG aggregates by BN 52021, a highly specific antagonist of PAF-acether. *Immunopharmacology* (1985), **10**, 69–75.
106 Beijer, L., Botting, J., Crook, P., Oyekan, A. O., Page, C. & Rylander, R. The involvement of PAF in endotoxin-induced pulmonary platelet recruitment in the guinea pig. *Br. J. Pharmacol.* (1987), **92**, 803–809.
107 Rola-Pleszczynski, M., Pignol, B., Pouliot, C. & Braquet, P. Inhibition of human lymphocyte proliferation and interleukin-2 production by platelet-activating factor (PAF-acether): reversal by a specific antagonist, BN 52021. *Biochem. Biophys. Res. Commun.* (1987), **142**, 754–760.
108 Rola-Pleszczynski, M., Pouliot, C., Pignol, B. & Braquet, P. Platelet-activating factor induces human suppressor cell activity. *Fed. Proc.* (1987), **46**, 444 (A743).
109 Pignol, B., Henane, S., Mencia-Huerta J.M., Rola-Pleszczynski M. & Braquet, P. Effect of PAF-acether (platelet-activating factor) and its specific antagonist, BN 52021, on interleukin-1 (IL-1) synthesis and release by rat monocytes. *Prostaglandins* (1987), **33**, 931–939.
110 Foegh, M. L., Khirabadi, B. S., Rowles, J. R., Braquet P & Ramwell, P. W. Prolongation of cardiac allograft survival with BN 52021, a specific antagonist of platelet-activity factor. *Transplantation* (1986), **42**, 86–88.
111 Pirotzky, E., Colliez, Ph., Guilmard, C., Schaeverbeke, J. & Braquet, P. Cyclosporin-induced nephrotoxicity: preventive effect of a PAF-acether antagonist, BN 52063. *Transplantation Proc.* (1988), **20**, 199–207.
112 Pignol, B., Henane, S., Pirotzky, E., Mencia-Huerta, J. M. & Braquet P. Potentiation of immunosuppressive action of cyclosporin A by platelet-activating factor antagonists: an approach of the mechanism of action of these drugs in graft rejection. *Transplantation Proc.* (1988), **20**, 259–265.
113 Gebhart, P. B., Bazan, H. E. P., Braquet, P. & Bazan, N. G. Platelet activating factor suppresses cell mediated immune reactions *in vivo*. In Braquet, P. (ed.) *New Trends in Lipid Mediator Research.* Vol. 1, (1988), pp. 99–107. Karger, Basel.
114 Farkas, G., Mandi, Y., Koltai, M. & Braquet, P. Graft protective effect of BN 52021: a specific PAF-acether antagonist in an *in vitro* Langerhans islet splenic lymphocyte model. In Braquet, (ed.) *Ginkgolides: Chemistry, Biology, Pharmacology and Clinical Perspectives* (1988), pp. 737–748. J.R. Prous Science Publishers, Barcelona.
115 Carter, S. K. & Livingston, R. B. Plant products in cancer chemotherapy. *Cancer Treat, Rep.* (1976), **60**, 1141–56.
116 Shen, T. Y., Hwang, S. B., Chang, M. N. *et al.* Characterization of a platelet-activating factor receptor antagonist isolated from haifenteng *(Piper futokadsura)*:

specific inhibition of *in vitro* and *in vivo* platelet-activating factor-induced effects. *Proc. Nat. Acad. Sci. (USA)* (1985), **82**, 672–676.
117 Godfroid, J. J., Broquet, C., Jouquey, *et al.* Structure–activity relationship in PAF-acether. 3. Hydrophobic contribution to the agonistic activity. *J. Med. Chem.* (1987), **30**, 792–797.
118 Hwang, S. B., Lam, M. H., Biftu, T., Beattie, T.R & Shen, T. Y. Trans-2,5-bis (3,4,5-trimethoxyphenyl)tetrahydrofuran. An orally active specific and competitive receptor antagonist of platelet activating factor. *J. Biol. Chem.* (1985), **260**, 15 639–15 645.
119 Levi, R., Burke, J. A., Guo, Z. G. *et al.* Acetyl glyceryl ether phosphorylcholine (AGEPC). A putative mediator of cardiac anaphylaxis in the guinea-pig. *Circ. Res.* (1984), **54**, 117–124.
120 Hwang, S. B., Li, C. L., Lam, M. H. & Shen, T. Y. Characterization of cutaneous vascular permeability induced by platelet-activating factor in guinea pigs and rats and its inhibition by a platelet-activating factor antagonist. *Lab. Invest.* (1985), **52**, 617–630.
121 Doebber, T. W., Wu, M. S., Robbins, J. C., Choy, B. M., Chang, M. N. & Shen, T. Y. Platelet activating factor (PAF) involvement in endotoxin-induced hypotension in rats. Studies with PAF-receptor antagonist, kadsurenone. *Biochem. Biophys. Res. Comm.* (1985) **29**, 799–808.
122 Thompson, D. L., Chang, M. N., Chabala, J. C. *et al.* Metabolism of kadsurenone and 9,10-dihydrokadsurenone in rhesus monkey and rat liver micromes. *Drug Met. Dis.* (1988), **16**, 737–743.
123 Hwang, S. B., Lam, M. H. & Chang, M. N. Specific binding of [^{3}H]dihydrokadsurenone to rabbit platelet membranes and its inhibition by the receptor agonists of platelet-activating factor. *J. Biol. Chem.* (1986), **261**, 13 720–13 726.
124 Ponpipom, M. M., Hwang, S. B., Doebber, W., *et al. Trans*-2-(3-methoxy-5-methyl-sulfonyl-4-propoxyphenyl)-5-(3,4,5-trimethoxyphenyl)tetrahydrofuran(L-659989), a novel potent PAF receptor antagonist. *Biochem. Biophys. Res. Comm.* (1988), **150**, 1213–1220.
125 Biftu, T., Gamble, N. F., Doebber, T. *et al.* Conformation and activity of tetrahydrofuran lignans and analogues, specific platelet-activating factor antagonists. *J. Med. Chem.* (1986), **29**, 1912–1921.
126 Chaing, Y-C.P., Biftu, T., Graham, D. W. *et al.* New 1,3-diaryl cyclopentanes and derivatives thereof as PAF antagonists. European Patent No. 257–921. A2 (1988).
127 Setchell, K. D., Lawson, A. M., Mitchell, F. L., Adlercreutz, H., Kirk, D. N. & Axelson, M. Lignans in man and in animal species. *Nature* (1980), **287**, 740–742.
128 Stitch, S. R., Toumba, J. K., Groen, M. B., *et al.* Excretion, isolation and structure of a new phenolic constituent of female urine. *Nature* (1980), **287**, 738–740.
129 Setchell, K. D., Lawson, A. M., Conway, E., *et al.* The definitive identification of the lignans *trans*-2,3-bis(3-hydrobenzyl)-γ-butyrolactone and 2,3-bis(3-hydroxybenzl) butane-1,4-diol in human and animal urine. *Biochem. J.* (1981), **197**, 447–458.
130 Braquet, P., Esanu, A., Etienne, A. & Robin, J. P. Endogenous mammalian lignans: a dual action on PAF-acether receptors and the Na^+, K^+-pump. In Winslow, C. M. & Lee, M. L. (eds). *Proceedings of the First Sandoz Research Symposium New Horizons in Platelet-activating Factor Research* (1987), John Wiley, London.
131 Aldercreutz, H., Fotsis, T., Heikkinen, R., *et al.* Excretion of the lignans enterolactone and enterodiol and of equol in omnivorous and vegetarian postmenopausal women and in women with breast cancer. *Lancet* (1982), **ii**, 1295–1299.

132 Braquet. P., Senn, N., Fagoo, M. *et al.* Lignanes de mammifères: une possible implication dans l'activité digitale endogène. *C.R. Acad. Sci. Paris* (1986), **302**, 443–447.
133 Mullbacher, A., Waring, P., Tiwari-Palni, U. & Eichner, R. D. Structural relationship of epipolythiodioxopiperazines and their immunomodulating activity. *Mol. Immunol.* (1986), **23**, 231–235.
134 Okamoto, M., Yoshida, K., Uchida, I., Nishikawa, M., Kohsaka, M. & Aoki, H. Studies of platelet activating factor (PAF) antagonists from microbial products. I. Bisdethiobis(methylthio)gliotoxin and its derivatives. *Chem. Pharm. Bull.* (1986), **34**, 340–344.
135 Okamoto, M., Yoshida, K., Uchida, I., Kohsaka, M. & Aoki, H. Studies of platelet activating factor (PAF) antagonists from microbial products. II. Pharmacological studies of FR-49175 in animal models. *Chem. Pharm. Bull. Tokyo* (1986), **34**, 345–348.
136 Okamoto, M., Yohida, K., Nishikawa, M. *et al.* Studies of platelet activating factor (PAF) antagonists from microbial products. 3. Pharmacological studies of FR-900-452 in animal models. *Chem. Pharm. Bull. Tokyo* (1986), **34**, 3005–3010.
137 Okamoto, M., Yoshida, K., Nishikawa, M., Kohsaka, M. & Aoki, H. Platelet activating factor (PAF) involvement in endotoxin-induced thrombocytopenia in rabbits: studies with FR-900452, a specific inhibitor of PAF. *Thromb. Res.* (1986), **42**, 661–671.
138 Yoshida, K., Okamoto, M., Shimazaki, N. & Hemmi, K. PAF inhibitors of microbial origin. Studies on Diketopiperazine. In Braquet, P. (ed.) *Progress in Biochemistry and Pharmocology. Biologically Active Ether Lipids*, Vol. 22, pp. 66–80 (1988). Karger, Basel.
139 Mimura, K., Yukawa, S., Goto, T. *et al.* Effect of FR-900452, a PAF inhibitor on experimental nephrotic disease in rats. *Lipids* (1986), **28**, 253–256.

Chapter 5
PAF and cell activation

Joseph T. O'Flaherty and Robert L. Wykle

Introduction

In 1971, Siraganian & Osler (reviewed in [1]) reported that leukocytes from sensitized rabbits released a platelet-activating factor (PAF) upon exposure to specific allergen. Since then, PAF has been found to activate not only platelets but also polymorphonuclear neutrophils (PMN) [2,3], eosinophils [4,5], basophils [6], monocytes [7–9], T-lymphocytes [9], vascular endothelium [10], renal juxtaglomerular [11] and mesangial [12] cells, macrophages [13,14], 3T3 fibroblasts [15], pancreatic and parotid exocrine cells [16], smooth muscle [17,18], cultured neurocytes [19], and amnionic membranes [20]. This list is certain to enlarge with future studies. In addition, PAF stimulates cells to release mediators that can activate other cells including those which may not be sensitive to PAF *per se*. Such transcellular interactions further expand the list of bioactivities ascribed to PAF. Thus, PAF directly or indirectly influences an extraordinarily large number of cell types. Studies into the mechanisms involved in these diverse effects has contributed to our fundamental understanding of cellular biochemistry, stimulus–response coupling and the pathophysiology of disease.

Biochemistry of PAF metabolism

As reviewed in Chapter 2, PAF is a *sn*-glycero-3-phosphocholine derivative containing principally a C_{16} or C_{18} straight chain, fatty alkyl ether at the *sn*-1 position and an acetate ester at the *sn*-2 position. A large variety of cells commonly form PAF from their membranous 1-O-alkyl-2-acylglycerophosphocholine by sequential deacylation and acetylation reactions (Fig. 5.1, pathway a). Deacylation is presumably mediated by phospholipase A_2. This enzyme may also release *sn*-2 fatty acid from other phospholipids (Fig. 5.1, pathway b) besides the alkyl ether precursor to PAF. Arachidonic acid is one of the major fatty acids released from the alkyl ether as well as other phospholipid pools. Following its release, the arachidonate generally is metabolized to hydroxyicosatetraenoates (HETEs), leukotrienes (LTs), thromboxanes (TXs) and/or prostaglandins (PGs). These metabolites are themselves bioactive and have effects that may overlap, complement or synergize those of PAF. Thus, PAF normally forms and operates in an environment rich with relevant co-products.

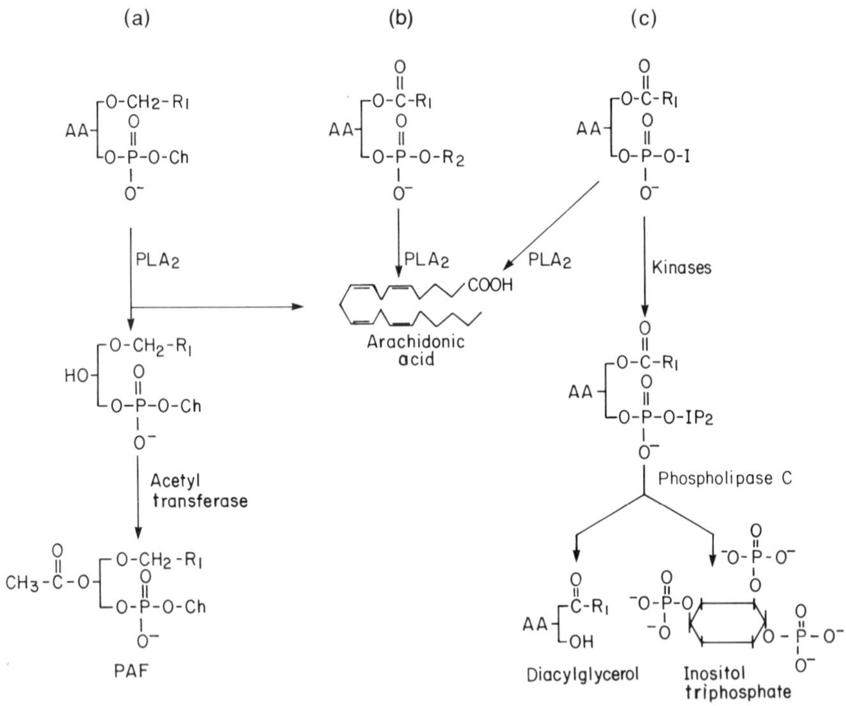

Fig. 5.1 Stimulus-induced phospholipid mobilization. Alkyl ether glycerophosphoclines are converted to PAF by phospholipase A_2 (PLA_2)-mediated deacylation followed by acetyl transferase-mediated acetylation, pathway (a). PAF inactivation proceeds by a reversal of this pathway: acetyhydrolase cleaves PAF and transacylase forms the acylated metabolite. In addition to the alkyl ether phospholipid, PLA_2 also removes fatty acid (commonly arachidonic acid) from 1-O-acyl phosholipids, pathway (b) and phosphatidylinositol. The latter phospholipid is also phosphorylated and then cleaved by phospholipase C to produce diacylglycerol and inositol triphophosphate, pathway (c).

Interactions between PAF and arachidonate metabolites may be critical to the responses examined in this review.

Cells also form PAF by a multi-step pathway utilizing 1-O-alkyl-2-lyso-*sn*-glycero-3-phosphate. In this pathway, the latter intermediate is formed from fatty alcohol and dihdroxyacetone phosphate. It is converted to PAF by *sn*-2 acetylation, with removal of the *sn*-3 phosphate group, and transfer of phosphocholine to the vacated *sn*-3 position. This pathway does not involve release of arachidonate; may operate in the constitutional (i.e. unstimulated) synthesis of PAF, and in certain cell types, may form PAF in concert with the deacylation–acetylation pathway described above.

Many cell types inactivate PAF. In general, this inactivation proceeds through a two-step sequence that, in effect, reverses the deacylation–acetylation synthetic pathway: PAF is deacetylated and the lyso-intermediate is transacylated (Fig. 5.1, pathway a). PAF catabolism appears to be induced by a variety of cellular stimuli, including PAF itself. It is both rapid and quantitative. For example, human PMN can inactivate PAF at rates as high as 100 000 molecules/min/cell.

Stimulus–response coupling

Mammalian cells often respond to exogenous, physiological stimuli through the following ordered sequence of reactions: (i) the stimulus binds with its plasmalemmal receptors; (ii) the ligand-bound receptors activate N-proteins; (iii) in turn, the N-proteins activate critical effector elements such as adenyl cyclase and phospholipase C; (iv) adenyl cyclase produces cAMP which activates protein kinase A; (v) phospholipase C cleaves phosphatidylinositol diphosphate into inositol triphosphate and diacyglycerol (Fig. 5.1, pathway c); (vi) inositol triphophate raises cytosolic Ca^{2+} by inducing the release of storage calcium; (vii) diacylglycerol, operating in concert with mobilized Ca^{2+}, activates protein kinase C (PKC); (viii) phospholipase A_2 is activated (perhaps directly by N-proteins or as a consequence of Ca^{2+} mobilization and PKC activation) and releases arachidonate from phospholipids (Fig. 5.1, pathways a and b) (ix) arachidonate is metabolized to HETE, LTs, TXs and PGs by enzymatic pathways which may themselves be induced during cell stimulation; and (x) phospholipase A_2-generated 1-O-alkyl-GPC is converted to PAF by acetyltransferase (Fig. 5.1, pathway a). The activated enzymes (e.g. protein kinase (PK) A, PKC), elevated cytosolic Ca^{2+}, and synthesized products (e.g. HETEs, LTs, TXs, PGs and PAF) proceed to trigger events that elicit or in other ways modulate cellular responses. They influence function in various ways. Some operate by binding to their own plasma-membrane receptors and stimulating the entire sequence anew. PAF acts in this manner.

PAF receptors

Early studies demonstrated specific, saturable uptake of PAF by PMN and platelets [21–23]. A large percentage of this uptake may have been due to ligand internalization and metabolism. More recent studies have examined PAF binding under non-metabolic conditions (i.e. at low temperature or with cells or organelles unable to process PAF). These studies have found that platelets [24–27], PMN [28–29], and cultured macrophages [30], as well as particulate fractions from these cells [28,31–33] and lung [34], liver [35], brain [36] and smooth muscle-containing tissues [31] reversibly bind PAF. PAF specific binding activity co-purifies with plasma membrane markers [28,31–36] and, in general, appears to involve a single class of homogeneous, high-affinity ($K_d \approx 0.2$–5 nM) receptors. PMN [28,29] and brain [36] may have low ($K_d \approx 30$–600 nM) along with high-affinity receptors. Chesney *et al.* have found three receptor affinity types in human platelets [26]. Nevertheless, most studies agree that the actions of PAF are transduced by high-affinity sites: In human PMN [37] and platelets [26], responses to PAF correlate with high-, but not low-, affinity binding.

High-affinity PAF receptors may rapidly down-regulate. For example, human platelets pretreated with even low concentrations of PAF quickly lose their PAF binding capacity [25,26] as well as their capacity to respond to a second PAF challenge [25,38]. The PAF-desensitized platelets respond fully to agonists acting through other plasmalemmal receptors. The platelets, therefore, have not exhausted their post-receptor, stimulus–transduction mechanism. PMN [2,3,29], monocytes [7], smooth muscle [17] and various other cell types pre-incubated with PAF also become unresponsive to PAF but not other agonists. These target cells may, like human platelets, down-regulate their PAF receptors. However, recent studies by Homma *et al.* [39] have found that PAF-pretreated rabbit platelets bind PAF normally. Consequently, PAF-induced unresponsiveness (or densitization) seems to have at least two origins: (i) it may reflect high-affinity receptor down-regulation; or (ii) alternatively, the uncoupling of these receptors from their normal linkages to the pathways involved in stimulus transduction. In either event, the development of desensitization may be critical in regulating function. PMNs challenged with PAF rapidly aggregate. Within 1–3 min the cells begin to disaggregate although their suspending medium contains stimulatory amounts of PAF [2,28]. Coincident with the onset of disaggregation, the PMNs lose their sensitivity to PAF. PAF receptors, therefore, seemed programmed to issue short-lived bursts of excitation and then to become inactive. This second phase of induced inactivity provides, in effect, a stop signal which limits, and allows reversal of, the cellular response. Similar events may occur *in vivo* and underlie, for example, the desensitization of allergic reactions (e.g. see [17,40]).

G-proteins

G-proteins are a series of dissociable hereotrimers with similar β-and γ-subunits but functionally and structually distinct α-subunits. Plasmalemmal receptors, when bound to their stimulating ligands, directly interact with these G-proteins. This produces three effects. First, the receptors' affinities for their ligands dramatically increase. In effect, low-affinity binding sites convert to a higher affinity state. Second, the G-protein subunits exchange their GDP for GTP and then dissociate from their β–γ-subunits. Third, the liberated, GTP-bound α-subunits move within the plasma membrane to interact with, and functionalize, adenyl cyclase (i.e. α- from G_s-proteins) or phospholipase C (α- from G_i- and G_o-proteins). However, the activated state is short-lived: subunits rapidly hydrolyze their GTP to GDP and then unite with their β–γ-subunits thereby reforming an inactive G-protein. The re-assembled G-protein can again associate with ligand-bound receptors and recycle repeatedly through the activated state. A single receptor, therefore, may activate many G-protein molecules to amplify its signalling capacity.

PAF receptors interact with this G-protein system. Thus, excess GTP (which dissociates G-proteins and, therefore, interferes with the G-protein-receptor association) dose dependently reduces high-affinity PAF binding to isolated plasma membranes of human PMN and platelets [41,42]. This suggests that G-proteins regulate the affinity state of PAF receptors. Furthermore, PAF stimulates GTPase activity in these membrane preparations [32,42–44]. This provides additional evidence of linkage between G-proteins and PAF receptors and suggests that these receptors induce G-protein subunit dissociation. Finally, PAF enhances phospholiphase C activity (see e.g. [45–47]), while blocking activation of adenyl cyclase [48,49], in intact cells. (However, in human PMN, PAF promotes net accumulation of cAMP [50], perhaps by raising cytosolic Ca^{2+} and thereby inhibiting cAMP degradation [51].) Thus, PAF receptors appear to activate G_1- or G_o-proteins without comparably influencing G_s-protein.

The conclusions made above are supported in studies using toxins which interfere with G-protein function. Pertussis toxin inactivates G_i and G_o proteins; it inhibits many functional responses of both rabbit and human PMN to PAF [52–56]). Cholera toxin continuously stimulates G_s-protein and, therefore, interferes with the receptor-mediated activation of G_s-protein. This toxin has relatively little effect on these same PAF-induced responses [55,57]. It should be emphasized, however, that human platelet responses to PAF seem to involve a novel (i.e. pertussis and cholera toxin-insensitive) G-protein [43]. Furthermore, the Ca^{2+}-mobilizing actions of PAF in rabbit [55] and human [47,57] PMN proceed, in part, either through a novel G-protein or, alternatively, through a pathway that bypasses G-proteins (see below). Currently, therefore, it appears that many, but not all, of the bioactions of PAF proceed through classically-defined G-proteins.

Phosphatidylinositol turnover

Cells stimulated with PAF cleave their membraneous phosphatidylinositol diphosphate into inositol triphosphate and diacyglycerol (Fig. 5.1, pathway c) [11,12,15,16,38,45,46,53,58–60]. This response occurs during the initial 15 s or so of cell challenge. Within 15–60 s, net accumulation of the two products begins to reverse as the cells: (i) dephosphorylate inositol triphosphate; (ii) phosphorylate diacylglycerol; and (iii) regenerate phosphatidylinositol phosphates. Desensitization also limits this cycle. For example, metabolism of phosphatidylinositols by PAF-challenged rabbit platelets decays rapidly (i.e. $t_{1/2} \approx 15$ s) and cannot be re-stimulated with PAF. The platelets, however, turnover their phosphatidylinositols anew in response to other agonists such as thrombin [38]. This finding suggests that the transduction defect in PAF-desensitized rabbit platelets (which bind PAF normally [39]) localizes between the PAF receptor–phospholiphase C linkage reactions.

Calcium (Ca^{2+})

Within seconds of PAF challenge, cells increase their cytosolic Ca^{2+}[11,12,16,19,20,25,47,53,55,57,61–77]. PAF elicits this response by (i) inducing the production of inositol triphosphate (which mobilizes storage Ca^{2+}[12,53–55,57,68,71–73] and (ii) opening plasmalemmal Ca^{2+} channels [11,12,16,19,25,47,53,55,61–63,67,68,72,73,75]. The relative contribution of these two alternate mechanisms varies with cell type. For example, PAF-induced calcium transients in cultured neurocytes seem completely dependent on extracellular Ca^{2+} and, therefore, presumably involve the opening of plasmalemmal Ca^{2+} channels rather than the mobilization of sub-cellular Ca^{2+}[19]. Contrastingly, human PMN Ca^{2+} transients, at least under some conditions (e.g., lower PAF concentrations), appear relatively independent of extracellular Ca^{2+} [57]. In most cell types and under many conditions, however, both mechanisms probably operate to varying extents [12,53,55,68,72,73]. Thus, in human PMN, high concentrations of PAF initially trigger release of storage Ca^{2+}. The attendant rises in cytosolic Ca^{2+} may then open plasma membrane, Ca^{2+}-sensitive, Ca^{2+} channels [72]. PAF-induced Ca^{2+} transients in rabbit PMN or human platelets also seem to involve both mechanisms although linkages between storage Ca^{2+} and membrane Ca^{2+} channels have not been directly demonstrated [53–55,61,67,68,73,75]. These two cells types raise cytosolic Ca^{2+} principally by increasing their plasma membrane Ca^{2+} permeability when challenged with lower concentrations of PAF

[55,61,67,68,73]. They mobilize storage Ca^{2+} only when challenged with high PAF concentrations.

The uptake of extracellar Ca^{2+} in PAF-stimulated rabbit platelets is dramatically inhibited by drugs that block the lipoxygenase-dependent metabolism of arachidonic acid to HETEs; agents blocking TX and PG production have relatively little effect on this response ([63], see also [68,71]). Hydroxylated arachidonate metabolites, then, may contribute to the regulation of Ca^{2+}-channel opening in rabbit platelets.

Contrasting with many other PAF-induced responses, PAF-induced uptake of extracellular Ca^{2+} is relatively insensitive to pertussis toxin ([47,53,55,57]; however, see [54] for conflicting results). This suggests that the link between PAF receptors and Ca^{2+} channels could involve either a novel G-protein or, perhaps, a G-protein-independent pathway. Naccache *et al.* [53] have considered the possibility that PAF receptors directly interact with, or are a part of, plasma membrane Ca^{2+} channels. Indeed Ca^{2+}-channel blockers inhibit PAF binding to human platelets [26,78]. Although the reason for this inhibition is unknown, it could indicate that there is a direct, physical association between Ca^{2+} channels and PAF receptors [78].

PAF-induced Ca^{2+} transients begin to reverse within 15–60 s; by 2–3 min, cytosolic Ca^{2+} levels return toward pre-stimulatory levels (e.g. see [57]). Restoration of normal Ca^{2+} levels reflects: (i) metabolic inactivation of inositol triphosphate; (ii) pumping of Ca^{2+} out of the cytosol by ATP-dependent mechanisms; (iii) closure of Ca^{2+} channels (in PAF-stimulated human platelets, the channels close with a $t_{1/2}$ of *c.* 1 min [69]); and (iv) desensitization of the cell to PAF [57,65,76,77].

Protein kinase C (PKC)

PKC exists as an inactive component of the cytosol in resting cells. During cell stimulation, it moves to plasmalemma, binds membranous diacylglycerol, and thereby becomes active in phosphorylating critical effector elements of the cellular response mechanism. Rises in cytosolic Ca^{2+} promote both the movement and activation of PKC [79]. Hence, Ca^{2+} and diacylglycerol serve as synergistic messengers in the regulation of PKC.

PAF stimulates the mobilization and activation of PKC in human PMN [80,81] and platelets[59]. It likewise induces rabbit [82] and human platelets [46,59] to phosphorylate a *c.* 40-kD protein (this phosphorylation appears mediated specifically by PKC [59]). The phospholipid induces these responses by an indirect [59,80,81], receptor-mediated [80] mechanism that requires responding cells to raise cytosolic Ca^{2+} [81,82]. Thus, PAF activates cellular PKC through the secondary messenger system outlined above.

The target proteins phosphorylated by PKC (e.g. myosin light-chain kinase), presumably, are thereby activated to promote events resulting in cellular responses [80,83–85]. However, the phosphorylated elements may also dampen function. For example, direct PKC activators inhibit human PMN [37], human platelet [64,66,70,73], rabbit PMN [53,75] and human vascular endothelium [84] responses to PAF. The PKC activators indirectly block the binding of PAF to high-affinity receptors on human PMN apparently by decreasing these receptors' availability [37]. Thus, activated PKC may down-regulate (or otherwise uncouple) PAF receptors. This effect could underlie desensitization. In this view, PAF-induced receptor activation results in the mobilization of PKC. The phosphorylating enzyme then feeds back upon these receptors to dampen their availability for ligand binding capacity (or linkages with, for example G-proteins). PKC, therefore, may operate as a stop signal to limit cellular responses initiated by PAF (see the above discussion on PAF receptors).

Phospholipid and arachidonate metabolism

PAF stimulates cells to release arachidonate from the *sn*-2 position of membranous phospholipids [12,15,58,86,87] and metabolize the fatty acid into HETEs, LTs, TXs, and PGs [13,50,86,88–93]. PAF appears to induce this release reaction by activating phospholipase A_2 [15,86] (Fig. 5.1, pathway b) through a mechanism dependent upon Ca^{2+}, calmodulin and PKC [94,95]. PAF also induces human and rat PMN to activate acetyltransferase [96,97] perhaps by stimulating cyclic AMP accumulation [98]. Thus, PAF influences both enzymes of the deacylation–acetylation pathway (Fig. 5.1, pathway a). Accordingly, PAF-challenged cells produce PAF [96,97] concurrently with various arachidonate metabolites.

Synergy and priming

PAF can interact with a second stimulus to induce cellular responses that far exceed in magnitude those elicited by either stimulus alone. Thus, 5-HETE increases, by as much as 100–1000-fold, the potency of PAF in stimulating human PMN to activate PKC [80], synthesize PAF [97], degranulate [99], and release superoxide anion (Braquet, P., unpublished). 5,15-diHETE and 5,20-diHETE are 30- and 100-fold weaker, respectively, than 5-HETE while other HETEs (e.g. 8-HETE and 15-HETE) are ineffective in promoting the bioactions of PAF [57,79]. Other examples of synergy include: PAF and PKC activators in human PMN and platelets [37,83,85]; PAF and chemotactic peptides in human PMN [2,100]; and PAF and either immunoglobulins [65] or epinephrine [101] in human platelets.

PAF may have an enduring effect on cellular responsiveness. Human PMN pre-incubated with PAF demonstrate remarkably enhanced responses to chemotactic peptides and PKC activators for up to 60 min [102–105]. Such sustained effects, which have been termed priming, occur at picomolar concentrations of PAF; they can result in enhanced PMN responses to various other agonists in assays of Ca^{2+} transients [104], assembly of actin [103], aggregation [2,104], degranulation [104], superoxide anion release [102,104–106], and endothelial cell injury [104]. It seems likely that these examples of synergy and/or priming reflect the selective recruitment of different, but cooperatively interacting, effector elements by the paired stimuli. For example, in the instance of PAF and PKC activators, PAF raises cytosolic calcium to increase the amount of PKC mobilized by a fixed amount of activator [37]. The 5-HETE–PAF synergy may have a similar basis. Recent studies find that 5-HETE raises cytosolic Ca^{2+} by a unique, possibly receptor-mediated mechanism [57]. This may promote the PKC-mobilizing actions of PAF [79,80] and thereby enhance PKC-dependent responses.

Inhibition of PAF effects

As shown above, PAF induces cells to form an expanding series of signalling molecules which elicit function. Interference with the formation or action of these signals can dampen the PAF-induced response. Indeed, a large number of studies show that competitive antagonists, inactivators of G-proteins, calcium antagonists, PKC blockers, and arachidonate antimetabolites inhibit PAF. Their effects, however, may vary with the cell type and response examined.

Responses in homogeneous tissues

As predicted by the transduction scheme, competetive antagonists of PAF reduce virtually all responses to PAF (see Chapter 4). Agents interfering with events occurring after the initial step of receptor binding have progressively more limited effects. Inactivation of G_i- or G_o-proteins inhibits many actions of PAF but seems less effective in reducing the influences of PAF on plasmalemmal calcium channels (see G-proteins). Interference with Ca^{2+} transients likewise reduces many platelet [68,73,82,107] and PMN [2,37,61,74,81,108] responses to PAF. PKC blockers, while not yet extensively examined, are reported to reduce human PMN degranulation induced with PAF [80].

Non-steroidal anti-inflammatory drugs (NSAID), which block TX and PG synthesis, weakly inhibit PAF-induced rabbit platelet aggregation and degranulation [89]. They have a much more substantial inhibitory effect on human platelet serotonin release without comparably inhibiting aggregation [68,90,91]. These drugs also block PMN adherence to nylon fibres stimulated by PAF [109]. However, many other PMN responses to PAF (e.g. autoaggregation, degranulation, superoxide anion generation, chemotaxis, etc.) are inhibited by lipoxygenase inhibitors rather than NSAID [50,86,92,108,111–114]. These latter responses, therefore, may be mediated by endogenously-formed HETEs and LTs.

Responses in heterogeneous tissues

Heterogeneous tissue responses to PAF may involve only a single type of cell. However, in such mixed-cell populations, PAF can stimulate specific target cells to release mediators which recruit other cell types into the final response. For example, isolated rat liver responds to PAF infusion by turning over its phosphatidylinositol stores and hydrolyzing glycogen [115]. NSAID inhibit the glycogenolytic actions of PAF. However, while PAF activates parenchymal vascular endothelium and macrophages, it does not appear to be capable of stimulating isolated hepatocytes. The data suggest that in liver some secondary cell (e.g. vascular endothelium or macrophage) responds to PAF by releasing TX or PG which, in turn, excites hepatocytes [116]. Other interesting examples of this transcellular mechanism exist. The vascular and spasmogenic effects of PAF in perfused rat lung are associated with the release of LTC_4; agents blocking the release or action of this LT inhibit lung responses to PAF [117]. In a platelet-perfused rabbit lung model, PAF-induced vasoconstriction and parenchymal oedema are inhibited by either platelet depletion or inhibitors of TX formation. Here, PAF appears to stimulate platelet release of TXA_2. This arachidonate metabolite may then constrict pulmonary veins thereby raising capillary pressure and producing a transudation of blood fluid into lung parenchyma [118]. Similarly, contractile responses of rabbit lung to PAF may be similarly mediated by the release of HETEs or LTs [119]. However, contraction of guinea-pig lung strips induced by PAF is blocked by tetrodotoxin and atropine while being enhanced with physostigmine. Spasmogenic responses to PAF in this system may result from stimulation of parasympathetic, cholinergic, post-synaptic neurons [120]. Finally, PAF inhibits mitogen-induced T-cell proliferation *in vitro* [9, 121]. This inhibition is partly reversed by a NSAID and, therefore, may be mediated through the release of TX or PG by PAF-stimulated monocytes [9]. (PAF may also act more directly to stimulate suppressor [9] and, perhaps other lymphocytic cells [121,122] in this system.)

In vivo responses

PAF was initially implicated in anaphylaxis because (i) leukocytes from sensitized rabbits release PAF when challenged with allergen; (ii) PAF circulates in the blood of animals undergoing classical anaphylactic reactions [127]; (iii) selected tissues from animals undergoing anaphylaxis are desensitized to PAF; and (iv) PAF mimics many aspects of the anaphylactic reaction [1,123]. To varying extents, PAF has been similarly implicated in rabbit serum sickness [124], rat endotoxaemia [125] and human cold urticaria [126]. Furthermore, PAF is detected in human amniotic fluid [18,128] and psoriatic scales [129]; consequently, it has been suggested that it is involved in nidation, parturition, and the inflammatory component of psoriasis. Finally, recent studies lead further support to a general role for PAF in disease. PAF-specific competitive antagonists dramatically ameliorate endotoxic shock in rats [125,130,131] and an agent that inhibits the release of PAF reduces human angioedema in cold urticaria [126]. While the target cells and mechanisms involved in these presumed effects of PAF have not yet been identified, studies on some of the more limited *in vivo* actions of the phospholipid have been reported.

PAF increases vascular permeability when injected cutaneously [17] or systemically [132–136]. The local effects of PAF on animal and human vascular permeability are synergistically enhanced by PGs [137] and, in guinea-pigs, inhibited by NSAID [135]. Thus, the oedematous reaction appears to involve, in part, the release of PG or TX from an unidentified (perhaps vascular endothelial) cell in response to PAF. The effects of PAF on vascular tone, contrastingly, are only minimally inhibited by NSAID [138,139]. Compounds inhibiting lipoxygenase or the actions of peptido-leukotrienes reduce the blood pressure-altering effects of PAF [116,117,138,139]. Pharmacological studies similarly implicate lipoxygenase-dependent but not cyclooxygenase-dependent products in the *in vivo* actions of PAF on the release of tissue plasminogen activator [140], induction of bowel ischemia [141] and cutaneous hyperalgesia [142].

PAF, when insufflated or intravenously injected, contracts the airways of guinea-pigs, dogs, rhesus monkeys and humans [143–148]. The effect is one of immediate but short-lived airways constriction followed by a sustained (e.g. up to 2 weeks in humans [145]) broncheolar hyper-reactivity. Thus, while the airways are unresponsive or desensitized to a second PAF challenge [143–145], they are overly responsive to other spasmogens [143,145–148]. These findings have been interpreted as indicating that PAF primes pulmonary airway smooth muscle to a state of generalized, asthma-like irritability. The bronchoconstrictive diathesis in hypoxia may similarly involve PAF [149]. Both the acute spastic and sustained priming effects of PAF on guinea-pig airways are platelet-dependent [144–146] and, in dogs, both effects are blocked with inhibitors of TX synthesis [148]. Blockers of LT synthesis also inhibit the bronchospastic actions of PAF [150–151]. The available data, therefore, suggest that PAF stimulates platelets and/or other non-smooth muscle cells to release spasmogens (e.g. TXA_2 and LTC_4) which contract and also prime smooth muscle. Furthermore, PAF challenge depletes human lung [152] and rat brain [153] of β-adrenergic receptors. These receptors dilate bronchi and may be responsible for promoting airway opening. Loss of such receptors, therefore, may leave lung airways with defective dilatory mechanisms and, consequently, an imbalanced tendency to contract when stimulated.

Conclusions

Cells respond to many stimuli through a mechanism involving specific receptors that link with G-proteins, adenyl cyclase, cAMP, protein kinase A, phospholipase C, phosphatidylinositol turnover, cytosolic Ca^{2+} transients, Ca^{2+}-dependent effector elements (e.g. calmodulin), PKC, phospholipase A_2, and the production of bioactive arachidonate metabolites as well as PAF. PAF activates its many target cells through this same mechanism and, therefore, is both a product and stimulator of the transduction cascade. The phospholipid may function normally in a positive feedback loop to amplify the activation of this cascade and thereby the cellular response to exogenous stimuli.

The *in vitro* and *in vivo* bioactions of PAF appear limited by receptor down-regulation or uncoupling from other elements of the stimulus–response mechanism. PKC may mediate these stop signals. Thus, the cascade of events transducing the bioactions of PAF appear to contain a negative-feedback loop that dampens cellular responses to the phospholipid. Pharmacological agents that interfere with the transduction mechanism also can inhibit PAF-induced responses. Competitive antagonists, calcium antagonists, PKC blockers, and arachidonate anti-metabolites demonstrate such inhibitory effects. Future studies will determine if these agents can interfere with PAF in humans and thereby serve as clinically useful drugs to ameliorate disease.

Acknowledgements

The authors wish to thank Ms Jean Kimbrell for her expert help in preparing the manuscript.

References

1 O'Flaherty, J. T. & Wykle, R. L. Biology and biochemistry of platelet-activating factor. *Clin. Rev. Allergy* (1983), **1,** 353–567.

2 O'Flaherty, J. T., Lees, C. J., Miller, C. H. *et al.* Selective desensitization of neutrophils: Further studies with 1-O-alkyl-*sn*-glycero-3-phosphocholine analogues. *J. Immunol.* (1981), **127**, 731–737.

3 Shaw, J. O., Pinckard, R. N., Ferrigni, K. S., McManus, L. M. & Hanahan, D. J. Activation of human neutrophils with 1-O-hexadecyl/octadecyl-2-acetyl-*sn*-glyceryl-3-phosphorylcholine (platelet activating factor). *J. Immunol.* (1981), **127**, 1250–1255.

4 Wardlaw, A. J., Moqbel, R., Cromwell, O. & Kay, A. B. Platelet-activating factor: a potent chemotactic and chemokinetic factor for human eosinophils. *J. Clin. Invest.* (1986), **78**, 1701–1706.

5 Kimani, G., Tonnesen, M. G. & Henson, P. M. Stimulation of eosinophil adherence to human vascular endothelial cells *in vitro* by platelet-activating factor. *J. Immunol.* (1988), **140**, 3161–3166.

6 Bochner, B. S., Peachell, P. T., Brown, K. E. & Schleimer, R. P. Adherence of human basophils to cultured umbilical vein endothelial cells. *J. Clin. Invest.* (1988), **81**, 1355–1364.

7 Yasaka, T., Boxer, L. A. & Baehner, R. L. Monocyte aggregation and superoxide anion release in response to formyl-methionyl-leucyl-phenylalanine (FMLP) and platelet-activating factor (PAF). *J. Immunol.* (1982), **128**, 1939–1944.

8 Czarnetzki, B. Increased monocyte chemotaxis towards leukotriene B_4 and platelet activating factor in patients with inflammatory dermatoses. *Clin. Exp. Immunol.* (1983), **54**, 486–492.

9 Rola-Pleszczynski, M., Pouliot, C., Turcotte, S., Pignol, B., Braquet, P. & Bouvrette, L. Immune regulation by platelet-activating factor. *J. Immunol.* (1988), **140**, 3547–3552.

10 Bussolino, F., Camussi, G., Aglietta, M., Braquet, P., Bosia, A., Pescarmona, G., Sanavio, F., D'Urso, N., Marchisio, P. C. Human endothelial cells are target for platelet-activating factor. *J. Immunol.* (1987), **139**, 2439–2446.

11 Pfeilschifter, J., Kurtz R., & Bauer, C. Inhibition of renin secretion by platelet activating factor (acetylglyceryl ether phosphorylcholine) in cultured rat renal juxtaglomerular cells. *Biochem. Biophys. Res. Commun.* (1985), **127**, 903–910.

12 Bonventre, J. V., Weber, P. C. & Gronich, J. H. PAF and PDGF increase cytosolic [Ca^{2+}] and phospholipase activity in mesangial cells. *Am. J. Physiol.* (1988), **254**, F87–F94.

13 Hartung, H-P, Acetyl glyceryl ether phosphorylcholine (platelet-activating factor) mediates heightened metabolic activity in macrophages. *FEBS Lett.* (1983), **160**, 209–212.

14 Hayashi, H., Kudo, I., Inove, K., Onozaki, K., Tsushima, S., Nomura, H. & Nojima, S. Macrophage activation by PAF incorporated into dipalmitoylphosphatidylcholine-cholesterol liposomes. *J. Biochem.* (1985), **97**, 1255–1258.

15 Kawaguchi, H. & Yasuda, H. Platelet-activating factor-stimulates phospholipase in quiescent Swiss mouse 3T3 fibroblast. *FEBS Lett.* (1984), **176**, 93–96.

16 Soling, H-D., Eibl, H. & Fest, W. Acetylcholine-like effects of 1-O-alkyl-2-acetyl-*sn*-glycero-3-phosphocholine (platelet-activating factor) and its analogues in exocrine secretory glands. *Eur. J. Biochem.* (1984), **144**, 65–72.

17 Stimler, N. P., Bloor, C. M., Hugli, T. E., Wykle, R. L., McCall, C. E., & O'Flaherty, J. T. Anaphylactic actions of platelet-activating factor. *Am. J. Pathol.* (1981), **105**, 54–69.

18 Nishihira, J., Ishibashi, T., Imai, Y. & Muramatsu, T. Mass spectrometric evidence for the presence of platelet-activating factor (1-O-alkyl-2-acetyl-*sn*-glycero-3-phosphocholine) in human amniotic fluid during labor. *Lipids* (1984), **19**, 907–910.

19 Kornecki, E. & Ehrlich, Y. H. Neuroregulatory and neuropathological actions of the ether-phospholipid platelet-activating factor. *Science* (1988), **240**, 1792–1794.

20 Johnston, J. M., Bleasdale, J. E. & Hoffman, D. R. Functions of PAF in reproduction and development: involvement of PAF in fetal lung maturation and parturition. In Snyder, F. (ed). *Platelet-Activating Factor and Related Lipid Mediators* (1987), pp. 375–401. Plenum Press, New York.

21 Camussi, G., Bussolino, F., Tetta, C., Brusca, R. & Racni, R. The binding of platelet-activating factor (PAF) to polymorphonuclear neutrophils (PMN) as a trigger for the immune-induced PMN aggregation. *Pan. Med.* (1980), **22**, 1–5.

22 Valone, F. H., Coles, E., Reinhold, V. R. & Goetzl, E. J. Specific binding of phospholipid platelet-activating factor by human platelets. *J. Immunol.* (1982), **129**, 1637–1641.
23 Valone, F. H. & Goetzl, E. J. Specific binding by human polymorphonuclear leucocytes of the immunological mediator 1-O-hexadecyl/octadecyl-2-acetyl-*sn*-glycero-3-phosphorylcholine. *Immunology* (1983), **48**, 141–148.
24 Kloprogge, E. & Akkerman, J. W. N. Binding kinetics of PAF-acether 1-O-alkyl-2-acetyl-*sn*-glycero-3-phosphocholine) to intact human platelets. *Biochem. J.* (1984), **223**, 901–909.
25 Inarrea, P., Gomez-Cambronero, J., Nieto, M. & Crespo, M. S. Characteristics of the binding of platelet-activating factor to platelets of different animal species, *Eur. J. Pharmacol.* (1984), **105**, 309–315.
26 Chesney, C. M., Pifer, D. D. & Huch, K. M. Desensitization of human platelets by platelet activating factor. *Biochem. Biophys. Res. Commun.* (1985), **127**, 24–30.
27 Kloprogge, E., Mommersteeg, M. & Akkerman, J. W. Kinetics of platelet-activating factor 1-O-aklyl-2-acetyl-*sn*-glycero-3-phosphocholine-induced fibrinogen binding to human platelets. *J. Biol. Chem.* (1986), **261**, 11 071–11 076.
28 O'Flaherty, J. T., Surles, J. R., Redman, J., Jacobson, D., Piantadosi, C. & Wykle, R. L. Binding and metabolism of platelet-activating factor by human neutrophils. *J. Clin. Invest.* (1986), **78**, 381–388.
29 O'Flaherty, J. T., Redman, J.F., Jr, Schmitt, J. D. Ellis, J. M., Surles, J. R., Marx, M. H., Piantadosi, C. & Wykle, R. L. 1-O-alkyl-2-N-methyl-carbamyl-glycero-phosphocholine: A biologically potent, non-metabolizable analog of platelet-activating factor. *Biochem. Biophys. Res. Commun.* (1987), **147**, 18–24.
30 Valone, R. H. Identification of platelet-activating factor receptors in P388D murine macrophages. *J. Immunol.* (1988), **140**, 2389–2394.
31 Hwang, S. B., Lee, C-S.C., Cheah, M. J. & Shen, T. Y. Specific receptor sites for 1-O-alkyl-2-O-acetyl-*sn*-glycero-3-phosphocholine (platelet activating factor) on rabbit platelet and guinea pig smooth muscle membranes. *Biochemistry* (1983), **22**, 4756–4763.
32 Hwang, S-B. Identification of a second putative receptor of platelet-activating factor from human polymorphonuclear leukocytes. *J. Biol. Chem.* (1988), **263**, 3225–3233.
33 Valone, F. H. & Ruis, N. M. Platelet-activating factor binding to human platelet membranes. *Biotech. Appl. Biochem.* (1986), **8,** 465–470.
34 Hwang, S-B., Lam, M-H. & Shen, T. Y. Specific binding sites for platelet activating factor in human lung tissues. *Biochem. Biophys. Res. Commun.* (1985), **128**, 972–979.
35 Hwang, S-B. Specific receptor sites for platelet activating factor on rat liver plasma membranes. *Arch. Biochem. Biophys.* (1987), **257**, 339–344.
36 Domingo, M. T., Spinnewyn, B., Chabrier, P. E. & Braquet, P. Presence of specific binding sites for platelet-activating factor (PAF) in brain. *Biochem. Biophys. Res. Commun.* (1988), **51**, 730–736.
37 O'Flaherty, J. T., Jacobson, D. P. & Redman, J. R. Bidirectional effects of protein kinase C activators. *J. Biol. Chem.* (1989), **264**, 6834–6836.
38 Morrison, W. J. & Shukla, S. D. Desensitization of receptor-coupled activation of phosphoinositide-specific phospholipase C in platelets: evidence for distinct mechanisms for platelet-activating factor and thrombin. *Mol. Pharmacol.* (1988), **33**, 58–63.
39 Homma, H., Tokumura, A. & Hanahan, D. J. Binding and internalization of platelet-activating factor 1-O-alkyl-2-acetyl-*sn*-glycero-3-phosphocholine in washed rabbit platelets. *J. Biol. Chem.* (1987). **262**. 10 582–10 587.

40 Halonen, M., Palmer, J. D., Lohman, I. C., McManus, L. M. & Pinckard, R. N. Respiratory and circulatory alterations induced by acetyl glyceryl ether phosphorylcholine, a mediator of IgE anaphylaxis in the rabbit. *Am. Rev. Resp. Dis.* (1980), **122**, 915–924.
41 Ng, D. S. & Wong, K. GTP regulation of platelet-activating factor binding to human neutrophil membranes. *Biochem. Biophys. Res. Commun.* (1986), **141**, 353–359.
42 Hwang, S-B., Lam, M-H. & Pong, S. S. Ionic and GTP regulation of binding of platelet-activating factor to receptors and platelet-activating factor-induced activation of GTPase in rabbit platelet membranes. *J. Biol. Chem.* (1986), **261**, 532–537.
43 Houslay, M. D., Bojanic, D. & Wilson, A. Platelet activating factor and U44069 stimulate a GTPase activity in human platelets which is distinct from the guanine necleotide regulatory proteins, N_s and N_i. *Biochem. J.* (1986), **234**, 737–740.
44 Matsumoto, T., Molski, T. F. P., Kanaho, Y., Becker, E. L. & Sha'afi, R. I. G-Protein dissociation, GTP–GDP exchange and GTPase activity in control and PMA treated neutrophils stimulated by fMet–Leu–Phe. *Biochem. Biophys. Res. Commun.* (1987), **143**, 489–498.
45 Lapetina, E. G. Platelet-activating factor stimulates the phosphatidylinositol cycle. *J. Biol. Chem.* (1982), **257**, 7314–7317.
46 Lapetina, E. G. & Siegel, F. L. Shape change induced in human platelets by platelat-activating factor. *J. Biol. Chem.* (1983), **258**, 7241–7244.
47 Verghese, M. W., Charles, L., Jakoi, L., Dillon, S. B. & Snyderman, R. Role of a guanine nucleotide regulatory protein in the activation of phospholipase C by different chemoattractants. *J. Immunol.* (1987), **138**, 4374–4380.
48 Haslam, R. J. & Vanderwel, M. Inhibition of platelet adenylate cyclase 1-O-aklyl-2-O-acetyl-*sn*-glyceryl-3-phosphorylcholine (platelet-activating factor). *J. Biol. Chem.* (1982), **57**, 6879–6885.
49 Williams, K. A. & Haslam, R. J. Effects of NaCl on the inhibition of platelet adenylate cyclase by 1-O-octadecyl-2-O-acetyl-*sn*-glyceryl-3-phosphorylcholine (synthetic platelet-activating factor). *Biochim. Biophys. Acta* (1984), **770**, 216–223.
50 Gorman, R. R., Morton, D. R., Hopkins, N. K. & Lin, A. H. Acetyl glyceryl ether phosphorylcholine stimulates leukotriene B_4 synthesis and cyclic AMP accumulation in human polymorphonuclear leukocytes. *Adv. Prost. Thromb. Leuk. Res.* (1983), **12**, 57–63.
51 Verghese, M. W., Fox, K., McPhail, L. C. & Snyderman, R. Chemoattractant-elicited alterations of cAMP levels in human polymorphonuclear leukocytes requires a Ca^{2+} dependent mechanism which is independent of transmembrane activation of adenyl cyclase. *J. Biol. Chem.* (1985), **260**, 6769–6776.
52 Lad, P. M., Olson, C. V. & Grewal, I. S. Platelet-activating factor mediated effects on human neutrophil function are inhibited by pertussis toxin. *Biochem. Biophys. Res. Commun.* (1985), **129**, 632–638.
53 Naccache, P. H., Molski, M. M., Volpi, M., Becker, E. L. & Sha'afi, R. I. Unique inhibitory profile of platelet activating factor induced calcium mobilization, polyphosphoinositide turnover and granule enzyme secretion in rabbit neutrophils towards pertusis toxin and phorbol ester. *Biochem. Biophys. Res. Commun.* (1985), **130**, 677–684.
54 Lad, P. M., Olson, C. V., Grewal, I. S. & Scott, S. J. A pertussis toxin-sensitive GTP-binding protein in the human neutrophil regulates multiple receptors, calcium mobilization, and lectin-induced capping. *Proc. Nat. Acad. Sci.* (1985), **82**, 8643–8647.

55 Naccache, P. H., Molski, M. M., Volpi, M., Shefcyk, J., Molski, T. F., Loew, L., Becker, E. L. & Sha'afi, R. I. Biochemical events associated with the stimulation of rabbit neutrophils by platelet-activating factor. *J. Leuk. Biol.* (1986), **40**, 533–548.
56 Sha'afi, R. I., & Molski, T. F. P. Signalling for increased cytoskeletal actin in neutrophils. *Biochem. Biophys. Res. Commun.* (1987), **145**, 934–941.
57 O'Flaherty, J. T., Jacobson, D. & Redman, J. Mechanism involved in the mobilization of neutrophil calcium by 5-hydroxyeicosatetraenoate. *J. Immunol.* (1988), **140**, 4323–4328.
58 Shukla, S. D. & Hanahan, D. J. AGEPC (platelet activating factor) induced stimulation of rabbit platelets: effect on phosphatidylinositol, di- and tri-phosphoinositides and phosphatidic acid metabolism. *Biochem. Biophys. Res. Commun.* (1982), **106**, 697–703.
59 Ieyasu, H., Takai Y., Kaibuchi, K., Sawamura, M. & Nishizuka, Y. A role of calcium-activated, phospholipid-dependent protein kinase in platelet-activating factor-induced serotonin release from rabbit platelets. *Biochem. Biophys. Res. Commun.* (1982), **108**, 1701–1708.
60 Mauco, G., Chap H. & Douste-Blazy, L. Platelet activating factor (PAF-acether) promotes an early degradation of phosphatidylinositol-4,5-biphosphate in rabbit platelets. *FEBS Lett.* (1983), **153**, 361–365.
61 O'Flaherty, J. T., Swendsen, C. L., Lees, C. J. & McCall, C. E. Role of extracellular calcium in neutrophil degranulation responses to 1-O-alkyl-2-O-acetyl-*sn*-glycero-3-phosphocholine. *Am. J. Pathol.* (1981), **105**, 207–213.
62 Lee, T-c., Malone, B., Blank, M. L. & Snyder, F. 1-Aklyl-2-acetyl-*sn*-glycero-3-phosphocholine (platelet-activating factor) stimulates calcium influx in rabbit platelets. *Biochem. Biophys. Res. Commun.* (1981), **102**, 1262–1268.
63 Lee, T-c., Malone B. & Snyder, F. Stimulation of calcium uptake by 1-alkyl-2-acetyl-*sn*-glycero-3-phosphocholine (platelet-activating factor (in rabbit platelets: possible involvement of the lipoxygenase pathway. *Arch. Biochem. Biophys.* (1983), **223**, 33–39.
64 MacIntyre, D. E., McNicol, A. & Drummond, A. H. Tumour-promoting phorbol esters inhibit agonist-induced phosphatidate formation and Ca^{2+} flux in human platelets. *FEBS Lett.* (1985), **180**, 160–64.
65 Valone, F. H. & Johnson, B. Modulation of cytoplasmic calcium in human platelets by the phospholipid platelet-activating factor 1-O-alkyl-2-acetyl-*sn*-glycero-3-phosphorylcholine. *J. Immunol.* (1985), 1120–1124.
66 Zavoico, G. B., Halenda, S. P. Phorbol myristate acetate inhibits thrombin-stimulated Ca^{2+} mobilization and phosphatidylinositol 4,5-bisphosphate hydrolysis in human platelets. *Proc. Nat. Acad. Sci. (USA)* (1985), **82**, 3859–3862.
67 Hallam, T. J. & Rink, T. J. Agonists stimulate divalent cation channels in the plasma membrane of human platelets. *FEBS Lett.* (1985), **186**, 175–179.
68 Hallam, T. J., Sanchez, A. & Rink, T. J. Stimulus–response coupling in human platelets. Changes evoked by platelet-activating factor in cytoplasmic free calcium monitored with the fluorescent calcium indicator quin-2. *Biochem. J.* (1984), **218**, 819–827.
69 Valone, F. H. & Johnson, B. Decay of the activating signal after platelet stimulation with 1-O-alkyl-2-acetyl-*sn*-glycero-3-phosphorylcholine: changes in calcium permeability. *Thromb. Res.* (1985), **40**, 385–392.
70 MacIntyre, D. E., Bushfield, M. & Shaw, A. M. Regulation of platelet cytosolic free calcium by cyclic nucleotides and protein kinase C. *FEBS Lett. et al.* (1985), **188**, 383–388.
71 Doyle, V. M., Creba, J. A. & Rüegg, U. T. Platelet-activating factor mobilises intracellular calcium in vascular smooth muscle cells. *FEBS Lett.* (1986), **197**, 13–16.

72 Von Tscharner, V., Prod'hom, B., Baggiolini, M. & Reuter, H. Ion channels in human neutrophils activated by a rise in free cytosolic calcium concentration. *Nature* (1986), **324**, 369–372.

73 Valone, F. H. & Johnson, B. Modulation of platelet-activating-factor-induced calcium influx and intracellular calcium release in platelets by phorbol esters. *Biochem. J.* (1987), **247**, 669–674.

74 Hartiala, K. T., Scott, I. G., Viljanen, M. L. & Ackerman, K. E. Lack of correlation between calcium mobilization and respiratory burst activation induced by chemotactic factors in rabbit polymorphonuclear leukocytes. *Biochem. Biophys. Res. Commun.* (1987), **144**, 794–800.

75 Molski, T. F. P., Tao, W., Becker, E. L. & Sha'afi, R. I. Intracellular calcium rise produced by platelet-activating factor is deactivated by fMet–Leu–Phe and this requires uninterrupted activation sequence: Role of protein kinase. C. *Biochem. Biophys. Res. Commun.* (1988), **151**, 836–843.

76 Brock, T. A. & Gimbrone, M. A., Jr. Platelet activating factor alters calcium homeostasis in cultured vascular endothelial cells. *Am. J. Physiol.* (1986), H1086–H1092.

77 Bussolino, F., Aglietta, M., Sanavio, F., Stacchini, A., Lauri, D. & Camussi, G. Alkyl-ether phosphoglycerides influence calcium fluxes into human endothelial cells. *J. Immunol.* (1985), **135 (2)**, 48–53.

78 Valone, F. H. Inhibition of platelet-activating factor binding to human platelets by calcium channel blockers. *Thromb. Res.* (1987), **45**, 427–435.

79 O'Flaherty, J. T. & Nishihira, J. 5-Hydroxyicosatetraenoate promotes Ca^{2+} and protein kinase C mobilization in neutrophils. *Biochem. Biophys, Res. Commun.* (1987), **148**, 575–581.

80 O'Flaherty, J. T. & Nishihira, J. Arachidonate metabolites, platelet-activating factor, and the mobilization of protein kinase C in human polymorphonuclear neutrophils. *J. Immunol.* (1987), **138**, 1889–1895.

81 Gay, J. C. & Stitt, E. S. Platelet-activating factor induces protein kinase activity in the particulate fraction of human neutrophils. *Blood* (1988), **71**, 159–165.

82 Shaw, J. O. & Lyons, R. M. Requirements for different Ca^{2+} pools in the activation of rabbit platelets. *Biochim. Biophys. Acta* (1982), **714**, 492–499.

83 O'Flaherty, J. T., Schmitt, J. D., McCall, C. E. & Wykle, R. L. Diacylglycerols enhance human neutrophil degranulation responses: relevancy to a multiple mediator hypothesis of cell function. *Biochem. Biophys. Res. Commun.* (1984), **123**, 64–70.

84 Brock, T. A., Griendling, K. K. & Gimbrone, M. A. Phorbol ester-induced desensitization of platelet activating factor effects on calcium flux in vascular endothelial cells. In Winslow, C. M. & Lee, M. L. (eds) *New Horizons in Platelet Activating Factor Research* (1987), pp. 197–205. John Wiley, New York.

85 Siess, W. & Lapetina, E. G. Phorbol esters sensitize platelets to activation by physiological agonists. *Blood* (1987), **70**, 1373–1381.

86 Chilton, F. H., O'Flaherty, J. T., Walsh, C. E. *et al.* Platelet activating factor. Stimulation of the lipoxygenase pathway in polymorphonuclear leukocytes by 1-O-alkyl-2-O-acetyl-*sn*-glycero-3-phosphocholine. *J. Biol. Chem.* (1982), **257**, 5402–5407.

87 Tou, J-S. Platelet-activating factor modulates phospholipid acylation in human neutrophils. *Lipids* (1987), **22**, 333–337.

88 Tou, J-S. Platelet-activating factor promotes arachidonate incorporation into phosphatidylinositol and phosphatidylcholine in neutrophils. *Biochem. Biophys. Res. Commun.* (1985), **127**, 1045–1051.

89 Shaw, J. O., Printz, M. P., Hirabayashi, K. & Henson, P. M. Role of prostaglandin synthesis in rabbit platelet activation induced by basophil-derived platelet-activating factor. *J. Immunol.* (1978), **121**, 1939–1945.

90 Marcus, A. J., Safier, L. B., Ullman, H. L. *et al.* Effects of acetyl glyceryl ether phosphorylcholine on human platelet function *in vitro*. *Blood* (1981), **58**, 1027–1031.
91 Dahl, M-L. Aggregating and prostanoid-releasing effects of platelet-activating factor and leukotrienes on human polymorphonuclear leukocytes and platelets. *Int. Arch. Allergy Appl. Immunol.* (1985), **76**, 145–150.
92 Lin, A. H., Morton, D. R. & Gorman, R. R. Acetyl glyceryl ether phosphorylcholine stimulates leukotriene B_4 synthesis in human polymorphonuclear leukocytes. *J. Clin. Invest.* (1982), **70**, 1058–1065.
93 Ingraham, L. M., Coates, T. D., Allen, J. M., Higgins, C. P., Baehner, R. L. & Boxer, L. A. Metabolic, membrane, and functional responses of human polymorphonuclear leukocytes to platelet-activating factor. *Blood* (1982), **59**, 1259–1266.
94 Billah, M. M., Bryant, R. W. & Siegel, M. I. Lipoxygenase products of arachidonic acid modulate biosynthesis of platelet-activating factor (1-O-alkyl-2-acetyl-*sn*-glycero- 3-phosphocholine) by human neutrophils via phospholipase A_2. *J. Biol. Chem.* (1985), **260**, 6899–6906.
95 McIntyre, T. M., Reinhold, S. L., Prescott, S. M. & Zimmerman, G. A. Protein kinase C activity appears to be required for the synthesis of platelet-activating factor and leukotriene B_4 by human neutrophils. *J. Biol. Chem.* (1987), **262**, 15 370–15 376.
96 Doebber, T. W. & Wu, M. S. Platelet-activating factor (PAF) stimulates the PAF-synthesizing enzyme acetyl-CoA:1-alkyl-*sn*-glycero-3-phosphocholine O-acetyl transferase and PAF synthesis in neutrophils. *Proc. Nat. Acad. Sci. (USA)* (1987), **84**, 7557–7561.
97 Tessner, T. G., O'Flaherty, J. T. & Wykle, R. E., (1989). Stimulation of platelet-activating factor synthesis by a non-metabolizable bioactive analog of platelet-activating factor and influence of arachidonic acid metabolites. *J. Biol. Chem.*, **264**, 4794–4799.
98 Nieto, M. L., Velasco, S. & Sanchez Crespo, M. Modulation of acetyl-CoA:1-alkyl-2-lyso-*sn*-glycero-3-phosphocholine (lyso-PAF) acetyltransferase in human polymorphonuclears. *J. Biol. Chem.* (1988), **263**, 4607–4611.
99 O'Flaherty, J. T. Neutrophil degranulation: evidence pertaining to its mediation by the combined effects of leukotriene B_4, platelet-activating factor, and 5-HETE. *J. Cell Physiol.* (1985), **122**, 229–239.
100 Dewald, B. & Baggiolini, M. Activation of NADPH oxidase in human neutrophils. Synergism between fMLP and the neutrophil products PAF and LTB_4. *Biochem. Biophys. Res. Commun.* (1985), **128**, 297–304.
101 Vargaftig, B. B, Fouque, F., Joseph, D., Odiot, J. & Benveniste, J. Synergized activation of human platelets by epinephrine and platelet-activating factor-acether is adenosine diphosphate and thromboxane A_2-independent. *Adv. Prost. Thromb. Leuk. Res.* (1983), **11**, 429–432.
102 Kojima, S., Hagiwara, H., Soga, W., Sekiya, F., Saito, Y. & Inada, Y. Cooperativity between platelet-activating factor and collagen in platelet aggregation. *Biochem. Biophys. Res. Commun.* (1987), **145**, 915–920.
103 Gay, J. C., Beckman, J. K., Zaboy, K. A. & Lukens, J. N. Modulation of neutrophil oxidative responses to soluble stimuli by platelet-activating factor. *Blood* (1986), **67**, 931–936.
104 Shalit, M., Dabiri, G. A. & Southwick, F. S. Platelet-activating factor both stimulates and 'primes' human polymorphonuclear leukocyte actin filament assembly. *Blood* (1987), **70**, 1921–1927.
105 Vercellotti, G. M., Yin H.Q., Gustafson, K. S., Nelson, R. D. & Jacob, H. S. Platelet-activating factor primes neutrophil responses to agonists: role in promoting neutrophil-mediated endothelial damage. *Blood*, (1988), **17**, 1100–1107.

106 Worthen, G. S., Seccombe, J. F., Clay, K. L. Guthrie, L. A. & Johnston, R. B., Jr. The priming of neutrophils by lipopolysaccharide for production of intracellular platelet-activating factor. *J. Immunol.* (1988), **140**, 3553–3559.
107 Shaw, J. O. & Lyons, R. M. Requirement for different Ca^{2+} pools in the activation of rabbit platelets. II. Phospholipase activity. *Biochim. Biophys. Acta.* (1982), **714**, 500–504.
108 O'Flaherty, J. T., Wykle, R. L., Lees, C. J., Shewmake, T., McCall, C. E. & Thomas, M. J. Neutrophil-degranulating action of 5,12-dihydroxy-6,8,10,14-eicosatetraenoic acid and 1-O-alkyl-2-O-acetyl-*sn*-glycero-3-phosphocholine. *Am. J. Pathol.* (1981), **105**, 264–269.
109 Valone, F. H. & Goetzl, E. J. Enhancement of human polymorphonuclear leukocyte adherence by the phospholipid mediator 1-O-alkyl-2-O-acetyl-*sn*-glycero-3-phosphorylcholine (AGEPC). *Am. J. Pathol.* (1983), **113**, 85–89.
110 Moodley, I. & Stuttle, A. Evidence for a dual pathway in platelet activating factor-induced aggregation of rat polymorphonuclear leucocytes. *Prostaglandins* (1987), **33**, 253–264.
111 Smith, R. J. & Bowman, B. J. Stimulation of human neutrophil degranulation with 1-O-octadecyl-2-O-acetyl-*sn*-glyceryl-3-phosphorylcholine: modulation by inhibitors of arachidonic acid metabolism. *Biochem. Biophys. Res. Commun.* (1982), **104**, 1495–1501.
112 Smith, R. J., Bowman, B. J. & Iden, S. S. Characteristics of 1-O-hexadecyl- and 1-O-octadecyl-2-O-acetyl-*sn*-glyceryl-3-phosphorylcholine- stimulated granule enzyme release from human neutrophils. *Clin. Immunol. Immunopathol.* (1983), **28**, 13–28.
113 Smith, R. J., Bowman, B. J. & Iden, S. S. Stimulation of the human neutrophil superoxide anion-generating system with 1-O-hexadecyl/octadecyl-2-acetyl-*sn*-glyceryl-3- phosphorylcholine. *Biochem. Pharmacol* (1984), **33**, 973–974.
114 Hopkins, N. K., Schaub, R. G. & Gorman, R. R. Acetyl glyceryl ether phosphorylcholine (PAF-acether) and leukotriene B_4 mediated neutrophil chemotaxis through an intact endothelial cell monolayer. *Biochim. Biophys. Acta.* (1984), **805**, 30–36.
115 Shukla, S. D., Buxton, D. B., Olson, M. S. & Hanahan, D. J. Acetylglyceryl ether phosphorylcholine. *J. Biol. Chem.* (1983), **258**, 10 212–10 214.
116 Mendlovic, F., Corvera, S. & Garcia-Sáinz, J. A. Possible involvement of cyclooxygenase products in the actions of platelet-activating factor and of lipoxygenase products in the vascular effects of epinephrine in perfused rat liver. *Biochem. Biophys. Res. Commun.* (1984), **123**, 507–514.
117 Voelkel, N. F., Worthen, S., Reeves, J. T., Henson, P. M. & Murphy, R. C. Nonimmunological production of leukotrienes induced by platelet-activating factor. *Science* (1982), **218**, 286–288.
118 Heffner, J. E., Shoemaker, S. A. & Canham, E. M. *et al.* Acetyl glyceryl ether phosphorylcholine-stimulated human platelets cause pulmonary hypertension and edema in isolated rabbit lungs. *J. Clin. Invest.* (1983), **71**, 351–357.
119 Camussi, G., Montrucchio, G., Antro, C., Bussolino, F., Tetta, C. & Manuelli, G. Platelet-activating factor-mediated contraction of rabbit lung strips: pharmacologic modulation. *Immunopharmacology* (1983), **6**, 87–96.
120 Stimler-Gerard, N. P. Parasympathetic stimulation as a mechanism for platelet-activating factor-induced contractile responses in the lung. *J. Pharmacol. Exp. Ther.* (1986), **237**, 209–213.
121 Dulioust, A., Vivier, E., Salem, P., Benveniste, J. & Thomas, Y. Immunoregulatory functions of PAF-acether. *J. Immunol.* (1988), **140**, 240–245.
122 Patrignani, P., Valitutti, S., Aiello, F. & Musiani, P. Platelet-activating factor

(PAF) receptor antagonists inhibit mitogen-induced human peripheral blood T-cell proliferation. *Biochem. Biophys. Res. Commun.* (1987), **148**, 802–810.

123 McManus, L. M., Shaw, J. O. & Pinckard, R. N. Thromboxane B_2 (T × B_2) release during IgE anaphylaxis in the rabbit. *J. Immun.* (1980), **125**, 1950–1954.

124 Camussi, C., Tetta, C., Deregibus, M. C., Bussolino, F., Segoloni, G. & Vercellone, A. Platelet-activating factor (PAF) in experimentally-induced rabbit acute serum sickness: role of basophil-derived PAF in immune complex deposition. *J. Immunol.* (1982), **128**, 86–94.

125 Doebber, T. W., Wu, M. S., Robbins, J. C., Choy, B. M., Chang, M. N. & Shen, T. Y. Platelet activating factor (PAF) involvement in endotoxin-induced hypotension in rats. Studies with PAF-receptor antagonist kadsurenone. *Biochem. Biophys. Res. Commun.* (1985), **127**, 799–808.

126 Grandel, K. E., Farr, R. S., Wanderer, A. A., Eisenstadt, T. C. & Wasserman, S. I. Association of platelet-activating factor with primary acquired cold urticaria. (1984), **313**, 405–409.

127 Caramelo, C., Fernandez-Gallardo, S., Marin-Cao, D. *et al.* Presence of platelet-activating factor in blood from humans and experimental animals. Its absence in anephric individuals. *Biochem. Biophys. Res. Commun.* (1984), **120**, 789–796.

128 Billah, M. M. & Johnston, J. M. Identification of phospholipid platelet-activating factor (1-O-alkyl-2-acetyl-*sn*-glycero-3-phosphocholine) in human amniotic fluid and urine. *Biochem. Biophys. Res. Commun.* (1983), **113**, 51–58.

129 Mallet, A. I. & Cunningham, F. M. Structural identification of platelet activating factor in proriatic scale. *Biochem. Biophys. Res. Commun.* (1985), **126**, 192–198.

130 Toyofuku, T., Kubo, K., Kobayashi, T. & Kusama, S. Effects of ONO-6240, a platelet-activating factor antagonist, on endotoxin shock in unanesthetized sheep. *Prostaglandins* (1986), **31**, 271–281.

131 Chang, S-W., Feddersen, C. O., Henson, P. M. & Voelkel, N. F. Platelet-activating factor mediates hemodynamic changes and lung injury in endotoxin-treated rats. *J. Clin. Invest.* (1987), **79**, 1498–1509.

132 Sanchez Crespo, A., Alonso, F., Iñarrea, P., Alvarez, V. & Egido, J. Vascular actions of synthetic PAF-acether (a synthetic platelet-activating factor) in the rat: evidence for a platelet independent mechanism. *Immunopharmacology* (1981), **4,** 173–185.

133 Humphrey, D. M., McManus L. M., Satouchi, K., Hanahan, D. J. & Pinckard, R. N. Vasoactive properties of acetyl glyceryl ether phosphorylcholine and analogues. *Lab. Invest.* (1982), **46**, 422–427.

134 Handley D.A., Arbeeny, C. M., Lee, M. L., Van Valen, R. G., Saunders, R. N. Effect of platelet activating factor in endothelial permeability to plasma macromolecules. *Immunopharmacology* (1984), **8,** 137–142.

135 Hwang, S-B., Li, C-L., Lam, M. H. & Shen, T. Y. Characterization of cutaneous vascular permeability induced by platelet-activating factor in guinea pigs and rats and its inhibition by a platelet-activating factor receptor antagonist. *Lab. Invest.* (1985), **52**, 617–630.

136 Inarrea, P., Alonso, F. & Sanchez Crespo, M. Platelet-activating factor: an effector substance of the vasopermeability changes induced by the infusion of immune aggregates in the mouse. *Immunopharmacology* (1983), **6,** 7–14.

137 Archer, C. B., Frohlich, W., Page, C. W., Paul, W., Morley, J. & Macdonald, D. M. Synergistic interaction between prostaglandins and PAF-acether in experimental animals and man. *Prostaglandins* (1984), **27**, 495–501.

138 Montrucchio, G., Alloatti, G., Mariano, F. *et al.* The pattern of cardiovascular alterations induced by infusion of platelet-activating factor in rabbit is modified by pretreatment with H_1–H_2 receptor antagonists but not by cyclooxygenase inhibition. *Agents & Actions* (1987), **21**, 72–78.

139 Kenzora, J. L., Perez, J. E., Bergmann, S. R. & Lange, L. G. Effects of acetyl glyceryl ether of phosphorylcholine (platelet activating factor) on ventricular preload, afterload, and contractility in dogs. *J. Clin. Invest.* (1984), **74**, 1193–1203.

140 Emeis, J. J. and Kluft, C. PAF-acether-induced release of tissue-type plasminogen activator from vessel walls. *Blood* (1985), **66**, 86–91.

141 Hsueh, W., Crussi-Gonzalez, F. & Arroyave, J. L. Platelet-activating factor-induced ischemic bowel necrosis. *Am. J. Pathol.* (1986), **122**, 231–239.

142 Dallob, A., Guindon, Y. & Goldenberg, M. M. Pharmacological evidence for a role of lipoxygenase products in platelet-activating factor (PAF)-induced hyperalgesia. *Biochem. Pharmacol.* (1987), **36**, 3201–3204.

143 Maridonneau-Parini, I., Lagente, V., Lefort, J., Randon, J., Russo-Marie, F. & Vargaftig, B. B. Desensitization to PAF-induced bronchoconstriction and to activation of alveolar macrophages by repeated inhalations of PAF in the guinea pig. *Biochem. Biophys. Res. Commun.* (1985), **131**, 42–49.

144 Vargaftig, B. B., Lefort, J., Chignard, M. & Benveniste, J. Platelet-activating factor induces a platelet-dependent bronchoconstriction unrelated to the formation of prostaglandin derivatives. *Eur. J. Pharmacol.* (1980), **65**, 185–192.

145 Cuss, F. M., Dixon, C. M. S. & Barnes, P. J. Effects of inhaled platelet activating factor on pulmonary function and bronchial responsiveness in man. *Lancet.* (1986), **ii**, 189–192.

146 Mazzoni L., Morley, J., Page, C. P. & Sanjar, S. Induction of airway hyper-reactivity by platelet activating factor in the guinea pig *J. Physiol.* (1985), **365**, 107P.

147 Patterson, R., Bernstein, P. R., Harris, K. E. & Krell, R. D. Airway responses to sequential challenges with platelet-activating factor and leukotriene D_4 in rhesus monkeys. *J. Lab. Clin. Med.* (1984), **104**, 340–345.

148 Chung, K. F., Aizawa, H., Leikauf, G. D., Ueki, I. F., Evans, T. W. & Nadel, J. A. Airway hyperresponsiveness induced by platelet-activating factor: Role of thromboxane generation. *J. Pharmacol. Exp. Ther.* (1985), 580–584.

149 Prevost, M-C., Cariven, C., Simon, M. F., Chap, H. & Douste-Blazy, L. Platelet activating factor (PAF-acether) is released into rat pulmonary alveolar fluid as a consequence of hypoxia. *Biochem. Biophys. Res. Commun.* (1984), **119**, 58–63.

150 Bonnet, J., Thibaudeau, D. & Bessin, P. Dependency of the PAF-acether induced bronchospasm on the lipoxygenase pathway in the guinea-pig. *Prostaglandins* (1983), **26**, 457–466.

151 Lewis, A. J., Dervinis, A. & Chang, J. The effects of antiallergic and bronchodilator drugs on platelet-activating factor (PAF-acether) induced bronchospasm and platelet aggregation. *Agents & Actions* (1984), **15**, 636–642.

152 Agrawal, D. K. & Townley, R. G. Effect of platelet-activating factor on beta-adrenoceptors in human lung. *Biochem. Biophys. Res. Commun.* (1987), **143**, 1–6.

153 Braquet, P., Etienne, A. & Clostre, F. Down-regulation of β_2-adrenergic receptors by PAF-acether and its inhibition by the PAF-acether antagonist BN 52021. *Prostaglandins* (1985), **30**, 721.

Chapter 6
PAF and the cardiovascular system

Giora Z. Feuerstein

Introduction

The primary aims of this chapter are: (i) to delineate the main effects of PAF on cardiovascular organs (heart, blood vessels, microcirculation); (ii) to identify the direct and indirect components of the cardiovascular effects of PAF; (iii) to identify key pathological processes in the cardiovascular system where PAF might play an important role; (iv) to summarize the pharmacological evidence which indicates that PAF antagonists reverse or prevent pathological processes in the cardiovascular system; and (v) to identify major areas where additional work is critically needed to confirm the role of PAF in diseases of the cardiovascular system.

In an attempt to fulfill the above goals it is clear that only representative reports of the extensive work done in these areas can be reviewed. Therefore, reference to recent review papers in this field will be made to facilitate access to work not specifically reviewed here. In addition, the chemical, biochemical and cellular aspects of PAF biology have been recently reviewed [1–3].

In general, the discussion on the role PAF might have in physiological or patho-physiological processes related to the cardiovascular system will address three issues: (i) the ability of PAF to modify haemodynamic variables or specific organs important in cardiovascular control; (ii) the presence of PAF in specific sites where cardiovascular functions are executed; (iii) whether PAF production/release takes place at proper temporal relationships to pathological events of the cardiovascular system; and (iv) the ability of specific PAF-antagonists to modify physiological variables or counteract some or all of the patho-physiological phenomena attributed to PAF.

Haemodynamic responses to PAF (Table 6.1)

Systemic effects of PAF

The most consistent haemodynamic response to systemically-administered PAF is reduction in the arterial blood pressure. This response is instantaneous and profound and can be shown in extremely small doses of PAF (picomoles). This phenomenon has been described in the mouse, rat, guinea pig, rabbit, cat, dog, pig, sheep and sub-human primates [4–8]. The hypotensive response to PAF is usually accompanied by increased heart rate due to a reflex response elicited by the hypotension. The increased sympathetic tone is evidenced by elevated plasma levels of catecholamines and the complete blockade of the tachycardia by β-adrenergic receptor blockers [7,9]. The lack of tachycardia in the pithed rat preparation where the central nervous system and spinal cord are completely disrupted [7] also supports a reflex origin for the accelerated heart rate during PAF-induced hypotension. However, in the conscious guinea pig, systemic

Table 6.1 Effect of PAF on selected blood vessels of various species*

Blood vessels	Guinea pig	Rat	Rabbit	Dog	Pig
Cerebral	N.D.	C[4]	N.E.	N.D.	N.D.
Coronary	C	C	C	D/C[3]	D/C[2]
Pulmonary	C	C[7]	C	C	C[6]
Renal	N.D.	D[1,7]	N.D.	C	N.D.
Mesenteric	N.D.	D[1,5,8]	N.D.	N.D.	N.D.
Muscle	N.D.	D[3]	N.D.	D.	N.D.
Skin	D	D	D	D	N.D.

* D = dilation; C = constriction; N.D. = not detected; N.E. = no effect.

[1] High doses of PAF (>20 nmol/kg) were shown to increase spleen and renal vascular resistance in intact rats [39].

[2] Constriction of pig coronary vessels follows an initial vasodilation [18].

[3] Brief coronary dilatation followed by constriction [106].

[4] Decreased cerebral blood flow by low doses of PAF in SHR [107].

[5] High doses of PAF which produce hypotension result in increased mesenteric flow [108].

[6] *In vitro*, pulmonary veins but not arteries are constricted by PAF [43].

[7] Vasodilatation of pre-constricted pulmonary vessels [41].

[8] Low doses of PAF 0.1–10 nmol/kg [23].

administration of large doses of PAF, which produces severe hypotension, produce bradycardia [10]; this paradoxical response might be the result of severe reduction in oxygen delivery to the heart due to pulmonary and coronary constriction. The mechanisms involved in PAF-induced hypotension are complex and include actions on several organs and cellular elements. Of primary importance are the heart, peripheral blood vessels and the microcirculation. The contribution of each of these elements to PAF induced hypotension and shock will be discussed below.

Effect of PAF on the heart

Cardiac function can be modified by direct action on the heart or through indirect effects such as systemic changes in pre-load and/or after-load pressures. Direct cardiac actions might be the result of actions on one of three major cardiac variables: (i) the coronary circulation; (ii) myocardial contractility; and (iii) the rhythm generating and conducting system. Each of these variables is discussed below.

Coronary circulation

The coronary effects of PAF have been demonstrated in both *in vitro* and *in vivo* models which have yielded complex responses and some controversy. *In vitro* studies using guinea pig, rat or rabbit hearts perfused with artificial physiological solutions have demonstrated that PAF leads to an increase in coronary vascular resistance [11–17]. However, in contrast to the coronary effects of PAF *in vitro*, direct bolus injections of PAF into the coronary circulation of the *in situ*, blood-perfused heart of the domestic pig produced an initial increase in flow, due to coronary dilation, followed by a decrease in flow due to coronary constriction [18]. These same observations were later confirmed in the coronary circulation of the intact dog heart [19,20]. The vasodilator effect of PAF preceded the vasoconstriction and was invoked by low doses of PAF which did not change systemic or other cardiac variables. The vasodilator phase produced by PAF in coronary vessels of the domestic pig, unlike the constrictor effect, was not blocked by cyclooxygenase inhibitors (e.g. indomethacin) or the cysteinyl-leukotriene antagonist FPL 55712 [18]. Furthermore, continuous infusion of PAF over several minutes into the coronary circulation of the domestic pig demonstrated that low doses of PAF produce a substantial reduction in myocardial contractility as evidenced by a $>50\%$ reduction in regional shortening fraction (Fig. 6.1). This reduction in myocardial performance was seen at times where no significant changes could be observed in coronary blood flow, systemic arterial pressure or left-ventricular end-diastolic pressure [8]. Furthermore, the effect of PAF was associated with selective increases in circulating levels of TXB_2 (the stable metabolite of

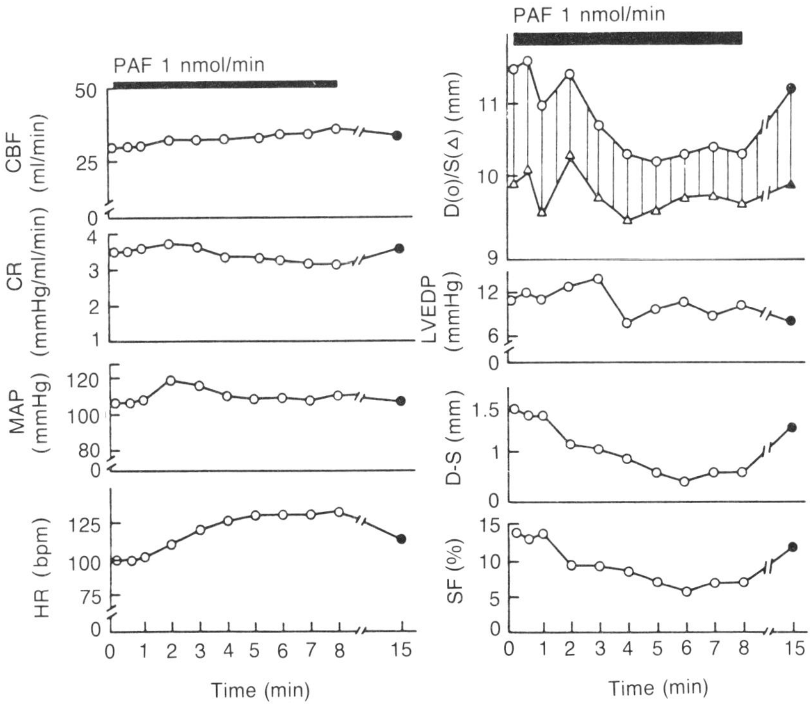

Fig. 6.1 Cardiac function during coronary infusion of PAF in the domestic pig. HR = heart rate; MAP = mean arterial pressure; CR = coronary resistance; CBF = coronary blood flow; SF = shortening fraction; D = diastole; S = systole; and LVEDP = left ventricular end diastolic pressure. The black bars indicate the time of PAF infusion. Note the reduction of SF 2–3 min after the onset of PAF infusion at a time where LVEDP and CBF are normal.

TXA_2), but not in 6-keto-$PGF_{1\alpha}$ (the stable metabolite of prostacyclin) or leukotriene C_4 immunoreactivity [8]. Of special interest are observations made which indicate that PAF-induced coronary dilation is mediated by a platelet-derived vasodilator factor [20]. However, larger doses of PAF ultimately result in a profound reduction of coronary blood flow, a response largely mediated by TXA_2 [18,21]. From a clinical point of view, a sudden increase in PAF release (anticipated in systemic anaphylaxis or septicaemia) might lead to severe coronary vasoconstriction, ischaemia and low cardiac output which are the hallmarks of cardiac anaphylaxis.

Myocardial function

Like many substances which affect systemic haemodynamic variables, as well as multiple cardiac functions, the question of whether or not a direct effect on myocardial contractility accounts for the overall reduction in cardiac output is also pertinent to PAF. In fact, a profound reduction in cardiac output during intra-coronary infusion of PAF together with reduction of regional 'shortening fraction' have been demonstrated in the anaesthetized domestic pig at PAF doses which had no substantial effect on systemic blood pressure [21,22]. In the rat, however, PAF reduces cardiac output only at doses which produce severe hypotension [23]. Such data, although suggestive of direct myocardial effects of PAF in some species, are inconclusive since it is impossible to completely isolate the haemodynamic status within different regions of the myocardium from the direct effects of PAF on the myocardium itself. Furthermore, a reduction in the force of contraction of *in vitro* perfused heart preparations [3,13–15,17] even if perfusion pressure is maintained, is not free of similar criticism regarding intra-mural flow maldistributions. However, evidence obtained from isolated strips of cardiac muscle suggest that PAF can exert a primary negative inotropic effect. For example, Robertson *et al.* [24] have shown a direct negative inotropic effect of PAF in the human myocardium. Furthermore, PAF was shown to decrease the force of contraction of electrically paced, non-coronary perfused left atrium and ventricular papillary muscle [13,25]. In addition, electrophysiological studies showed that relatively high doses of PAF have direct effects on the canine Purkinje fibres (e.g. abnormal automaticity, decreased action potential amplitude) and the guinea-pig papillary muscle (e.g. decrease in action potential amplitude and duration); yet, in this latter preparation, a positive inotropic response was observed [26]. A transient inotropic effect in guinea-pig papillary muscle was also observed by Camussi *et al.* [25]. Since in such preparations it is possible to exclude neural, humoral, blood-cell or haemodynamic factors, a direct myocardial effect is suggested.

Additional evidence in support for the role PAF might have in direct cardiac dysfunction was obtained by Mickelson *et al.* [27] who used a rabbit myocardial ischaemia and reperfusion model; PAF infusion at the post-ischaemic period exacerbated the haemodynamic status and decreased cardiac performance at doses which had no consistent effect on a normal heart. These data are supported by the studies obtained by Lepran & Lefer [28] who showed an aggravating effect of PAF infused in a cat myocardial ischaemia model *in vivo*. Moreover, the production and release of PAF from *in vitro* perfused hearts has also been demonstrated in response to antigen challenge of sensitized rabbit [29] and guinea-pig [13] heart and the ischaemic baboon heart [30]. More recently, a role for PAF in mediation of the 'stunned myocardium' syndrome after ischaemia and reperfusion was also suggested by using PAF antagonists [31].

The mechanisms by which PAF affects myocardial contractility are poorly understood. Interference by PAF with Na^+ conductance in guinea-pig papillary muscle has been suggested [32] but other studies conducted on human [33] or guinea-pig papillary muscle suggested that PAF affects

Ca^{2+} fluxes via the slow Ca^{2+} channels [25, 34]. Interference in ion fluxes is strongly suggested by the appearance of multiple forms of rhythm disturbances (for a review see [35] and [36]).

Peripheral vascular effects of PAF

The effects of PAF on specific blood vessels is largely dependent on the species, the experimental conditions (*in vivo* versus *in vitro*) and the doses of PAF utilized. Therefore, it is difficult to predict the ultimate effect of PAF on a given organ blood flow *in vivo* from *in vitro* studies or between species (e.g. dog versus rat). However, the common response to small doses of PAF directly applied on blood vessels is vasodilation. This suggestion is primarily drawn from studies where extremely low doses of PAF were administered directly into the coronary circulation of the domestic pig and dog [18,20] or the systemic circulation of the rat [23,37], a species where PAF effects are independent of platelets [3,38,39]. In the rat, picomole doses of PAF, which produced no systemic changes, reduced vascular resistance and increased blood flow in the hindquarters (primarily skeletal muscle), the kidney and mesenteric vessels (see Fig. 6.2). Such responses could be observed by using the directional pulsed Doppler flowmetry which allows on-line, instantaneous recording of blood flow in the conscious state. The vasodilatory action of PAF in the rat renal circulation has also been confirmed in *in vitro* studies using intact rat kidneys [40]. However, constriction of blood vessels by PAF has been shown in both *in vitro* and *in vivo* preparations such as the pig pulmonary vessels [22,41–45]. However, it seems that the constricting effect of PAF shown *in vivo* and in some cases *in vitro* (e.g. rat coronary and pulmonary circulation) is mediated by arachidonate metabolites such as thromboxane A_2 and peptido-leukotrienes [16,46].

Cerebral vascular effects of PAF

The brain is an organ rich in enzymes for synthesis and metabolism of alkyletherphospholipids [47] and PAF has been isolated from the normal bovine brain [48–50]. The potential involvement of PAF in cerebral blood flow (CBF) regulation is inferred from studies where PAF antagonists (e.g. BN 52021) were shown to improve CBF after brain ischaemia and reperfusion [51] along with improved neurological/motor function [52]. In addition, the PAF antagonist kadsurenone was shown to improve cortical neural recovery as evidenced by cortical somato-sensory evoked potentials of dogs subjected to focal ischaemia by air emboli [53]. Furthermore, direct infusion of PAF into the carotid artery was shown to reduce CBF in the anaesthetized rat [54] while systemic administration of PAF to rabbits reduced spinal cord blood flow [55].

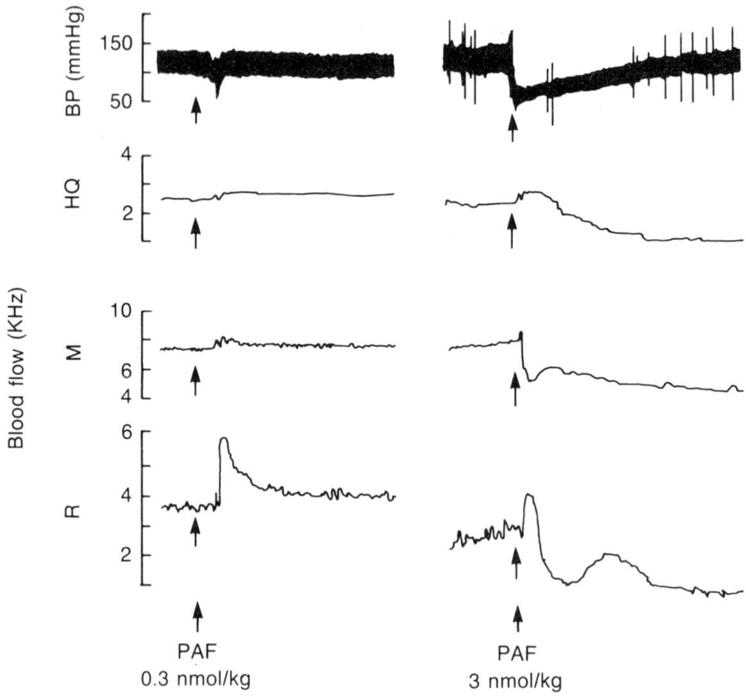

Fig. 6.2 Effect of PAF on organ blood flow in the conscious rat. The authentic recording shows the arterial blood pressure (BP), the hindquarter blood flow (HQ), superior mesenteric blood flow (M) and renal blood flow (R). The recordings were obtained by the directional pulsed Doppler velocimetry. Note the marked increase in M blood flow by the low dose of PAF which had no effect on the mean arterial pressure; the high dose of PAF showed marked vasodilation (increase in flow) even at the nadir of the hypotension.

It is important to note that even if PAF produces vasodilation in some vascular beds, the overall net result of systemic administration of large quantities of PAF is always a severe reduction in blood flow even in organs where vasodilation and increased blood flow is demonstrated by low doses of PAF.

Microcirculatory effects of PAF

Parallel to the discovery that PAF is a potent hypotensive agent, PAF was also found to induce a haemoconcentration and increased permeability of the microcirculation leading to a decrease in plasma volume [35,56–59]. The increase in the permeability of the microcirculation was shown by discrete injections of PAF into the skin of several species [60] including humans [61]. Direct microscopic examination of the microcirculation of the hamster cheek pouch revealed that PAF produced increased permeability at the post-capillary venules [62].

The cellular and humoral basis of the effects of PAF on the microcirculation are still poorly understood. While low doses of PAF seem to increase permeability independently of white blood cells (WBC), the effect of high doses seems to be associated with polymorphorphonuclear leukocyte adhesion and activation [62]. Direct damage by PAF to endothelial cells is construed by disruption of endothelial cell junctions and vacuolization [60]. Overall, PAF is the most potent substance known to date to increase the permeability of the microcirculation. Generally, PAF effects on the microcirculation, although amplified by secondary mediators (e.g. prostaglandins), are independent of blood cells and involve direct interaction with endothelial cell receptors [57,63]. Direct actions of PAF on endothelial cells are associated with activation of arachidonate metabolism such as enhanced release of PGI_2 [64] and increased Ca^{2+} fluxes [65].

In addition to the direct and indirect effects of PAF on endothelial cells, the endothelium was also shown to produce [66] and metabolize [67] PAF. The synthesis of PAF by endothelial cells seems to be down-regulated by prostacyclin (PGI_2) as treatment with indomethacin (a potent cyclooxygenase inhibitor) potentiated PAF synthesis in endothelial cells [66]. Of special interest are the similarities in the synthesis of PAF and endothelium-derived relaxing factor (EDRF, [68]); the synthesis of both these factors is increased by thrombin, ATP, histamine and inhibition of cyclooxygenase metabolites. Furthermore, enhanced synthesis and release of PAF from endothelial cells stimulated by the monokine interleukin-1 (IL-1, [69]) support the view that PAF might serve as a link between monocyte-endothelial cell interactions and thereby promote adhesion, which is the initial and crucial step for the pro-inflammatory actions of WBC. It would be of interest to further explore the possible significance of PAF and EDRF interactions in view of regulation of endothelial-cell adhesion receptors and pro-coagulant activity, two major mechanisms in the thrombotic features of endothelial cells.

PAF and patho-physiological processes of cardiovascular significance

Septic and endotoxic shock

While the literature is replete with reports demonstrating the pharmacological effects of PAF on the heart, lung, blood vessels and the microcirculation, only a few studies have shown generation of PAF in biological fluids and organs in normal or pathological situations. This unfortunate situation is the result of extreme difficulties in securing the isolation and definitive assay of PAF in tissues and biological fluids. Nevertheless, several studies have provided data in favour of PAF production during cardiovascular stress situations such as endotoxaemia and immune reactions. Doebber *et al.* [70] found an increase in circulating levels of PAF in anaesthetized rats treated with a highly toxic dose of endotoxin. These studies are supported by *in vitro* experiments performed on splenocytes and peritoneal macrophages isolated from rats exposed to sepsis [59]; in each of these cell types, high concentrations of PAF were found during sepsis and the formation of PAF preceded the increase in vascular permeability. It is important to note that PAF was also identified in cell-free supernatants indicating early release of PAF from activated monocytes/macrophages. A more complete proof for PAF generation during endotoxaemia was obtained by Chang *et al.* [71] who demonstrated accumulation of PAF in the systemic circulation as well as in lung tissue of rats treated with endotoxin. In this latter study, persistent elevated levels of PAF in the circulation strongly suggest that multiple organs might be exposed to PAF over a prolonged period of time; such organs could be affected by PAF even though no direct production of PAF took place in the specific organ. Of special importance in this regard are the observations negating a neutorphil source for the accumulation of PAF in the lungs [71]. The endothelial cells were suggested to be the cellular element in which PAF accumulation occurs since endothelial cells were shown to synthesize large amounts of PAF in response to injury [72,73].

Immune reactions and anaphylaxis

Systemic anaphylaxis is another situation of grave cardiovascular consequences. Release of PAF from sensitized cells [74] or systemic allergic reaction *in vivo* [75,76] have been demonstrated in both IgE and IgG immune reactions [73]. The demonstration of PAF release from sensitized guinea pig heart or lung challenged *in vitro* by the antigen supports the possibility of organ-specific release of PAF [13,77] in addition to circulating blood cells. However, temporal relationships of PAF release and the haemodynamic consequences of anaphylactic shock as well as the specific cell types in each organ which might be involved in PAF production are still unknown. Nevertheless, a partial protective effect of PAF antagonists in anaphylactic reactions *in vivo* was demonstrated by Darius *et al.* [78]. Furthermore, PAF antagonists were repeatedly shown to prevent or reverse many of the haematological and cardiovascular consequences produced by immune complexes [79–81].

Hypoxia

Hypoxia is an acute stress situation which results in typical haemodynamic responses and most notably pulmonary hypertension [82, 83]. As mentioned above, PAF is the most potent substance in constricting pulmonary vessels and eliciting pulmonary hypertension [42]. Some biochemical evidence supports the possibility of PAF production during hypoxia-induced pulmonary hypertension. For example, lung alveolar lavage obtained from rats exposed to hypobaric hypoxia showed a decrease in phosphatidylcholine concomitant to an increase in lysophosphatidylcholine and phospholipase A_2. More recent data demonstrated the presence of PAF in lung alveolar lavage fluid obtained from rats exposed to 4 h of hypobaric hypoxia [84] and in lung lavage fluid obtained from chronically hypoxic calves [85]. However, Chang *et al.* [71] failed to detect PAF in lung alveolar lavage fluid obtained from rats treated with lipopolysaccharide endotoxin at a time where PAF levels in the lung and plasma were extremely high. Thus, it might be possible that the presence of PAF in lung lavage fluid might not reflect lung tissue production in all circumstances or that different stimuli such as hypoxia and endotoxin might elicit PAF production in different cell populations, e.g. endothelial cells versus lung macrophages, which vary in the releasable fraction of PAF. These issues remain however unresolved at present.

Hypertension

Although PAF is a most potent agent capable of modifying vascular tone and cardiac function, no real attempts have been made to study its role in the modulation of cardiovascular function in models of hypertension. Of special interest in this regard are the known observations that platelets from spontaneously hypertensive rats (SHR) are quite different from those of normotensive rats, and display enhanced turnover and activation [86]. Several pharmacological studies have shown enhanced vasodilator responses of venules and arterioles of SHR as compared to normotensive rats. Such data are consistent with the observations that systemic administration of PAF to SHR produced greater hypotension than in normotensive rats [7]. Interestingly, in both SHR and normal rats, plasma TXB_2 levels were markedly elevated by PAF yet indomethacin failed to modify the hypotensive effect of PAF. In addition, plasma acetylhydrolase activity (the key enzyme in the degradation of PAF in the circulation) is significantly higher in SHR than normotensive rats [9]; the significance of this finding is still unknown.

PAF antagonists

Numerous PAF antagonists have been developed in recent years which demonstrate both high affinity and specificity to PAF binding sites. The rapidly growing field in the pharmacology of PAF has been repeatedly reviewed [1,80,81]. Three different types of experiments are traditionally performed where PAF antagonists are used to support the view that PAF might have a role in a patho-physiological process. The most common experiments are *in vitro* or *in vivo* studies where the antagonist is tested aganst synthetic PAF; the second type of experiments utilize PAF antagonists in situations where exogenous stimuli produce PAF, e.g. administration of immune complexes or endotoxins; and the third, and least common are experiments where disease processes are stimulated (e.g. septic shock) while the therapeutic capcity of a PAF antagonist is tested *in vivo*. The ultimate test for efficacy of PAF antagonists should be clinical studies in patients suffering from disease.

Reversal of cardiovascular effects of PAF

Since numerous PAF antagonists were already tested in many systems the reader is referred to recent reviews [79,81,87]. In brief, the most common parameters used to test blockade of PAF effects are hypotension, haemoconcentration, WBC and platelet depletion, bronchoconstriction, and survival; only few studies evaluated more discrete haemodynamic and cardiac functions *in vivo*. Of particular importance in this regard are studies showing the complete protection by BN 52021 of cardiac function in the conscious rat administered with high doses of PAF which otherwise produced a severe reduction in cardiac output [23]. It is also noteworthy that PAF-induced hypotension can be reversed by compounds which have absolutely no antagonistic action at the PAF receptors, e.g. thyrotropin releasing hormone (TRH), which effectively activates the physiological responses, which counteract the effects of PAF [10]. In accord with this latter study, TRH was also found to prevent or reverse IgE-mediated anaphylactic shock [88].

Septic and endotoxic shock

Since endotoxaemia is one of the few pathological states where elevated circulating levels of PAF have been found repeatedly, it is only natural that many PAF antagonists have been tested in models of endotoxaemia. For example, kadsurenone, a potent and specific PAF antagonist [87] was found to reverse the hypotension produced by endotoxin [70]. A similar capacity to block endotoxin induced hypotension was also demonstrated with other PAF antagonists such as CV-3988 [71,89], BN 52021 [1,90], SRI 63-441 [80], ONO-6240 [91] or FR-900412 [92]. It is also noteworthy that PAF antagonists e.g. BN 52021 [81] reserve not only *Escherichia coli* lipopolysaccharide-induced shock but also other endotoxins such as the *Salmonella typhimurium* endotoxin. While several studies using a large variety of PAF antagonists have shown protection or reversal of endotoxin-induced hypotension, a haemoconcentration or blood-cell depletion, only few have extended their study to end points which included survival rate. Most notably are studies conducted by Etienne *et al.* [93]

showing increased survival of rats exposed to endotoxaemia and treated with BN 52021, and the protective effect of CV-3988 [71].

Furthermore, the protective effect of CV-3988 was also shown in an *E. coli* sepsis model where the PAF antagonist alleviated the cardiovascular depression during the early sepsis period (3 h). The beneficial effect of this PAF antagonist included protection against low cardiac output and the increase in total peripheral resistance; in addition, blood flow to essential areas such as heart, kidney and the splanchnic organs were substantially improved over the non-treated septic group [94].

Traumatic and haemorrhagic shock

Recent studies conducted on anaesthetized rats have shown the accumulation of PAF in the peritoneal fluid of rats subjected to the Noble–Collip trauma procedure [95]. In this same traumatic shock model, PAF antagonists such as WEB 2086, L-652731 or CV-6209 were shown to provide partial protection [96,97]. In addition, salutary consequences of pharmacological blockade of PAF was also demonstrated in a haemorrhagic shock model [98], although no evidence is available as yet on the release of PAF in this model of shock.

Mycotoxic shock

Trichothecenes are a family of fungal toxins of which T-2 is one of the most toxic members. Administration of T-2 toxin to rats results in severe toxaemia characterized by low cardiac output, haemoconcentration and high mortality. The PAF antagonist BN 52021 was shown to substantially increase the survival rate of rats exposed to a highly lethal dose (LD_{90}) of T-2 toxin [99].

Future directions

PAF is a unique example of a natural compound which shortly after its discovery has been recognized as one of the potentially most important mediators of inflammatory and tissue injury reactions. These events have been propelled by ever growing demonstrations of the potency of PAF to initiate complex biological phenomena which far surpass traditional mediators such as serotonin, histamine and prostaglandins. Furthermore, the rapid availability of potent and specific receptor antagonists of PAF has fuelled the research into extensive work on animal models of disease processes and more recently into clinical trials.

However, one should keep in mind that much of the present information suggesting a role for PAF in human diseases is derived from pharmacological studies where exogeneous PAF is administered to experimental animals or animal models where patho-physiological processes were antagonized by PAF antagonists. Very little information is available on the production, release and metabolism of PAF in humans. Only a handful of studies are available where PAF was measured in biological material such as blood [100], urine [39], amniotic fluid [101], saliva [102] or disease processes such as cold urticaria [103], psoriasis [104] or systemic lupus erythematosus [105]. Evidently, a major effort should be made to advance the technical capability for sensitive and accurate methods for PAF assay in normal humans and during disease processes.

Major cardiovascular areas most promising for PAF involvement in disease processes and therapeutic potential for PAF antagonists/synthesis inhibitors are: (i) adult respiratory distress syndrome (ARDS); (ii) septic shock; (iii) tissue injury, trauma; and (iv) ischaemia and reperfusion. In each of these areas, it is essential to focus on identification of PAF in the relevant organs and cellular elements which produce PAF. Furthermore, the relationships of PAF to other cellular mediators such as leukotrienes, TXA_2 and peptides must be clarified.

Acknowledgement

This work was supported by USUHS Protocol No. GM9229. The opinions or assertions contained herein are the private ones of the author(s) and are not to be construed as official or as necessarily reflecting the view of the Department of Defense or the Uniformed Services University of the Health Sciences. There is no objection to its presentation and/or publications. The experiments reported herein were conducted according to the principles set forth in the Guide for Care and Use of Laboratory Animals, Institute of Laboratory Animal Medicine, National research Council, DHEW Publication No (NIH) 80-23, 1980. We thank Miss Diane Bailey and Mrs Pamela Leader for preparing this manuscript.

References

1 Braquet, P., Shen, T. Y., Touqui, L, & Vargaftig, B. B. Perspectives in platelet-activating factor research. *Pharmacol. Rev.* (1987), **39**, 97.

2 Braquet, P., Mencia-Huerta, J. M., Chabrier, P. E., Touqui L. & Vargaftig, B. B. The promise of platelet-activating factor. *ISI Atlas of Science: Pharmacol.* (1987), **1**, 187–197.

3 Benveniste, J. & Chignard, M. A role for PAF-acether (platelet-activating factor) in platelet-dependent vascular disease. *Circulation* (1985), **72**, 713–717.

4 Vargaftig, B. B., Lefort, J., Chignard, M. & Benveniste, J. Platelet activating factor induce a platelet dependent bronchoconstriction unrelated to the formation of prostaglandin derivatives. *Eur. J. Pharmacol.* (1980), **65**, 185–192.

5 McManus, L. M., Hanahan, D. J., Demopoulos, C. A. & Pinckard, R. N. Pathobiology of the intravenous infusion of acetylglyceryletherphosphorylcholine (AGEPC), a synthetic platelet activating factor (PAF) in the rabbit. *J. Immunol.* (1980), **124**, 2919–2924.
6 Blank, M. L., Snyder, F., Byers, L. W. & Brooks B. Antihypertensive activity of an alkyl ether analog of phosphatidylcholine. *Biochem. Biophys. Res. Commun.* (1979), **90**, 1194–1200.
7 Feuerstein, G., Zukowska-Grojec, L., Krausz, M., Blank, M. L., Snyder, F., & Kopin, I. T. Cardiovascular and sympathetic effects of 1-O-hexadecyl-2-acetyl-*sn*-glycero-3-phosphorylcholine in conscious SHR and WKY rats. *Clin. Expt. Hyperten.* (1982), **4,** 1335–1350.
8 Feuerstein, G., Ezra, D., Ramwell, P. W., Letts, G. & Goldstein, R. Platelet-activating factor as a modulator of cardiac and coronary functions. In Bailey, J. M. (ed.) *Prostaglandins, Leukotrienes and Lipoxins* (1985), pp. 301–310. Plenum Press, New York.
9 Zukowska-Grojec, Z., Blank, M. L., Snyder, F. and Feuerstein, G. The adrenergic system and the cardiovascular effects of platelet activating factor (1-O-hexadecyl-2-acetyl-*sn*-glycero-3-phosphocoline) in SHR and WKY rats. *Clin. Exp. Hypertens.* (1985), **7,** 1015–1031.
10 Feuerstein, G., Lux, W. E., Ezra, D., Hayes, E. C., Snyder, F. & Faden, A. I. Thyrotropin releasing hormone blocks the hypotensive effect of platelet activating factor in the unanesthetized guinea pig. *J. Cardiovasc. Pharmacol.* (1985), **7,** 335–340.
11 Benveniste, J., Boullet, C., Brink, C., & Labat, C. The action of PAF-acether (platelet activating factor) on guinea pig isolated heart preparations. *Br. J. Pharmacol.* (1983), **80**, 81–83.
12 Kenzora, J. L. Perez, J. E., Bermann, S. R., & Large, L. Effects of acetylglyceryl-etherphosphorylcholine (platelet activating factor) on ventricular preload, after-load and contractility in dogs. *J. Clin. Invest.* (1984), **74**, 1193–1203.
13 Levi, R., Burke, J. A., Guo Z. G. *et al.* Acetylglyceryletherphosphorylcholine (AGEPC). A putative mediator of a cardiac anaphylaxis in the guinea pig. *Circ. Res.* (1984), **54**, 117–124.
14 Saeki, S., Masugi, F., Ogihara, R. *et al.* Effects of 1-O-alkyl-acetyl-glycero-3-phosphorylcholine (platelet activating factor) on cardiac function in perfused guinea pig heart. *Life Sci.* (1985), **37**, 325–330.
15 Stahl, G. L., Lefer, D. J. & Lefer, A. M. PAF-acether induced cardiac dysfunction in the isolated perfused guinea pig heart. *Arch. Pharmacol.* (1987), **336**, 459.
16 Piper, P. & Stewart, A. G. Coronary vasoconstriction in the rat isolated perfused heart induced by platelet-activating factor is mediated by leukotriene C_4. *Br. J. Pharmacol.* (1986), **881**, 595–605.
17 Piper, P. & Stewart, A. G. Antagonism of vasoconstriction induced by platelet activating factor in guinea pig perfused hearts by a selective platelet activating factor receptor antagonist. *Br. J. Pharmacol.* (1987), **90**, 771–783.
18 Feuerstein, G., Boyd, L. H., Azra, D. & Goldstein, R. E. Effect of platelet activating factor on coronary circulation of the domestic pig. *Am. J. Physiol.* (1984), **246**, H466–H471.
19 Mehta, J., Wargovich, T. & Nichols, W. W. Biphasic effects of platelet-activating factor on coronary blood flow in the anesthetized dog. *Prostaglandins Leukotrienes Med.* (1986), **21**, 87–95.
20 Jackson, C. V. Schumacher, W. A., Kunkel, S. L., Drisoll, E. M., Pope, T. K. & Lucchesi, B. P. Platelet activating factor release of a platelet-derived coronary artery vasodilator substance in the canine. *Circ. Res.* (1986), **58**, 218–229.

21 Ezra, D., Laurindo, F. R. M., Czaja, J. F., Snyder, F., Goldstein, R. E. & Feuerstein, G. Cardiac and coronary consequences of intracoronary platelet activating factor infusion in the domestic pig. *Prostaglandins* (1987), **34**, 41–57.
22 Goldstein, R., Ezra, D., Laurindo, F. R. M. & Feuerstein, G. Coronary and pulmonary vascular effects of leukotrienes and PAF-acether. *Pharmacol. Res. Commun.* (1986), **18**, 151–162.
23 Siren, A-L & Feuerstein, G. Effects of platelet activating factor and its antagonist, BN 52021, on cardiac function and regional blood flow in the conscious rat. *Am. J. Physiol.* (1989), in press.
24 Robertson, D. A., Wang, D.-Y., Lee, C. O. K. & Levi, R. Negative inotropic effect of platelet-activating factor: association with a decrease in intracellular sodium activity. *J. Pharmacol. Exp. Ther.* (1988), **245**, 124–128.
25 Camussi, G., Alloatti, G., Montrucchio, G., Meda, M. & Emmanuelli, G. Effect of platelet-activating factor on guinea-pig papillary muscle. *Experientia* (1984), **40**, 357–361.
26 Nakaya, H. & Tohse, N. Electrophysiological effects of acetylglyceryletherphosphorylcholine on cardiac tissue. Comparison with lysophosphatidylcholine and long chain acyl carnitine. *Br. J. Pharmacol.* (1986), **89**, 749–757.
27 Mickelson, J. K., Simpson, P. J. & Lucchesi, B. R. Myocardial dysfunction and coronary vasoconstriction induced by platelet-activating factor in post-infarcted isolated heart. *J. Mol. Cell. Cardiol.* (1988), **20**, 547–561.
28 Lepran I. & Lefer, A. M. Ischemia aggrevating effects of platelet-activating factor in acute myocardial ischemia. *Basic Res. Cardiol.* (1985), **80**, 135–141.
29 Camussi, G. M, Nielsen, N., Tetta, C., Saunders, R. N. & Nilgrom, F. Release of platelet-activating factor from rabbit kidney perfused *in vitro* by sera with transplantation alloantibodies. *Transplantation* (1987), **44**, 113–118.
30 Annable, C. R., McManus, L. M., Carey, K. D. & Pinckard, R. N. Isolation of platelet-activating (PAF) from ischemic baboon myocardium. *Fed. Proc.* (1988), 1271. (Abstract).
31 Schroeder, E., Van Mechelan, H., Maldague, P. *et al.* Increased coronary vascular resistance in the stunned myocardium: role of the platelet activating factor. In *Proceedings of the 61st Scientific Session of the American Heart Association* (1988), II-77. (Abstract).
32 Robertson, D. A., Genovese, A. & Levi, R. Negative inotropic effect of platelet-activating factor on human myocardium: a pharmacological study. *J. Pharmacol. Exp. Ther.* (1987), **243**, 834–839.
33 Alloatti, G., Montrucchio, G., Marino, G. *et al.* Effect of platelet-activating factor (PAF) on human cardiac muscle. *Int. Arch. Allergy Appl. Immun.* (1986), **79**, 108–114.
34 Tamargo, J., Tejerina, T., Delgado, C. & Barrigon, S. Electrophysiological effects of platelet-activating factor (PAF-acether) in guinea pig papillary muscles. *Eur. J. Pharmacol.* (1985), **109**, 219–227.
35 Bessin, P., Bonnet, J., Apffel, D. *et al.* Acute circulatory collapse caused by platelet activating factor (PAF-acether) in dogs. *Eur. J. Pharmacol.* (1983), **85**, 403–413.
36 Feuerstein, G. & Goldstein, R. E. Effect of PAF on the cardiovascular system. In Snyder, F. (ed.) *Platelet Activating Factor and Related Lipid Mediators* (1987), pp. 403–424. Plenum Press, New York.
37 Lai, F. M., Sheperd, C. A. Cervoni, P. & Wissner, A. Hypotensive and vasodilatory activity of (+)-1-O-octadecyl-2-acetyl-glyceryl-3-phosphorylcholine in the normotensive rat. *Life Sci.* (1983), **32**, 1159–1166.
38 Sanchez Crespo, M., Alonso, F. & Egido, J. Non-platelet mediated vascular actions of 1-O-alkyl-2-acetyl-*sn*-3-glyceryl-phosphorylcholine (a synthetic PAF). *Agents & Actions* (1981), **11**, 565–566.

39 Sanchez Crespo, M., Alonso, F., Inarrea, P., Alvarez, V., & Egido, J. Vascular actions of synthetic PAF-acether (a synthetic-platelet-activating factor) in the rat: evidence for a platelet independent mechanism. *Immunopharmacology* (1982), **4,** 173–185.

40 Schwertschlag, U., Scherf, H., Gerber, J. G., Mathias, M., & Nies, A. S. L. Platelet-activating factor induces changes on renal vascular resistance, vascular reactivity and renin release in isolated perfused rat kidney. *Circ. Res.* (1987), **60**, 534–539.

41 Gillespie, M. & Bowdy, B. Impact of platelet activating factor on vascular responsiveness in isolated rat lungs. *J. Pharmacol. Exp. Ther.* (1986), **23**, 396–402.

42 Bradley, L., Feuerstein, G. & Goldstein, R. E. The role of lipid mediators in hypoxic pulmonary hypertension. In Schror, K. (ed). *Eicosanoids and the Cardiovascular System* (1989), Allan R. Liss, New York.

43 Pritze, S., Simmet, T. H. & Preskar, B. A. Effects of platelet-activating factor (PAF) on porcine pulmonary vessels *in vitro. Proceedings of the IVth International Symposium on Prostaglandins and the Cardiovascular System, Dusseldorf, FRG, October 4–7 1988*, p. 72.

44 Vemulapalli, S., Chiu, P. J. S. & Barnett, A. Cardiovascular and renal action of platelet-activating factor in anesthetized dogs. *Hypertension* (1984), **6,** 489–493.

45 Scherf, H., Nies, A., Schwertschlag, U., Hughes, M. & Gerber, J. Hemodynamic effects of platelet activating factor in the dog kidney *in vivo. Hypertension* (1986), **8,** 737–741.

46 Voelkel, N., Worthen, S., Reeves, J., Henson, P. & Murphy, R. Non-immunologic production of leukotrienes induced by platelet activating factor. *Science* (1985), **218**, 286–288.

47 Clark, N. G. & Dawson, R. M. C. Alkaline O → N transacylation. *Biochem. J.* (1981), **195**, 301–306.

48 Tokumura A. & Tsukatani, H. Determination of molecular species of platelet-activating factor in bovine brain lipid extract. *Proceedings of the 2nd International Conference on PAF and Structurally Related Alkyl Ether Lipids, Gatlinburg, TN, October 1986*, p. 121.

49 Tokumura, A., Kamiyasu, K., Takauchi, K. & Tsukatani, H. M. Evidence for existence of various homologues and analogues and platelet activating factor in lipid extract of bovine brain. *Biochem. Biophys. Res. Comm.* (1987), **145**, 415–425.

50 Yoshida, J.-I. Tokumura, A., Fukezawa, K., Terao, M., Takaudri, K. & Tsukatani, H. A platelet aggregating and hypotensive phospholipid isolated from bovine brain. *J. Pharm. Pharmacol.* (1986), **38**, 878–882.

51 Panetta, T., Marchesetti, N.-L., Braquet, P., Spinnewyn, B. & Bazan, N. Effects of the platelet activating factor antagonist (BN 52021) on free fatty acids, diacylglycerols, polyphosphoinositides and blood flow in the gerbil brain. Inhibition of ischemia reperfusion induced cerebral injury. *Biochem. Biophys. Res. Commun.* (1987), **149**, 580–587.

52 Spinnewyn, B., Blavet, N., Clostre, F., Bazan N. & Braquet P. Involvement of platelet-activating factor (PAF) in cerebral post-ischemic phase in Mongolian gerbils. *Prostaglandins* (1987), **34**, 337–349.

53 Kochanek, P. M., Dutka, A. J., Kumaroo, K. K. & Hallenbeck, J. M. Platelet activating factor receptor blockade enhances early neuronal recovery after multifocal brain ischemia in dogs. *Life Sci.* (1987), **41**, 2639–2644.

54 Kochanek, P. M., Nemoto, E. M., Melick, J. A., Evans, R. W. & Burke, D. F. Cerebrovascular and cerebrometabolic effects of intracarotid infused platelet-activating factor in rats. *J. Cereb. Blood Flow Metab.* (1988), **8,** 546–551.

55 Lindsberg, P., Jacobs, T. P., Paakari, I. A., Hallenbeck, J. M. & Feuerstein, G. Effect of PAF-acether on spinal cord microcirculation. *FASEB J.* (1988). (Abstract).

56 McManus, L. M., Pinckard, R. N., Fitzpatrick, F. A., O'Rourke, R. A., Crawford, M. A. & Hanahan, D. J. Acetylglyceryletherphosphorylcholine. Intravascular alterations following intravenous infusion into the baboon. *Lab. Invest.* (1981), **45**, 303–309.

57 Handley, D. A., Lee, M. L. & Saunders, R. N. Evidence for a direct effect on vascular permeability of platelet-activating factor induced hemoconcentration in the guinea-pig. *Thromb. Hemost.* (1985), **54**, 756–759.

58 Inarrea, P., Alonso, F. & Sanchez Crespo, M. Platelet-activating factor: an effector substance of the vasopermeability changes induced by the infusion of immune aggregates in the mouse. *Immunopharmacology* (1983), **6**, 7–14.

59 Inarrea, P., Gomez-Cambronero, J., Pascual, J., Carmen Ponte, M. del-Hernañdo, L. & Sanchez Crespo, M. Synthesis of PAF-acether and blood volume changes in Gram-negative sepsis. *Immunopharmacology* (1985), **9**, 45–52.

60 Humphrey, D. M., McManus L. M., Hanahan, D. J. & Pinckard R N. Morphological basis of increased vascular permeability induced by acetyl-glyceryl ether phosphorylcholine. *Lab. Invest.* (1984), **50**, 16–25.

61 Archer, C. B., Page, C. P., Paul, W., Morley, J. & McDonald, D. M. Inflammatory characteristics of platelet activating factor (PAF-acether) in human skin. *Br. J. Dermatol.* (1984), **110**, 45–52.

62 Bjork, J. & Smedegard, G. Acute microvascular effects of PAF-acether as studied by intravital microscopy. *Eur. J. Pharmacol.* (1985), **96**, 87–93.

63 Kerth, R., Hirafungi, M. & Benveniste, J. Comparison of human endothelial cells in culture and platelets for ^{3}H-PAF-acether binding. *Fed. Proc.* (1987), **46**, 44. (Abstract).

64 D'Humieres, S., Russo-Marie, F. & Vargaftig, B. B. PAF-acether-induced synthesis of prostacyclin by human endothelial cells. *Eur. J. Pharmacol.* (1986), **131**, 13–19.

65 Brock, T. A. & Gimbrone, M. A. Platelet activating factor alters calcium homeostasis in cultured endothelial cells. *Am. J. Physiol.* (1986), **250**, H1086–H1092.

66 Zimmerman, G. A., McIntyre, T. M. & Prescott, S. M. Production of platelet activating factor by human vascular endothelial cells: evidence for a requirement for specific agonists and modulation by prostacyclin. *Circulation* (1985), **72**, 718–727.

67 Tan, E.-L. & Snyder, F. Metabolism of platelet activating factor (1-alkyl-2-acetyl-*sn*-glycero-3-phosphocholine) by capillary endothelial cells isolated from rat epididymal adipose tissue. *Thromb. Res.* (1985), **38**, 713–717.

68 DeFeudis, F. V. Possible relationship between the synthesis of endothelium-derived relaxing factor (EDRF) and PAF-acether. *Gen. Pharmacol.* (1986), **17**, 129–131.

69 Bussolino, F., Breviario, F., Tetta, C., Algietta, M. & Dejana, E. Interleukin-I stimulates platelet activating factor production in cultured human endothelial cells. *Pharmacol. Res. Commun.* (1985), **18**, 133–137.

70 Doebber, T. W., Wu, M. S., Robbins, J. C., Choy, R. M., Chang, M. N. & Shen, T. Y. Platelet activating factor (PAF) involvement in endotoxin-induced hypotension in rats. Studies with PAF-acether antagonist kadsurenone. *Biochem. Biophys. Res. Comm.* (1988), **127**, 799–808.

71 Chang, S-W, Feddersen, C. O., Henson, P. M. & Voelkel, N. F. Platelet-activating factor mediates hemodynamic changes and lung injury in endotoxin-treated rats. *J. Clin. Invest.* (1987), **79**, 1498–1509.

72 Camussi, G., Aghetta, M., Malavasi, F. The release of platelet-activating factor from human endothelial cells in culture. *J. Immunol.* (1983), **31**, 2397–2403.

73 Camussi, G., Pawlowski, I., Bussolino, F., Caldwell, P. R. B., Brentjens, J. & Anders, G. Release of platelet-activating factor in rabbits with antibody-mediated injury of the lung: the role of leukocytes and of pulmonary endothelial cells. *J. Immunol.* (1983), **131**, 1802–1807.

74 Mencia-Huerta, J.-M., Lewis, R. A., Razin, E. & Austen, K. F. Antigen-initiated release of platelet-activating factor (PAF-acether) from mouse bone marrow-derived mast cells sensitized with monoclonal IgE. *J. Immunol.* (1983), **131**, 2958–2964.

75 Camussi, G. M., Tetta, C. M., Deregibus, C., Bussolino, F., Segoloni, G. & Vercellone, A. Platelet-activating factor (PAF) in experimentally-induced rabbit acute serum sickness: role of basophil-derived PAF in immune complex deposition. *J. Immunol.* (1982), **128**, 86–94.

76 Pinckard, R. N., Farr, R. S. & Hanahan, D. J. Physicochemical and functional identity of rabbit platelet-activating factor (PAF) released *in vivo* during IgE anaphylaxis with PAF released *in vitro* from IgE sensitized basophils. *J. Immunol.* (1979), **123**, 1847–1857.

77 Fitzgerald, M. F., Moncada, S. & Parente, L. The anaphylactic release of platelet-activating factor from perfused guinea pig lung. *Br. J. Pharmacol.* (1986), **88**, 149–153.

78 Darius, H., Lefer, D. J., Smith, B. & Lefer, A. M. Role of platelet activating factor-acether in mediating guinea pig anaphylaxis. *Science* (1986), **232**, 58–60.

79 Saunders, R. N. & Handley, D. A. Platelet-activating factor antagonists. *Ann. Rev. Pharmacol. Toxicol.* (1987), **27**, 237–255.

80 Handley, D. A., Anderson, R. C. & Saunders, R. N. Inhibition by SRI 63–072 and SRI 63–119 of PAF-acether and immune complex effects in the guinea pig. *Eur. J. Pharmacol.* (1987), **141**, 409–416.

81 Braquet, P. *The ginkgolides: Potent Platelet-Activating Factor Antagonists Isolated from* Ginkgo bilola *L. Chemistry Pharmacology and Clinical Applications* (1988), Vol. I. J. R. Prous Science, Barcelona.

82 Cohn, M. A., Baier, H. & Wanner, A. Failure of hypoxic pulmonary vasoconstriction in canine asthma model. Effect of prostaglandin inhibitors. *J. Clin. Invest.* (1978), **611**, 1463–1470.

83 Bjertnaes, L. J., Hauge, A & Torgrimsen, T. The pulmonary vasoconstrictor response to hypoxia and the hypoxia-sensitive site studied with a volatile inhibitor. *Acta Physiol. Scand.* (1980), **109**, 447–462.

84 Prevost, M.-C. Cariven, C., Simon, M. F., Chap, H. & Douste Blazy, L. Platelet activating factor (PAF-acether) is released into rat pulmonary alveolar fluid as a consequence of hypoxia. *Biochem. Biophys. Res. Comm.* (1984), **119**, 58–63.

85 Fasules, J., Stenmark, K. R., Henson, P. M., Voelkel, N. E., Tucker, A. & Reves, J. T. Platelet activating factor in lung lavage of chronically hypoxic neonatal calves. *Am. Rev. Resp. Dis.* (1986), **133**, A277. (Abstract).

86 Clerck, De F., Gorp, L. V., Xhonneux, B., Sommers, Y. & Wouters L. Enhanced platelet turnover and prostaglandin production in spontaneously hypertensive rats. *Thromb. Res.* (1982), **27**, 243–249.

87 Shen, T. Y., Hwang, S.-B., Doebber, T. W. & Robbins, J. C. The chemical and biological nature of PAF agonists/antagonists and biosynthetic inhibitors. In Snyder, F. (ed.) *Platelet Activating Factor and Related Lipid Mediators* (1987), pp.153–190. Plenum Press, New York.

88 Lux, Jr W. E., Feuerstein, G. & Faden A. I. Thyrotropin-releasing hormone reverses experimental anaphylactic shock through a non-endorphin-related mechanism. *Eur. J. Pharmacol.* (1983), **90**, 301–302.

89 Terashita, Z. -I., Imura, Y., Nishikawa, K. & Sumida S. Is platelet activating factor (PAF) a mediator of endotoxin shock? *Eur. J. Pharmacol.* (1985), **109**, 257–261.

90 Adnot, S., Lefort, J., Braquet, P. & Vargaftig, B. B. Interference of PAF-acether antagonist BN 52021 with endotoxin-induced hypotension in the guinea pig. *Prostaglandins* (1986), **32**, 791–802.

91 Toyofuku, T., Kubo, K., Kobayashi, T. & Kusama, S. Effects of ONO-6240, a platelet-activating factor antagonist on endotoxin shock in unanesthetized sheep. *Prostaglandins* (1986), **31**, 271–281.

92 Okamoto, M., Yoshida, K., Nishikawa, M. Platelet-activating factor (PAF) involvement in endotoxin-induced thrombocytopenia in rabbits: studies with FR-900412, a specific inhibitor of PAF. *Thromb. Res.* (1986), **42**, 661–671.

93 Etienne, A., Hecquet, F., Soulard, C., Spinnewyn, B., Clostre, F. & Braquet, P. *In vivo* inhibition of plasma protein leakage and *Salmonella enteritidis*-induced mortality in the rat by a specific PAF-acether antagonist BN 52021. *Agents & Actions* (1985), **17**, 386–370.

94 Minei, J., Shires, G. T. III & Shires, G. T. PAF antagonist CV-3988 improves cardiac performance during live *E. coli* bacteremia. *Circ. Shock* (1988), **24**, 253. (Abstract)

95 Stahl, G. L., Craft, D. V., Lento, P. H. & Lefer, AM. Detection of platelet-activating factor during traumatic shock. *Circ. Shock* (1988), **26**, 237–244.

96 Stahl, G. L., Bitterman, H., Terashita, Z. & Lefer, A. M. Beneficial effects of platelet activating factor receptor antagonist in traumatic shock. *Circ. Shock* (1988), **24**, 214. (Abstract).

97 Terashita, Z.-I., Stahl, G. L. & Lefer, A. M. Protective effect of platelet activating factor (PAF) antagonist and its combined treatment with prostaglandin (PGE_1) in traumatic shock. *J. Cardiovasc. Pharmacol.* (1988), **12**, 505–511.

98 Stahl, G. L., Bitterman, H., Terashita, Z.-I. & Lefer, A. M. Salutary consequences of platelet-activating factor in hemorrhagic shock. *Eur. J. Pharmacol.* (1988), **149**, 233–240.

99 Feuerstein, G., Leader, P., Siren, A.-L. & Braquet, P. Protective effect of a PAF-acether antagonist, BN 52021, in trichothecene toxicosis. *Toxicol. Lett.* (1987), **38**, 271–274.

100 Caramelo, C., Fernandez-Gallardo, S., Marin-Cao, D. *et al.* Presence of platelet activating factor in blood from humans and experimental animals. Its absence in anephric individuals. *Biochem. Biophys. Res. Commun.* (1984), **120**, 789–796.

101 Nishihira, J., Ishibashi, T., Imai, Y. & Muramatsu, J. Mass spectrometric evidence for the presence of platelet activating factor (1-O-alkyl-2-acetyl-*sn*-glycerol-phosphocholine) in human amniotic fluid during labor. *Lipids* (1984), **19**, 907–910.

102 Cox, C. P., Wardlow, M. L., Jorgensen, R. & Farr, R. S. The presence of platelet-activating factor (PAF) in normal human mixed saliva. *J. Immunol.* (1981), **127**, 46–50.

103 Grandel, K. E., Farr, R. S., Wanderer, A. A., Eisenstadt, T. C. & Wasserman, S. Association of platelet-activating factor with primary acquired cold urticaria. *New Engl. J. Med.* (1985), **313**, 405–409.

104 Mallet, A. I. & Cunningham, F. M. Structural identification of platelet activating factor in psoriatic scales. *Biochem. Biophys. Res. Commun.* (1985), **126**, 192–198.

105 Camussi, G. M., Tetta, C., Coda, R. & Benveniste, J. Release of platelet-activating factor in human pathology. I. Evidence for the occurrence of basophil degranulation and release of platelet-activating factor in systemic lupus erythematosus. *Lab. Invest.* (1981), **44**, 241–251.

106 Sybertz, E. J., Watkins, R. W., Baum T., Pula, K. & Rivelli, M. Cardiac, coronary

and peripheral vascular effects of acetyl glyceryl phosphoryl choline in the anesthetized dog. *J. Pharmacol. Exp. Ther.* (1985), **232**, 156–162.

107 Goldstein, B. M., Gabel, R. A., Huggins, F. J., Cervoni, P. & Grandall, D. I. Effect of platelet activating factor (PAF) on blood flow distribution in the spontaneously hypertensive rat. *Life Sci.* (1984), **35**, 1373–1378.

108 Bessin, P. PAF-acether and leukotriene participation in acute circulatory shock. *Pharmacol. Res. Comm.* (1986), **18**, 139–150.

Chapter 7
PAF and lung disease

Peter J. Barnes, K. Fan Chung and Clive P. Page

Introduction

Platelet activating factor (PAF) has been implicated in several lung diseases, and in particular asthma [1,2] and 'shock lung' or adult respiratory distress syndrome [3]. There has therefore been considerable interest in the potential of PAF antagonists in these conditions. Indeed, asthma is one of the primary targets for newly developed PAF antagonists and may be the first common clinical condition in which these drugs are tested. This chapter reviews the effects of PAF on various target cells in the lung, the evidence which implicates PAF in airway and pulmonary vascular disease, and the potential therapeutic uses for PAF antagonists in lung disease.

Asthma

The pathogenesis of asthma remains uncertain, but recent studies have emphasized that there is a complex and distinctive inflammatory process in the airway which is associated not only with contraction of airway smooth muscle, but also with microvascular leakiness, oedema and plasma extravasation, with mucus hypersection and with epithelial damage [4]. Many inflammatory mediators have been implicated in asthma [5] and these may account for many of the pathological features of asthma. However, it has been difficult to account for bronchial hyper-responsiveness, which is the hallmark of asthma. PAF is the only mediator so far described which causes sustained bronchial hyper-responsiveness, and has several other properties which may be relevant to asthma.

Bronchial hyper-responsiveness

Asthma is characterized by increased responsiveness of the airways to a wide variety of unrelated stimuli, including pharmacological agents such as histamine, cholinergic agonists, prostaglandins and leukotrienes, and physical stimuli, such as cold air and dusts [6]. The degree of bronchial hyper-responsiveness (BHR) is more closely related to the frequency of symptoms, the clinical severity of asthma and the need for anti-asthmatic medication than is baseline lung function [7,8]. Understanding the mechanism of BHR is, therefore, of fundamental importance in elucidating the pathophysiology of asthma and in the development of logical therapy. There is now increasing evidence that BHR is associated with airway inflammation [9,10], although the relationship between BHR, inflammation and asthma symptoms is by no means certain.

It has long been known that the airways of patients dying in status asthmaticus demonstrate acute inflammatory changes that are characterized by airway oedema secondary to an increase in vascular permeability, by cellular infiltration with eosinophils, neutrophils, lymphocytes and mononuclear cells, and by epithelial shedding [11]. Increased numbers of inflammatory cells have been found in broncho-alveolar lavage fluid of asthmatics [12], and inflammatory changes are present in the bronchial biopsies of patients whose asthma is in remission [13]. Although there are no data as to whether the degree of airways inflammation is related to the severity of asthma, there is compelling experimental evidence to suggest that increases in airways responsiveness can result from the induction of an acute inflammatory response [9]. Thus, there is a temporal association between either the acute exudative phase or the cellular infiltrative phase of acute inflammation and the peak period of BHR induced by inflammatory agents, such as ozone, cigarette smoke and antigen. After antigen challenge of allergic asthmatic subjects, the number of eosinophils in broncho-alveolar lavage fluid increases in subjects who developed a late-phase response [14,15]. Eosinophil infiltration is a distinctive and specific feature of the inflammation in asthmatic airways [11,13], and suggests that the eosinophil may play a critical role in its pathogenesis [16]. Indeed, there is a direct relationship between peripheral and broncho-alveolar lavage eosinophil counts and BHR [17,18].

Inflammatory mediators

Many inflammatory mediators have been implicated in the pathogenesis of asthma [5]. These include histamine, prostaglandins, leukotrienes, adenosine and bradykinin, which all induce several effects, such as acute broncho-constriction, microvascular leakage and mucus secretion. However, it is difficult to account for the sustained BHR seen in asthma. Prostaglandin D_2 (probably acting via thromboxane receptors) induced an increase in bronchial responsiveness in man, but the effect is transient [19]. Neither leukotrienes B_4, D_4 nor bradykinin increase histamine responsiveness [19–21]. On the other hand, PAF is able to induce sustained BHR in guinea pig [22], dog [23], primate [24], sheep [25], and man [26,27], and to induce several of the inflammatory features reported in asthmatic airways [28].

Sources of PAF in asthma

PAF may be formed from several types of cell which have been implicated in the pathogenesis of asthma. PAF is released from sensitized guinea-pig lungs after intra-tracheal antigen challenge, although the cellular source is not certain [29]. Release of PAF has been demonstrated from neutrophils, platelets and some types of mast cell (although not yet human lung mast cells) [2]. Of particular interest is the demonstration that PAF may be released from pulmonary macrophages [12,30]. Alveolar macrophages removed from broncho-alveolar lavage fluid of asthmatic patients release PAF, whereas those from non-asthmatic subjects do not. Eosinophils are the richest cellular source of PAF, and eosinophils isolated from asthmatic patients release more PAF than those from non-asthmatic subjects [31]. As PAF also activates eosinophils (see below) the release of PAF from eosinophils provides a possible mechanism for amplifying the involvement of eosinophils in allergic inflammation.

Inflammatory effects of PAF

When instilled into the airways of rabbits, PAF causes an inflammatory response consisting of desquamation of epithelial cells into the lumen with accumulation of polymorphonuclear cells and macrophages [32]. Similar changes have been reported after intravenous PAF in guinea pigs [33], with sub-mucosal oedema and infiltration of eosinophils and neutrophils. These changes mimic the inflammatory changes seen after allergen exposure in this species. In baboons, intra-tracheal PAF causes a selective accumulation of eosinophils in broncho-alveolar lavage [34], which may persist for up to two weeks [24]. PAF is chemotactic for human eosinophils *in vitro* [35,36]. In normal and atopic subjects PAF inhalation is associated with an increase in neutrophils rather than eosinophils in broncho-alveolar lavage fluid. Interestingly, this correlates negatively with the increase in airway responsiveness [37], although such studies have yet to be undertaken in allergic asthmatics. However, intra-dermal administration of PAF to atopic subjects but not normal subjects induces an infiltration of eosinophils into the skin [38]. This ability of PAF to act as a chemotactic agent for eosinophils *in vivo* only in allergic subjects raises the possibility that PAF may also be responsible for the influx of eosinophils into the airways of allergic asthmatic subjects. PAF also enhances the adhesion of eosinophils to endothelial cells [39], which may be an important step in the recruitment of eosinophils into tissues.

Effects on microvascular permeability

Increased vascular permeability, allowing the formation of airway oedema and extravasation of plasma into the airway lumen, may be important in asthma [40]. Several mediators can induce increased microvascular leakage [5]. PAF causes a dose-dependent increase in airway vascular permeability, as measured by the extravasation of Evans blue dye which binds to plasma albumin, having effects at doses as low as 1 ng/kg in guinea pigs, which makes PAF the most known potent mediator of microvascular leakage (Fig. 7.1) [41]. The site of leakage, as for other mediators, is in post-capillary venules [42]. The effect of PAF on leakage is not inhibited by severe depletion of circulating platelets with anti-platelet serum [41]. However, the increase in vascular permeability is blocked in a dose-dependent manner by specific PAF receptor antagonists, such as BN 56203 [41] and WEB 2086 [43]. Cyclooxygenase inhibition by

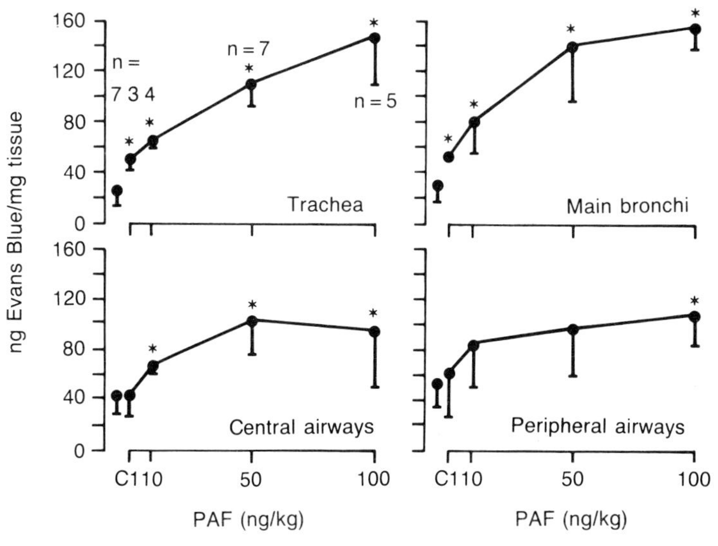

Fig. 7.1 Effect of intravenous PAF on microvascular leakage in guinea pig airways. Leakage was measured by extravasation of Evans blue dye. From Evans *et al.* [41].*, $P < 0.05$.

indomethacin or lipoxygenase inhibition by BW 755C does not alter PAF-induced increase in vascular permeability [41], suggesting that this effect of PAF is mediated directly on the endothelial cells of post-capillary venules. Antigen-induced microvascular leakage in guinea pig airways (at least that induced by i.v. antigen) is not reduced by prior treatment with a PAF antagonist, however, suggesting that PAF cannot account for the immediate microvascular leakage which occurs after allergen [44]. Although PAF effects on the microvasculature of human airways cannot be studied directly, PAF produces a wheal-and-flare response when injected into human skin [45, 46]. Both responses are inhibited in a dose-dependent manner by oral administration of the PAF antagonist BN 52063 [46].

Effects on airway smooth muscle

PAF is a potent broncho-constrictor in the guinea pig *in vivo*, yet has little effect on airway smooth muscle *in vitro*, suggesting that its effect is indirect [47]. In guinea pig, the broncho-constrictor effect is dependent on platelets after i.v. administration [47], but not when given by aerosol [48]. Guinea-pig lung strips show a consistent contractile response to PAF, which is partly mediated by acetylcholine release [49]. Human airways *in vitro* are unresponsive to PAF, but show variable contractile responses in the presence of platelets [50].

Administration of high doses of PAF (0. 04–1.2 mg/kg) by intratracheal instillation in artificially-ventilated humans with cerebral death has been reported to cause broncho-constriction associated with hypoxaemia and a fall in cardiac output [51]. In normal subjects inhaled PAF causes a dose-dependent broncho-constriction, but there is rapid tachyphylaxis [26,27] (Fig. 7.2). By giving two appropriate doubling amounts of PAF, the provocative dose needed to cause a 40% fall in the partial expiratory flow rate at 30% vital capacity (PD_{40}) can be calculated. The mean PD_{40} for PAF (0.13 μmol) is lower than the PD_{40} for methacholine (7.1 μmol), but there is no significant correlation between the PD_{40} for methacholine and the PD_{40} for PAF. This is unlike any other broncho-constrictor mediator which has been studied. The discrepancy is even more striking in asthmatic patients who are no more sensitive to the broncho-constrictor action of PAF than normal subjects, although they have an increased responsiveness to methacholine [52].

A single inhalation of PAF, at a dose equivalent to the predetermined PD_{40}, causes maximal broncho-constriction within 5 min, and spontaneously reverses over 2 h, with no evidence of late-phase broncho-constriction [26] (Fig. 7.3). All subjects experience transient facial flushing, an increase in heart rate and a decrease in diastolic blood pressure, suggesting

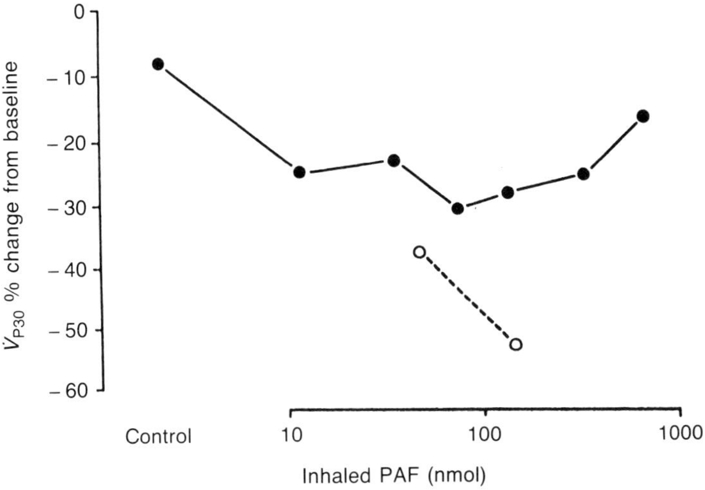

Fig. 7.2 The effect of inhaled PAF on airway function in a normal human subject. Cumulative doses were given and the bronchoconstrictor response recovered at higher doses, indicating the development of tachyphylaxis. ○---○ = control.

systemic vasodilatation. Lyso-PAF, the biologically inactive major precursor and metabolite of PAF, has no systemic or airway effects [26].

PAF-induced broncho-constriction must be indirect, since PAF has no consistent effect on human airways *in vitro*. The broncho-constriction is reduced but not completely blocked by an inhaled β-agonist at a dose which completely blocks other spasmogens [53], raising the possibility that part of the acute response to inhaled PAF may be due to narrowing of

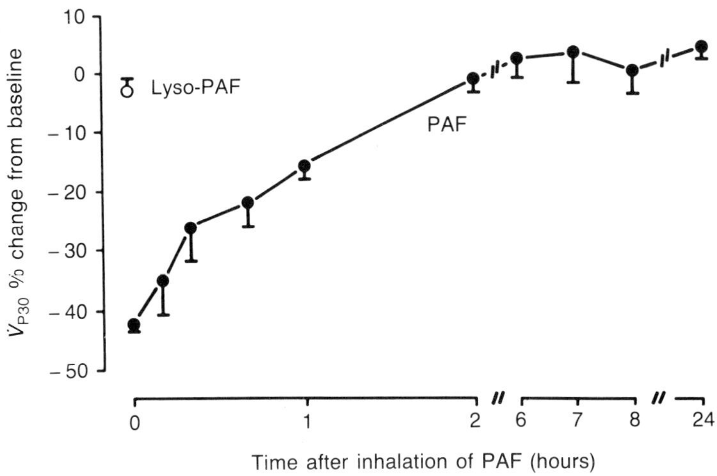

Fig. 7.3 PAF-induced bronchoconstriction in nine normal subjects. From Cuss *et al.* [26].

the airways by oedema. This would then account for the lack of correlation between the PC_{40} for PAF and the direct contractile effects seen after methacholine.

PAF-induced broncho-constriction is not reduced by an antihistamine ketotifen [54], although in another study chlorpheniramine was reported to reduce the broncho-constrictor effect [55]. PAF-induced broncho-constriction in man is unaffected by indomethacin, suggesting that cyclo-oxygenase products are not involved [55], but whether lipoxygenase products are relevant is not yet known.

Effects on bronchial responsiveness

In several species PAF has been shown to cause a sustained increase in BHR [22–27]. In guinea pig the increase in bronchial responsiveness is platelet-dependent [22], but the cell dependency in other species is not certain. In human subjects methacholine responsiveness is increased at 6 h after inhaled PAF and is maximal at 3 days. The increased responsiveness induced by PAF is sustained and may last for up to 4 weeks after inhalation (Fig. 7.4) [26]. In asthmatic subjects increased bronchial responsiveness to methacholine is also seen, although to a lesser extent than that found in normal subjects [52], possibly indicating that endogenously released PAF may have already had an effect on bronchial responsiveness.

Mechanisms of PAF-induced BHR

There are several mechanisms by which PAF might induce an increase in bronchial responsiveness.

Effect on airway receptors

PAF might induce changes in receptors in airway smooth muscle. However, in guinea pigs showing increased responsiveness to histamine or methacholine after inhaled PAF, the *in vitro* responses of airway smooth muscle to both of these spasmogens are not increased. Furthermore, there is no change in histamine H_1-receptors or muscarinic receptors as assessed by direct receptor binding, nor any change in phosphoinositide hydrolysis to these agonists, indicating no change in coupling of receptors [56]. This suggests that PAF-induced hyper-responsiveness cannot be due to any effect on these spasmogenic receptors.

Another possibility is that PAF may induce a reduction in β-receptor function, particularly since PAF is able to reduce β-receptor density in cerebral tissue *in vitro* [57] and to reduce β-receptor density in lung *in vitro* [58]. Although infused PAF reduces the bronchodilator response to infused isoprenaline in guinea pigs, there is no reduction in the relaxant

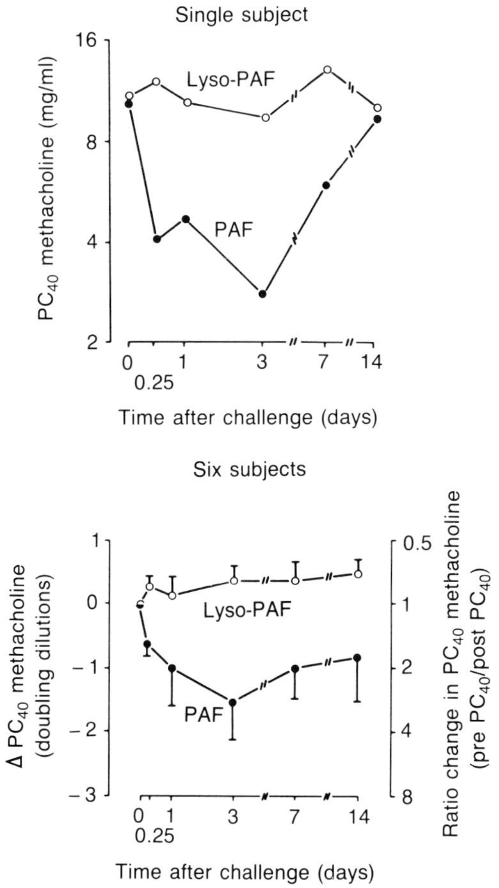

Fig. 7.4 PAF-induced increase in bronchial responsiveness to inhaled methacholine in six normal subjects. A similar dose of lyso-PAF had no effect. Mean $\pm$ SEM; $n = 6$. From Cuss *et al.* [26].

response to isoprenaline *in vitro*, nor any reduction in β-receptor binding characteristics [59]. This might indicate that the reduced bronchodilator response to isoprenaline is unlikely to be due to any defect in β-receptor function, and perhaps may be due to an effect of PAF on mucosal oedema resulting in airway narrowing which cannot be readily decreased by a bronchodilator.

Effect on circulating cells

Inhalation of PAF is accompanied by a marked fall in the circulating white-cell count (predominantly neutrophils) but the platelet count is unchanged. This effect is maximal at 5 min, returning to baseline values by 15 min, but in some subjects a rebound neutrophilia is observed [52,53].

The transient leukopaenia is tachyphylactic to further doses of inhaled PAF. These observations are similar to those reported by Gateau *et al.* [51], who found leukopaenia at a low dose of PAF instilled into the trachea; at higher doses, both leukopaenia and thrombocytopaenia were observed. Because the neutropaenia is transient, these changes may be secondary to the slowing of the pulmonary circulation with pulmonary vasoconstriction due to PAF. It is possible that the transient increase in margination of neutrophils (and eosinophils) in the pulmonary and bronchial circulations is the initial step for chemotaxis. After infusion of prostacyclin (PGI_2) there is a significant abrogation of the neutropaenic response to inhaled PAF, possibly due to a reduction in margination and adhesion to endothelial cells [60].

Interaction with eosinophils

Since PAF is rapidly inactivated in airways, its prolonged effect on airway responsiveness must be indirect. It seems likely that PAF initiates a series of inflammatory events in the airway. Eosinophils, which are prominent inflammatory cells in the asthmatic airway, may be recruited by a direct chemotactic effect of PAF, perhaps involving an interaction with endothelial cells in the bronchial circulation. Eosinophils themselves are a rich source of further PAF which may serve to perpetuate the inflammation. Stimulation of eosinophils may release mediators that are toxic to the airway epithelium, such as major basic protein, eosinophil cationic protein and eosinophil-derived neurotoxin [16] and may account for the denudation of the epithelium observed in asthma (Fig. 7.5). Eosinophils are potently activated by PAF to release basic proteins [61] and have a high density of PAF receptors [62]. Furthermore, eosinophils from asthmatic patients appear to be more sensitive to the stimulatory effects of PAF than cells from non-asthmatic subjects [63]. Because airway epithelium has been shown to elaborate a putative smooth muscle relaxant factor [64,65], loss of epithelial cells or epithelial cell function may directly underlie airway hyper-responsiveness. Recent studies have demonstrated that eosinophil-derived major basic protein will induce hyper-responsiveness of guinea pig tracheal muscle *in vitro* through some interaction with epithelium [66].

Epithelial damage may also result in the exposure of C-fibre afferent nerve endings which may in turn be stimulated by mediators such as bradykinin to release sensory neuropeptides such as substance P, neurokinin A and calcitonin gene-related peptide [67]. This axon reflex may amplify the inflammatory responses in asthmatic airways with mucus hypersecretion and bronchial oedema. The development of epithelial damage after PAF may take some time to develop and will presumably taken even longer to recover, and so could account for the duration of the increased responsiveness seen after PAF. Whether PAF can account for

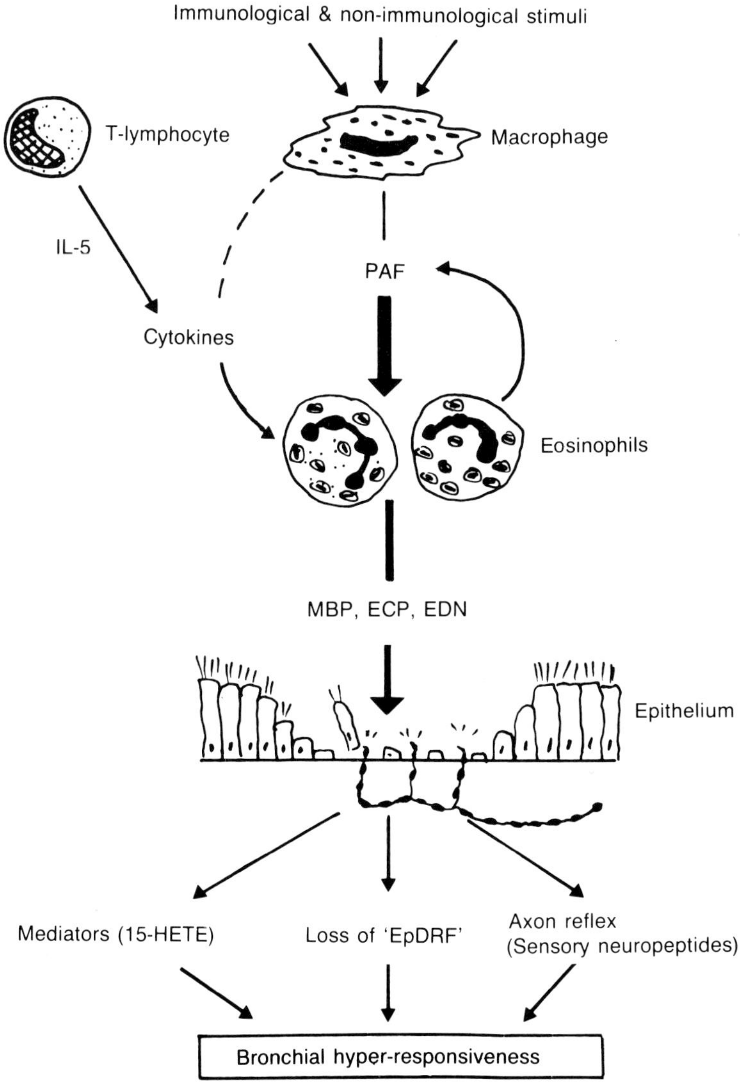

Fig. 7.5 Possible mechanisms of PAF-induced bronchial hyper-responsiveness. Adapted from Barnes *et al.* [5]. MBP = major basic protein; ECP = eosinophil cationic protein; EDN = eosinophil derived neurotoxin; and 'EpDRF' = epithelial derived relaxant factor.

the increased responsiveness which follows allergen will remain uncertain until the effects of specific PAF-antagonists have been studied in man.

Airway secretions

Few studies have investigated the effects of PAF on airway secretion. PAF increases airway secretions in animal airways *in vitro* and *in vivo* [68, 69].

In isolated human airways, PAF weakly stimulates mucus secretion *in vitro*, and this effect may depend upon the generation of leukotrienes [70]. In guinea-pig, PAF given intravenously increases the protein content of airway secretions, presumably as a result of plasma extravasation [71]. When given directly into the airway PAF causes a marked slowing of mucociliary transport [72]. This suggests that, if PAF is released in asthmatic airways, it may contribute to the mucus hypersecretion and impaired mucociliary clearance which results in luminal plugging of peripheral airways.

Role of PAF in asthma?

Because of the powerful inflammatory effects of PAF and of its capacity to induce prolonged increases in airway responsiveness, its possible role in the patho-physiology of asthma is of great interest. The measurement of PAF release in biological fluids remains a problem as PAF is very rapidly metabolized and specific and sensitive assays are difficult. However, the development of specific antagonists (see Chapter 4) now makes it possible to evaluate the role of PAF in asthma [73].

PAF antagonists have now been used in a variety of experimental animal models of asthma. PAF antagonists reduce allergen-induced contraction of lung strips from sensitized guinea pigs *in vitro* [74]. In sensitized guinea pig the hyper-responsiveness induced by allergen exposure is inhibited by prior treatment with BN 52021 (Fig. 7.6) [75]. Furthermore, PAF antagonists also block the eosinophil infiltration in the airways which follows allergen exposure in this species [76]. In allergic sheep WEB 2086 reduces the late response and the subsequent increase in bronchial reactivity following allergen inhalation, while having no effect on the early broncho-constrictor response [77]. Similar results have been obtained in IgE-producing rabbits [78,79].

The availability of PAF antagonists for human use now makes it possible to study the role of PAF in human asthma. The ginkgolide mixture, BN 52063, in a dose which effectively blocks the skin response to PAF [46], has no effect on the flare response to allergen but reduces the late onset cutaneous response to allergen (Fig. 7.7) [80]. Since the late skin response to allergen is associated with eosinophil infiltration, this might indicate that PAF is an important signal for eosinophil influx. PAF release has recently been demonstrated in blister fluid from allergic patients with late-onset inflammatory responses to intra-dermal allergen when eosinophil infiltration has been demonstrated [81]. Such studies have yet to be done in asthmatics. However, oral BN 52063, in a dose which is effective in blocking skin responses to PAF, has only a modest inhibitory effect on the broncho-constriction induced by inhaled PAF [82], so more potent antagonists, or antagonists given by inhalation, will be needed in asthma.

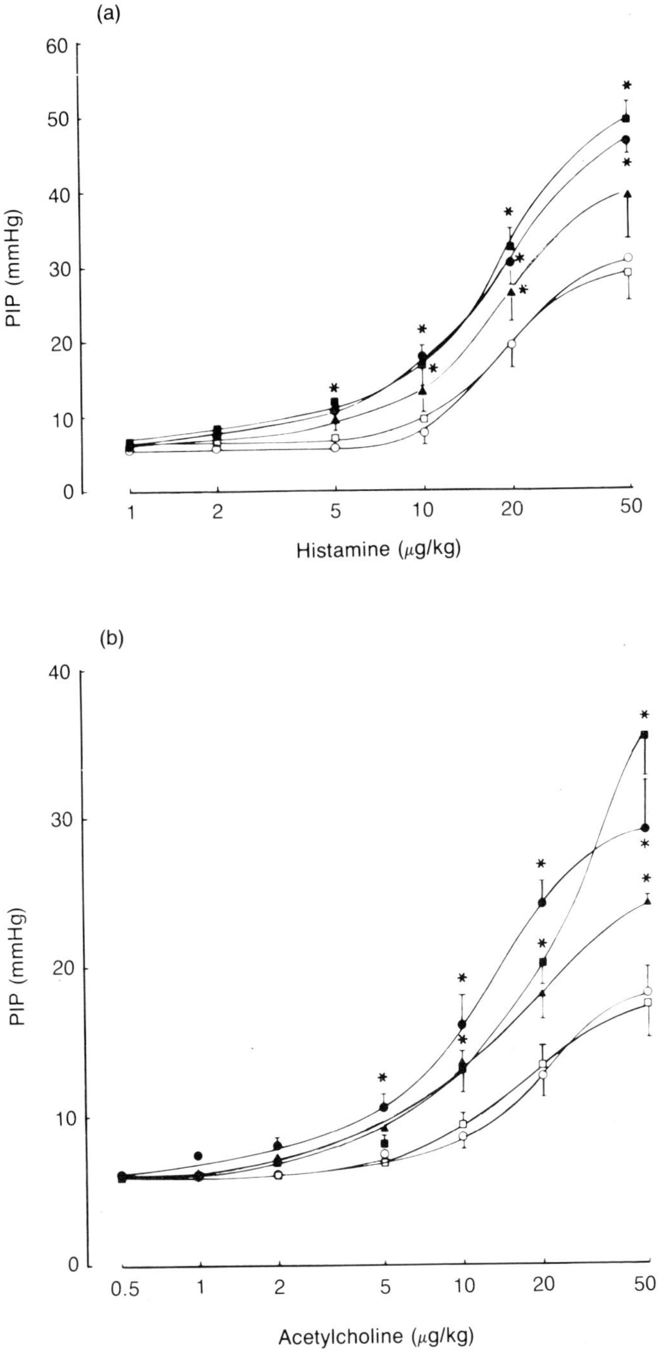

Fig. 7.6 Effect of BN 52021 on the increase in airway reactivity which follows allergen challenge in guinea pig PIP = pulmonary inflation pressure. From Coyle *et al.* [75].

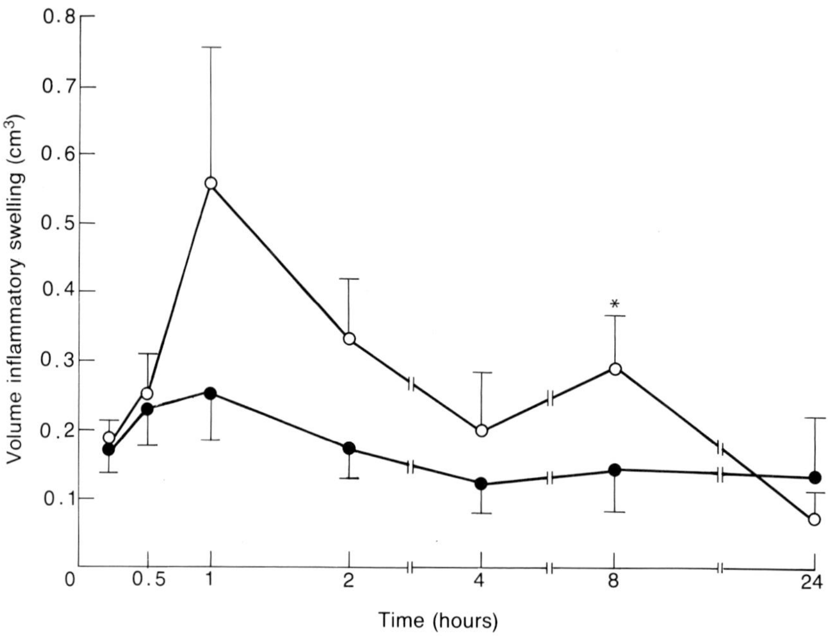

Fig. 7.7 The effect of an oral PAF antagonist (BN 52063) on the skin responses to allergen in atopic subjects. BN 52063 significantly blocks the late (inflammatory) response, but not the early weal and flare reactions. From Roberts *et al.* [80].*, $P < 0.05$.

Other allergic diseases

Although the case for the involvement of PAF in asthma looks convincing, it may also play a part in other allergic diseases [2].

Anaphylactic shock

The release of PAF intravenously in an allergic reaction may contribute to the hypotension seen in anaphylactic shock [83]. In guinea pigs a number of PAF antagonists, such as BN 52021 or WEB 2086, effectively inhibit the cardiovascular and bronchoconstrictor changes resulting from intravenous allergen exposure in sensitized animals [84,85]. Cardiac dysfunction, characterized by decreased ventricular contractility, which may be seen in anaphylactic shock in humans, is mimicked by PAF in experimental animals and on isolated human heart preparations [86] (see Chapter 6).

Allergic rhinitis

PAF induces a dose-dependent vasoconstriction when administered topically to the human nose [87], which can be inhibited by the anti-allergic drug, sodium cromoglycate [88]. PAF has little effect on nasal reactivity, however [89]. The precise role of PAF in allergic rhinitis will only be known after studies with PAF antagonists.

Extrinsic allergic alveolitis

The pathological changes in this group of diseases, which include farmer's lung and bird fancier's lung, suggest a form of Arthus reaction. In experimental Arthus reactions, which involve immune complexes, PAF antagonists have an inhibitory effect [90], raising the possibility that PAF release may be contributory to some of the pathological events in extrinsic allergic alveolitis.

Pulmonary vascular disease

PAF has potent effects on pulmonary vascular tone and may therefore play a role in some pulmonary vascular disorders. *In vitro* PAF has variable effects on pulmonary vascular smooth muscle preparations, partly determined by the resting tone. In isolated perfused rat lung PAF has a dual effect: at low doses PAF vasodilates the pulmonary vascular bed, whereas at higher doses constriction occurs [91]. Infusion of PAF in the sheep increases pulmonary vascular resistance, an effect which is partially inhibited by indomethacin, suggesting the involvement of a cyclooxygenase product, such as thromboxane [92].

Since pulmonary endothelial cells may be a source of PAF [93], and PAF is released into broncho-alveolar lavage fluid in experimental animals during hypoxia [94], it is possible that PAF might be involved in hypoxic vasoconstriction. In isolated perfused rat lung hypoxic vasoconstriction is reduced by the PAF antagonist WEB 2086 at doses which have little effect on the direct vasoconstrictor effect of angiotensin-II [95]. This might indicate that PAF is contributory to the hypoxic vasoconstriction, although another PAF antagonist, BN 52021, is without effect (unpublished), indicating that WEB 2086 might have some additional effect, or that there are sub-types of PAF receptor on pulmonary vascular smooth muscle, as has been postulated elsewhere [96]. The role of PAF in pulmonary vascular diseases must await clinical studies with PAF antagonists.

Acute lung injury and adult respiratory distress syndrome

One of the major clinical features of acute lung injury and adult respiratory distress syndrome (ARDS) is pulmonary oedema, resulting from endothelial cell dysfunction. Lungs isolated from PAF-treated animals exhibit oedematous changes evidenced by accumulation of markers of plasma proteins, such as Evans Blue dye or radiolabelled plasma proteins

[97,98]. PAF induces oedema formation in isolated perfused lung populations even in the presence of circulating blood elements [99]. This suggests that PAF-induced vascular permeability in the pulmonary vasculature is a direct effect on endothelial cells, as has been suggested for other vascular beds [100]. Histopathologically, lungs taken from PAF-treated animals also reveal frank endothelial cell damage in addition to vascular permeability [101].

Another prominent feature of acute lung injury and ARDS is the intravascular accumulation of platelets and neutrophils within the pulmonary vasculature. Such pathological changes can be minicked by systemic administration of PAF, assessed both histologically [102] or radioisotopically [103,104]. Recently, it has been shown that WEB 2086 affects the increase in lung fluid and solute exchange in awake sheep following administration of intravenous endotoxins [105]. Furthermore, SRI-63 441 has been shown to reduce the hypoxaemia and leukopenia associated with endotoxin infusion in sheep, suggesting a role for PAF in certain aspects of the pathogenesis of ARDS.

Acknowledgement

We would like to thank Madeleine Wray for her careful preparation of this manuscript.

References

1 Barnes, R. J. Platelet-activating factor and asthma. *J. Allergy Clin. Immunol.* (1988), **81**, 152–161.

2 Barnes, R. J., Chung, K. F. & Page, C. P. Platelet-activating factor as a mediator of allergic disease. *J. Allergy. Clin. Immunol.* (1988), **81**, 919–934.

3 Page, C. P. & Robertson, D. N. A role for platelet activating factor in shock and acute lung injury. In Paubert-Braquet, M. (ed.) *Lipid Mediators in Immunology and Shock* (1987), pp.197–208. Plenum Press, New York.

4 Barnes, P. J., Rodger, I. W. & Thomson, N. C. *Asthma: Basic Mechanisms and Clinical Management* (1988). Academic Press, London.

5 Barnes, P. J., Chung, K. F. & Page, C. P. Inflammatory mediators in asthma. *Pharmacol. Rev.* (1988), **40**, 49–84.

6 Boushey, H. A., Holtzman, M. J., Sheller, J. R. & Nadel, J. A. Bronchial hyperreactivity. *Am. Rev. Resp. Dis.* (1980), **121**, 398–413.

7 Juniper, E. F., Frith, P. A. & Hargreave, F. E. Airway responsiveness to histamine and methacholine: relationship to minimum treatment to control symptoms of asthma. *Thorax* (1981), **36**, 575–579.

8 Britton, J. R., Burney, P. G. J., Chinn, S., Papacosta, A. O. & Tattersfield, A. E. The relation between changes in airway reactivity and change in respiratory symptoms and medication in respiratory symptoms and medication in a community survey. *Am. Rev. Resp. Dis.* (1988), **138**, 530–534.

9 Chung, K. F. Role of inflammation in the hyperreactivity of the airways in asthma. *Thorax* (1986), **41**, 657–662.

10 Barnes, P. J. New concepts in the pathogenesis of bronchial hyperresponsiveness and asthma. *J. Allergy Clin. Immunol.* (1989), in press.
11 Dunnill, M. S. The pathology of asthma with special reference to changes in the bronchial mucosa. *J. Clin. Path.* (1960), **13**, 27–33.
12 Godard, P., Chaintreuil J., Damon, M. *et al.* Functional assessment of alveolar macrophages: comparison of cells from asthmatics and normal subjects. *J. Allergy Clin. Immunol.* (1982), **70**, 88–93.
13 Laitinen, L. A., Heino, M., Laitinen, A., Kava, T. & Haahtela, T. Damage of the airway epithelium and bronchial reactivity in patients with asthma. *Am. Rev. Resp. Dis.* (1985), **131**, 599–606.
14 De Monchy, J. G. R., Kauffman, H. F., Venge, P., *et al.* Bronchoalveolar eosinophilia during allergen-induced late asthmatic reactions. *Am. Rev. Resp. Dis.* (1985), **131**, 373–376.
15 Metzger, W. J., Zavala, D., Richerson, H. B. *et al.* Local allergen challenge and bronchoalveolar lavage of allergic asthmatic lungs. *Am. Rev. Resp. Dis.* (1987), **135**, 433–440.
16 Frigas, E. & Gleich, G. J. The eosinophil and the pathology of asthma. *J. Allergy Clin. Immunol.* (1986), **77**, 527–537.
17 Taylor, K. J. & Luksza, A. R. Peripheral blood eosinophil counts and bronchial responsiveness. *Thorax* (1987), **42**, 452–456.
18 Wardlaw, A. J., Dunnette, S., Gleich, G. J., Collins, J. V. & Kay, A. B. Eosinophils and mast cells in bronchoalveolar lavage in subjects with mild asthma. *Am. Rev. Resp. Dis.* (1988), **88**, 62–69.
19 Fuller, R. W., Dixon, C. M. S., Dollery, C. T. & Barnes, P. J. Prostaglandin D_2 potentiates airway responses to histamine and methacholine. *Am. Rev. Resp. Dis.* (1986), **133**, 252–254.
20 Barnes, N. C., Piper, P. J. & Costello, J. F. Actions of inhaled leukotrienes and their interactions with other allergic mediators. *Prostaglandins* (1984), **28**, 629–631.
21 Black, P. N., Fuller, R. W., Taylor, G. W., Barnes, P. J. & Dollery, C. T. Bronchial reactivity is not increased after inhalation of leukotriene B_4 and prostaglandin D_2. *Br. J. Clin. Pharmacol.* (1988), **25**, 667.
22 Mazzoni, L., Morley, J., Page, C. P. & Sanjar, S. Induction of airway hyperreactivity by platelet activating factor in the guinea-pig. *J. Physiol.* (1985), **365**, 107p.
23 Chung, K. F., Aizawa, H., Leikauf, G. D., Ueki, I. F., Evans, T. W. & Nadel, J. A. Airway hyperresponsiveness induced by platelet-activating factor: role of thromboxane generation. *J. Pharmacol. Exp. Ther.* (1986), **236**, 580–584.
24 Denjean, A., Arnoux, B. & Benveniste, J. Long-lasting effect of intratracheal administration of PAF-acether in baboons. *Am. Rev. Resp. Dis.* (1988), **137**, A283.
25 Christman, B. W., Lefferts, P. L. & Snapper, J. R. Effect of platelet activating factor on aerosol histamine responses in awake sheep. *Am. Rev. Resp. Dis.* (1987), **135**, 1267–1270.
26 Cuss, F. M., Dixon, C. M. S. & Barnes, P. J. Effects of inhaled platelet activating factor on pulmonary function and bronchial responsiveness in man. *Lancet* (1986), ii, 189–192.
27 Rubin, A.-H., Smith, L. J. & Patterson, R. The bronchoconstrictor properties of platelet-activating factor in humans. *Am. Rev. Resp. Dis.* (1987), **136**, 1145–1151.
28 Barnes, P. J. & Chung, K. F. PAF closely mimics the pathology of asthma. *Trends Pharmacol. Sci.* (1987), **8**, 285–287.
29 Fitzgerald, M. F., Moncada, S. & Parente, L. The anaphylactic release of platelet-activating factor from perfused guinea pig lungs. *Br. J. Pharmacol* (1986), **88**, 149–153.

30 Arnoux, B., Joseph, M., Simoes, M. H., *et al.* Antigenic release of PAF-acether and beta-glucuronidase from alveolar macrophages of asthmatics. *Bull. Eur. Physiopathol. Respir.* (1987), **23**, 119–124.

31 Lee, T. C., Lenihan, D. J., Malone, B., Roddy, L. L. & Wasserman, S. I. Increased biosynthesis of platelet activating factor in activated human eosinophils. *J. Biol. Chem.* (1984), **259**, 5526–5530.

32 Camussi, G., Pawlowski, I., Tetta, C. *et al.* Acute lung inflammation induced in the rabbit by local instillation of 1-O-octadecyl-2-acetyl-*sn*-glyceryl-3-phosphorylcholine or of native platelet activating factor. *Am. J. Pathol.* (1983), **112**, 78–88.

33 Lellouch-Tubiana, A., Lefort, J., Pirotzky, E., Vargaftig, B. B. & Pfister, A. Ultrastructural evidence for extravascular platelet recruitment in the lung upon intravenous injection of platelet activating factor (PAF-acether) to guinea-pigs. *Br. J. Exp. Pathol.* (1985), **66**, 345–355.

34 Arnoux, B., Denjean, A., Page, C. P., Nolibe, D., Morley, J. & Benveniste, J. Accumulation of platelets and eosinophils in baboon lung after PAF-acether challenge: inhibition by ketotifen. *Am. Rev. Resp. Dis.* (1988), **137**, 855–860.

35 Wardlaw, A. J., Moqbel, R., Cromwell, O. & Kay, A. B. Platelet-activating factor. A potent chemotactic and chemokinetic factor for human eosinophils. *J. Clin. Invest.* (1986), **78**, 1701–1706.

36 Tamura, N., Agrawal, D. K. & Townley, R. G. Effects of platelet activating factor on the chemotaxis of normodense eosinophils from normal subjects. *Biochem. Biophys. Res. Commun.* (1987), **142**, 638–644.

37 Wardlaw, A. J., Chung, K. F., Moqbel, R. *et al.* Cellular changes in blood and bronchoalveolar lavage (BAL) and bronchial responsiveness after inhaled PAF in man. *Am. Rev. Resp. Dis.* (1988), **137**, A283.

38 Henocq, E. & Vargaftig, B. B. Accumulation of eosinophils in response to intracutaneous PAF-acether and allergens in man. *Lancet* (1986), **i**, 1378–1379.

39 Kimani, G., Tonnesen, M. G. & Henson, P. G. Stimulation of eosinophil adherence to human vascular endothelial cells *in vitro* by platelet activating factor. *J. Immunol.* (1988), **140**, 3161–3166.

40 Persson, C. G. A. Role of plasma exudation in asthmatic airways. *Lancet* (1986), **ii**, 1126–1128.

41 Evans, T. W., Chung, K., Rogers, D. F. & Barnes, P. J. Effect of platelet-activating factor on airway vascular permeability: possible mechanisms. *J. Appl. Physiol.* (1987), **63**, 479–484.

42 O'Donnell, S. R. & Barnett, C. J. K. Microvascular leakage to platelet activating factor in guinea-pig trachea and bronchi. *Eur. J. Pharmacol.* (1987), **138**, 385–396.

43 Evans, T. W., Dent, G., Rogers, D. F., Aursudkij, B., Chung, K. F. & Barnes, P. J. Effect of a PAF antagonist, WEB 2086, on airway microvascular leakage in the guinea pig and platelet aggregation in man. *Br. J. Pharmacol.* (1988), **94**, 164–168.

44 Evans, T. W., Rogers, D. F., Aursudkij, B., Chung, K. F. & Barnes, P. J. Microvascular leakage associated with antigen-induced bronchial anaphylaxis is inhibited by nedocromil sodium or BW 755C in the guinea pig. *Am. Rev. Resp. Dis.* (1988), in press.

45 Archer, C. B., Page, C. P., Morley, J. & MacDonald, D. M. Accumulation of inflammatory cells in response to intracutaneous platelet-activating factor (PAF-acether) in man. *Br. J. Dermatol.* (1985), **112**, 285–290.

46 Chung, K. F., Dent, G., McCusker, M., Guinot, Ph, Page, C. P. & Barnes, P. J. Effect of a ginkgolide mixture (BN 52063) in antagonising skin and platelet responses to platelet activating factor in man. *Lancet* (1987), **i**, 248–251.

47 Vargaftig, B. B., Lefort, J., Chignard, M. & Benveniste, J. Platelet-activating factor

induces a platelet-dependent bronchoconstriction unrelated to the formation of prostaglandin derivatives. *Eur. J. Pharmacol.* (1980), **65**, 185–192.

48 Lefort, J., Rotilio, D. & Vargaftig, B. B. The platelet-independent release of thromboxane A_2 by PAF-acether by guinea-pig lungs involves mechanisms distinct from those for leukotriene C_4 and bradykinin. *Br. J. Pharmacol.* (1984), **82,** 525–531.

49 Stimler-Gerard, N. P. Parasympathetic stimulation as a mechanism for platelet-activating factor-induced contractile responses in lung. *J. Pharmacol. Exp. Ther.* (1986), **237**, 209–213.

50 Schellenberg, R. R., Walker, B. & Snyder, F. Platelet-dependent contraction of human bronchus by platelet activating factor. *J. Allergy Clin. Immunol.* (1983), **71,** 145.

51 Gateau, O., Arnoux, B., Deriaz, H., Viars, P. & Benveniste, J. Acute effects of intratracheal administration of PAF-acether (platelet-activating factor) in humans. *Am. Rev. Resp. Dis.* (1984), **3,** A129.

52 Chung, K. F. & Barnes, P. J. Effects of platelet activating factor on airway calibre, airway responsiveness and circulating cells in asthmatic subjects. *Thorax* (1989), **44**, 108–115.

53 Chung, K. F. & Barnes, P. J. Effect of a beta-adrenoceptor agonist on airway responses to platelet activating factor. *Thorax* (1989), **44**, 102–107.

54 Chung, K. F., Minette, P., McCusker, M. & Barnes, P. J. Ketotifen inhibits the cutaneous but not the airway responses to platelet-activating factor in man. *J. Allergy. Clin. Immunol.* (1988), **81**, 1192–1198.

55 Smith, L. J., Rubin, A.-H. & Patterson, R. Mechanism of platelet activating factor-induced bronchoconstriction in humans. *Am. Rev. Resp. Dis.* (1988), **137**, 1015–1019.

56 Robertson, D. N., Rhoden, K. J., Grandordy, B., Page, C. P. & Barnes, P. J. The effect of platelet activating factor on histamine and muscarinic receptor function in guinea-pig airways. *Am. Rev. Resp. Dis.* (1988), **137**, 1317–1322.

57 Braquet, P., Etienne, A. & Clostre, F. Down-regulation of beta$_2$-adrenergic receptors by PAF-acether and its inhibition by the PAF-acether antagonist BN 52021 *Prostaglandins* (1985), **30**, 721–726.

58 Agrawal, D. K. & Townley, R. D. Effects of platelet activating factor on beta-adrenoceptors in human lung. *Biochem, Biophys, Res. Commun.* (1987), **143**, 1–6.

59 Barnes, P. J., Grandordy, B. M., Page, C. P., Rhoden, K. J. & Robertson, D. N. The effect of platelet activating factor on pulmonary beta-adrenoceptors. *Br. J. Pharmacol.* (1987), **90**, 709–715.

60 Lammers, J.-W., Kioumis, I., McCusker, M., Chung, K. F. & Barnes, P. J. Effect of prostacyclin (PGI_2) on bronchoconstriction induced by platelet-activating factor (PAF) in man. *Am. Rev. Respir. Dis.* (1988), **137**, A373.

61 Kroegel, C., Yukawa, T., Dent, G., Chanez, P., Chung, K. F. & Barnes, P. J. Platelet activating factor induces eosinophil peroxidase release from purified human eosinophils. *Immunology* (1988), **64**, 559–562.

62 Dent, G., Ukena, D., Chanez, P., Sybrecht, G. W. & Barnes, P. J. Characterization of platelet-activating factor (PAF) receptors in human neutrophils and eosinophils using the new competitive PAF antagonist WEB 2086. *Am. Rev. Resp. Dis.* (1988), **137**, 236.

63 Chanez, P., Dent, G., Yukawa, T., Chung, K. F. & Barnes, P. J. Increased eosinophil responsiveness to platelet-activating factor in asthma. *Clin. Sci* (1988), **74**, 5.

64 Cuss, F. M. & Barnes, P. J. Epithelial mediators. *Am. Rev. Resp. Dis.* (1987), **136,** S32–S35.

65 Vanhoutte, P. M. Epithelium-derived relaxing factor: myth or reality. *Thorax* (1988), **43**, 665–668.
66 Flavahan, N. A., Slitman, N. R., Gleich, G. J. & Vanhoutte, P. M. Human eosinophil major basic protein causes hyperreactivity of respiratory smooth muscle. *Am. Rev. Resp. Dis.* (1988), **135**, 685–688.
67 Barnes, P. J. Asthma as an axon reflex. *Lancet* (1986), **i**, 242–245.
68 Lang, M., Hansen. D. & Hahn, H. L. Effect of the PAF antagonist CV-3988 on PAF-induced changes in mucus secretion and in respiratory and circulatory variables in ferret. *Agents & Actions* (1987), Suppl. 21, 245–251.
69 Steiger, J., Bray, M. A. & Subramanian, N. Platelet activating factor (PAF) is a potent stimulator of porcine tracheal fluid secretion *in vitro*. *Eur. J. Pharmacol.* (1987), **142**, 367–372.
70 Goswami, S. K., Ohashi, M., Panagiotis, G. & Marom, Z. Platelet activating factor enhances mucous glycoprotein release from human airways *in vitro*. *Am. Rev. Resp. Dis.* (1987), **135**, A159.
71 Rogers, D. F., Aursudkij, B., Evans, T. W., Belvisi, M. G., Chung, K. F. & Barnes, P. J. Platelet activating factor increases protein exudation but not mucus secretion in guinea-pig trachea *in vivo*. *Am. Rev. Resp. Dis.* (1987), **135**, 160.
72 Aursudkij, B., Rogers, D. F., Evans, T. W., Alton, E. W. F. W., Chung, K. F. & Barnes, P. J. Reduced tracheal mucus velocity in guinea pig *in vivo* by platelet activating factor. *Am. Rev. Resp. Dis.* (1987), **35**, 160.
73 Chung, K. F. & Barnes, P. J. PAF antagonists: their therapeutic potential in asthma. *Drugs* (1988), **35**, 93–103.
74 Darius, H., Lefer, D. J., Smith, B. & Lefer, A. M. Role of platelet-activating factor-acether in mediating guinea pig anaphylaxis. *Science* (1986), **232**, 58–60.
75 Coyle, A. J., Urwin, S. C., Page, C. P., Touvay, C., Villain, B. & Braquet, P. The effect of the selective antagonist BN 52021 on PAF and antigen-induced bronchial hyperreactivity and eosinophil accumulation. *Eur. J. Pharmacol.* (1988), **148**, 51–58.
76 Lellouch-Tubiana, A., Lefort, J., Simon, M.-T., Pfister, A. & Vargaftig, B. B. Eosinophil recruitment into guinea pig lungs after PAF-acether and allergen administration: modulation by prostacyclin, platelet depletion, and selective antagonists. *Am. Rev. Resp. Dis.* (1988), **137**, 948–954.
77 Stevenson, J. S., Tallent, M., Blinder, L. & Abraham, W. M. The effect of the PAF antagonist WEB 2086 on the early and late response in allergic sheep. *Fed. Proc.* (1987), **46**, 6683.
78 Coyle, A., Sjoerdsma, K., Page, C. P., Brown, L. & Metzger, W. J. Modification of the late asthmatic response and bronchial hyperreactivity by BN 52021, a platelet activating factor antagonist. *Clin. Res.* (1987), **35**, 254.
79 Smith, H. R., Henson, P. M., Clay, K. L. & Larsen, G. L. Effect of the PAF-antagonist L-659-989 on the last asthmatic response and increased airway reactivity in the rabbit. *Am. Rev. Resp. Dis.* (1988), **137**, A283.
80 Roberts, N. M., Page, C. P., Chung, K. F., Barnes, P. J. The effect of a specific PAF antagonist, BN 52063, on antigen-induced cutaneous responses in man. *J. Allergy Clin. Immunol.* (1988), **82**, 2136–2241.
81 Michel, L., Denizot, Y., Thomas, Y., Benveniste, J. & Dubertret, L. Release of PAF-acether and precursors during allergic cutaneous reactions. *Lancet* (1988), **ii**, 404.
82 Roberts, N. M., McCusker, M., Chung, K. F. & Barnes, P. J. The effect of PAF antagonist, BN 52063, on PAF-induced bronchoconstriction and neutropenia in man. *Br. J. Clin. Pharmacol.* (1988), **26**, 65–72.
83 Henson, P. M. & Pinckard, R. N. Basophil-derived platelet-activating factor

(PAF) as an *in vivo* mediator of acute allergic reactions: demonstration of specific densitization of platelets to PAF during IgE-induced anaphylaxis in the rabbit. *J. Immunol.* (1977), **119**, 2179–2184.

84 Sanchez Crespo, M., Fernandez-Gallardo, S., Nieto, M. L., Baranes, J. & Braquet, P. Inhibition of the vascular actions of IgG aggregates by BN 52021, a highly specific antagonist of PAF-acether. *Immunopharmacology* (1985), **10**, 69–75.

85 Pretolani, M., Lefort, J., Malenchere, E. & Vargaftig, B. B. Interference by the novel PAF-acether antagonist WEB 2086 with the bronchopulmonary responses to PAF-acether and to active and passive anaphylactic shock in guinea pigs. *Eur. J. Pharmacol.* (1987), **140**, 311–321.

86 Levi, R., Shen, T.-Y. Yee, S. J. *et al.* Platelet activating factor: effects on human and guinea pig heart preparations. In Winslow, C. M. & Lee, M. L. (eds) *New Horizons in Platelet Activating Factor Research* (1987), pp. 255–267. John Wiley, Chichester.

87 Pipkorn, U., Karlsson, G. & Bake, B. Effect of platelet activating factor on the human nasal mucosa. *Allergy* (1984), **39**, 141–145.

88 Karlsson, G. & Pipkorn, U. Effect of disodium cromoglycate on nasal airway resistance induced by platelet activating factor. *Eur. J. Clin. Pharmacol.* (1984), **27**, 1142–1144.

89 Andersson, M. & Pipkorn, U. The effect of platelet activating factor on nasal hypersensitivity. *Eur. J. Clin. Pharmacol.* (1988), **35**, 231–235.

90 Hellewell, P. G. & Williams, T. J. A specific antagonist of platelet-activating factor suppresses oedema formation in an Arthus reaction but not oedema induced by leukocyte chemoattractants in rabbit skin. *J. Immunol.* (1986), **137**, 302–307.

91 McMurtry, I. F. & Morris, K. G. Platelet-activating factor causes pulmonary vasodilation in the rat. *Am. Rev. Resp. Dis.* (1986), **134**, 757–762.

92 Burhop, R. E., van der Zee, H., Bisios, R. *et al.* Pulmonary vascular responses to platelet-activating factor in awake sheep and the role of cyclooxyenase metabolites. *Am. Rev. Resp. Dis.* (1986), **134**, 548–554.

93 Prescott, S. M., Zimmerman, G. A. & McIntyre, T. M. Human endothelial cells in culture produce platelet-activating factor (1-alkyl-2-acetyl-*sn*-glycero-3-phosphocholine) when stimulated with thrombin. *Proc. Nat. Acad. Sci.* (USA) (1984), **81**, 3534–3538.

94 Prevost, M.-C. Cariven, C., Simon, M.-F., Chap, H. & Douste-Blazy, L. Platelet activating factor (PAF-acether) is released into rat pulmonary alveolar fluid as a consequence of hypoxia. *Biochem. Biophys. Res. Commun.* (1984), **119**, 58–63.

95 McCormack, D. M., Barnes, P. J. & Evans, T. W. Evidence for platelet-activating factor as a mediator of hypoxic pulmonary vasoconstriction. *Clin. Sci.* (1988), **75**, 21P.

96 Hwang, S. B. Identification of a second putative receptor of platelet-activating factor from human polymorphonuclear leukocytes. *J. Biol. Chem.* (1988), **263**, 3235–3233.

97 Page, C. P., Paul, W., Dewar, A., Wood, L. E., Basran, C. S. & Morley, J. PAF-acether: a putative mediator of asthma and inflammation. Morley, J. & Rainsford, K. D. (eds) *Pharmacology of Asthma, Agents & Actions* (1982), **13** (Supplement 13), pp. 177–183. Birkhauser-Verlag, Basle.

98 Mojarad, M., Hamasaki, Y. & Said, S. I. Platelet activating factor increases pulmonary microvascular permeability and induces pulmonary oedema. *Bull. Eur. Physiopathol Resp.* (1983), **19**, 253–257.

99 Heffner, J. E. Shoemaker, S. A., Canham, E. M. *et al.* Acetyl glyceryl ether phosphorylcholine-stimulated human platelets cause pulmonary hypertension and edema in isolated rabbit lungs. *J. Clin. Invest.* (1983), **71**, 351–357.

100 Pirotzky, E., Page, C. P., Roubin, R. *et al.* PAF-acether-induced plasma exudation in rat skin is independent of platelets and neutrophils. *Microcirc. Endothelium Lymphatics* (1984), **1,** 107–122.

101 Lewis, J. C., O'Flaherty, J. T., McCall, C. E., Wykle, R. L. & Bond, M. G. Platelet activating factor effects on pulmonary ultrastructure in rabbits. *Exp. Mol. Pathol.* (1983), **38**, 100–108.

102 Dewar, A., Archer, C. B., Paul, W., Page, C. P., MacDonald, D. M. & Morley, J. Cutaneous and pulmonary histopathological responses to platelet activating factor (PAF-acether) in the guinea-pig. *J. Pathol.* (1984), **144**, 25–34.

103 Robertson, D. N. & Page, C. P. Effect of platelet agonists on airway reactivity and intrathoracic platelet accumulation. *Br. J. Pharmacol.* (1987), **92**, 105–111.

104 Walker, J. R., Sweatman, W. J. F., Brandon, D. R., Cranstom, S. & Gooderham, R. Histological and radiological assessment of neutrophil and platelet responses to PAF *in vivo. Prostaglandins* (1989), in press.

105 Purvis, A. W., Christman, B. W., McPherson, C. D., Miller, R. F., Lefferts, P. L. & Snapper, S. R. WEB-2086, a platelet activating receptor antagonist, attenuates the response to endotoxin in awake sheep. *Am. Rev. Respir. Dis.* (1988), **137** (Suppl.), 99.

Chapter 8
PAF and renal disease

Giovanni Camussi, Giuseppe Montrucchio, Gennaro Salvidio and Ciro Tetta

Introduction

The initiation and expression of immune vascular injury involves the complex array of inflammatory mediators including complement, coagulation proteins, neutrophils, macrophages, platelets and resident glomerular cells. Recently, a new class of lipid chemical mediators, the acetylated alkyl phosphoglycerides with a wide spectrum of biological and pharmacological activities has been identified and recognized as potent autacoids [1–7].

In addition to its activity on platelets, platelet activating factor (PAF) promotes the aggregation, chemotaxis and granule secretion of polymorphonuclear neutrophils (PMN) and monocytes, produces the contraction of smooth muscle, and has negative inotropic and arrhythmogenic effects. When injected *in vivo*, PAF induces a systemic haemoconcentration, oedema, vasoconstriction, vasodilation and increased vascular permeability. Finally, PAF has a strong hypotensive action. Since target cells or tissues respond to PAF by a receptor-mediated mechanism, the recent availability of specific antagonists for PAF has provided a sensitive tool for research on the role of PAF in disease. PAF is implicated in the regulation of the immune response and host defence (reviewed in [6]). At fentomolar concentrations, PAF enhances the production of interleukin-1 (IL-1) from lipopolysaccharide (LPS)-stimulated rat monocytes, with higher concentrations being inhibitory [8]. PAF also regulates IL-2 production and lymphocyte proliferation [9]. The effect of PAF on the immune response may greatly vary depending on the type of cellular subset with which it interacts. While PAF inhibits T-cell proliferation independently of IL-2 production [10], it activates suppressor cells via an indomethacin-independent mechanism [11,12].

The multiple biological activities of PAF are frequently associated with, or dependent on, the generation of arachidonate metabolites generated via the cyclooxygenase or lipoxygenase-mediated pathways and prostaglandins and leukotrienes have been demonstrated to participate in a number of biological activities induced by PAF in several experimental *in vitro* and *in vivo* systems [13,14].

The cellular origins of PAF are numerous [2,3,7]; cells which participate in the inflammatory response release PAF both following immunological and non-immunological stimulation [15–22]. Sensitized basophils and mastocytes release PAF in response to antigen or anti-IgE challenge, suggesting that PAF might be involved in the pathogenesis of anaphylactic reactions (see also Chapter 7). PMN, monocytes and macrophages may produce and release PAF in *in vitro* experimental conditions mimicking the immune complex-mediated hypersensitivity reaction or the anti-infectious response. In fact, PMN, monocytes and macrophages respond to phagocytic stimuli such as bacteria, IgG or complement-opsonized particles or immune complexes. PMN also respond to the chemotactic agents C5a, C5a des arg and to PMN-derived cationic proteins. Eosinophils respond also to the eosinophil chemotactic factor of anaphylaxis (ECF-A). Results of experiments involving the binding of antibodies to surface antigens or endothelial cells implicate PAF in certain antibody and complement-dependent cytotoxic hypersensitivity reactions [21–23]. In addition, endothelial cells produce PAF in response to thrombin, vasopressin, angiotensin-II, histamine and bradykinin [21,24]. No direct information is available on PAF release in cell-mediated hypersensitivity reactions. In fact, lymphocytes are generally unable to produce PAF. However, cells including macrophages, endothelial cells and even PMN produce PAF when stimulated with cytokines such as IL-1 and tumour necrosis factor (TNF) [25,26] which may be involved in cell-mediated hypersensitivity reactions. In addition, a lymphocyte subset, the large granular lymphocytes with natural killer activity, produces PAF after Fc receptor stimulation [27].

These multiple biological activities make PAF a potential mediator of inflammation, hypersensitivity reactions, endotoxin shock, and graft rejection. In this review, the available direct and indirect evidence for a role of PAF in renal pathophysiology will be discussed.

PAF production in the kidney

PAF may be produced locally in the kidney (i) by inflammatory cells recruited during glomerular or interstitial inflammatory injury or (ii) by renal cells. In addition to inflammatory cells which are known to produce

PAF under appropriate stimulation, renal cells are potential sources of PAF. Rabbit renal slices produce PAF when incubated at pH 10.6 or with calcium ionophore A23187 [15]. *In vitro* challenge of renal slices from pre-sensitized rats with the specific antigen [15] induces the release of PAF, suggesting an immunological mechanism. Similarly, antigen stimulation of isolated perfused kidney from pre-sensitized rats induces the production and release of PAF as well as leukotrienes, histamine and serotonin [28].

Glomeruli and suspensions of renal medullary cells but not cortical tubular cells produce PAF after A23187 stimulation [28–32]. In glomeruli, mesangial cells are the major source of PAF [30,32]. Isolated human and rat glomeruli [31] as well as cultured mesangial cells [33] synthesize PAF after stimulation with endotoxin suggesting a possible role of PAF in the endotoxin-induced acute renal injury [34]. In addition, mesangial cells produce PAF in response to phagocytosis of immune complexes [35], to stimulation with angiotensin-II [36] and with monokines such as IL-l and TNF. Furthermore, complement-derived anaphylatoxin (C3a, C5a) and platelet-derived growth factor (PDGF) are potent inducers of enzymes involved in the PAF biosynthetic pathway [37].

Although in *in vitro* or culture conditions, PAF remains undetectable in the absence of stimuli, *in vivo* PAF is present in the rat kidney inner medulla at a basal level of 0.044 pmol/mg of tissue [38]. The finding of PAF-like biological activity in human urine [39] suggests that renal tissue may generate PAF even under physiological conditions. Kidney from various animal species possesses the complete enzymatic repertoire known to be necessary for PAF biosynthesis (for review see [40]).

Effects of PAF on cultured glomerular cells

PAF enhances prostaglandin and thromboxane A_2 production in isolated perfused rat [41] and rabbit [42] kidney. In primary cultures of rat [43] and human [44] glomerular mesangial cells, PAF causes a rapid and dose-dependent stimulation of prostaglandin synthesis which is inhibited by PAF receptor antagonists [45]. Since PAF, like angiotensin-II, induces contraction of mesangial cells in culture [43,44] and of human cultured endothelial cells [46], it is likely that in the absence of inflammatory cells, PAF acts directly on glomerular cells. Indeed, PAF causes a decrease in planar surface area of isolated glomeruli as a consequence of mesangial cell contraction [43]. Modification of the shape of cultured mesangial cells stimulated by PAF is enhanced by blockade of prostaglandin synthesis and partially reversed by readdition of exogenous PGE_2 [43]. Schlondorff *et al.* [43] interpreted these results as indicating that PGE_2 generated in response to PAF could serve as a feedback inhibition for the PAF-induced contraction of the mesangial cells. PAF has also been reported to release reactive oxygen species from cultured mesangial cells [47] and could therefore be implicated in the production of oxygen free radicals and the ensuing lipid peroxidation during re-flow in ischaemic acute renal failure in the rat [48]. Furthermore, glomeruli from ischaemic rat kidneys produce increased amounts of PAF [49].

Renal effects of PAF

Systemic infusion of PAF produces a marked reduction in renal plasma flow, glomerular filtration rate and urine formation as a consequence of the systemic hemodynamic effects [50]. However, PAF may directly modify renal haemodynamics. In fact, PAF infusion into the renal artery of anaesthetized dogs induces a dose-dependent decrease in blood flow, glomerular filtration rate, urinary flow and sodium excretion in the absence of systemic effects [51]. These results suggest that PAF determines renal vasoconstriction.

PAF infusion in the abdominal aorta as well as injection into the renal artery induces an increase in glomerular permeability (Fig. 8.1) associated with accumulation of platelets and PMN in the capillary lumina (Fig. 8.2a) and with deposition of both platelet- (Fig. 8.2b) and PMN-derived cationic proteins in the glomerular capillary walls [52]. The concomitant loss of fixed negative charges of the glomerular capillary wall, that maintain normal glomerular selectivity, may suggest an indirect action of PAF on glomerular structures due to the release of inflammatory mediators from platelets and PMN and neutralization and/or destruction of glomerular anionic charges leading to an increased glomerular permeability. Increased glomerular permeability (Fig. 8.2c), accumulation of inflammatory cells and localization of cationic proteins are prevented by PAF receptor antagonists indicating the specificity of PAF action (Fig. 8.1).

However, a modest increase in permeability associated with ultrastructural changes in glomerular endothelial cells was observed in platelet- and PMN-depleted rabbits suggesting a concomitant direct action of PAF on renal vascular structures [7] (Fig. 8.1; Fig. 8.3a, b, c). This direct action is confirmed by recent experiments of Perico *et al.* [53] performed on blood-free isolated perfused rabbit kidney showing that infusion of PAF increases urinary protein excretion independently of renal haemodynamic alterations or loss of anionic charges. An increase in glomerular permeability is also observed in isolated perfused rat kidney [54]. In this model, however, PAF induces renal vasodilation, decreased glomerular filtration rate, decreased renal vasculature resistance and increased glomerular permeability. PAF does not alter the glomerular pattern of sialo-glycoproteins in isolated kidneys perfused with PAF. Since PAF

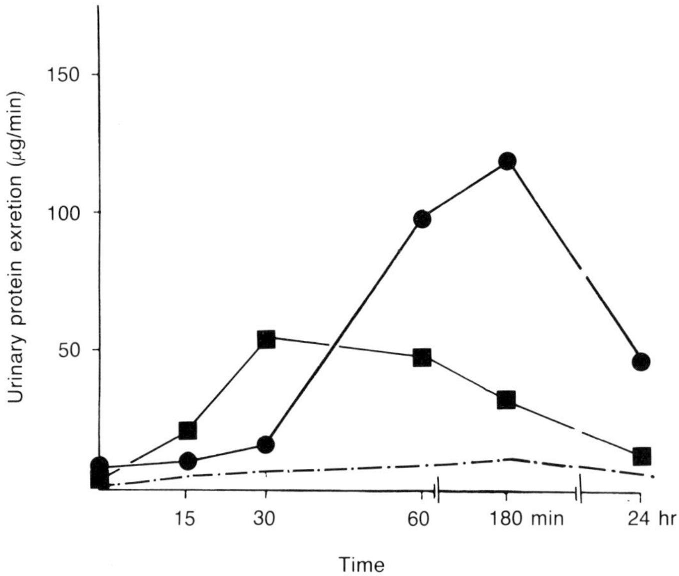

Fig. 8.1 Effect on the urinary protein excretion of PAF infusion into the renal artery of rabbits. After volume expansion performed as described in [52] 0.6 μg of PAF were infused and the urinary protein excretion was monitored for a 24 h period in: normal rabbits (●); rabbits pretreated with PAF specific receptor antagonist (SRI 63-072, 1 mg/kg) —·—; and PMN- and platelet depleted rabbits (■—■). PAF induces an increase in urinary protein excretion that begins after 30 min, progressively increases up to 180 min, decreases 24 h after infusion and is abrogated by pretreatment with a PAF-specific receptor antagonist. In PMN- and platelet-depleted rabbits, PAF produces an early (after 30 min), transient, modest increase in urinary protein excretion. These results suggest that *in vivo* the increase in glomerular permeability in the rabbit is related only to a minor extent to a direct effect of PAF.

induces contraction of mesangial cells in culture [43] and of human cultured endothelial cells [46], it is likely that, in the absence of inflammatory cells, PAF acts directly on glomerular cells. In fact, PAF causes a decrease in planar surface area of isolated glomeruli as a consequence of mesangial cell contraction [43]. In addition, PAF is able to increase albumin transport across an endothelial monolayer *in vitro* [46]. The possible explanations for the reduction of glomerular filtration rate are therefore post-glomerular vasodilation, contraction of mesangial cells and increased permeability. Thus it is possible that two different mechanisms of PAF-induced increase in glomerular permeability may be operating *in vivo* via the release of inflammatory mediators and through its direct vasoactive properties.

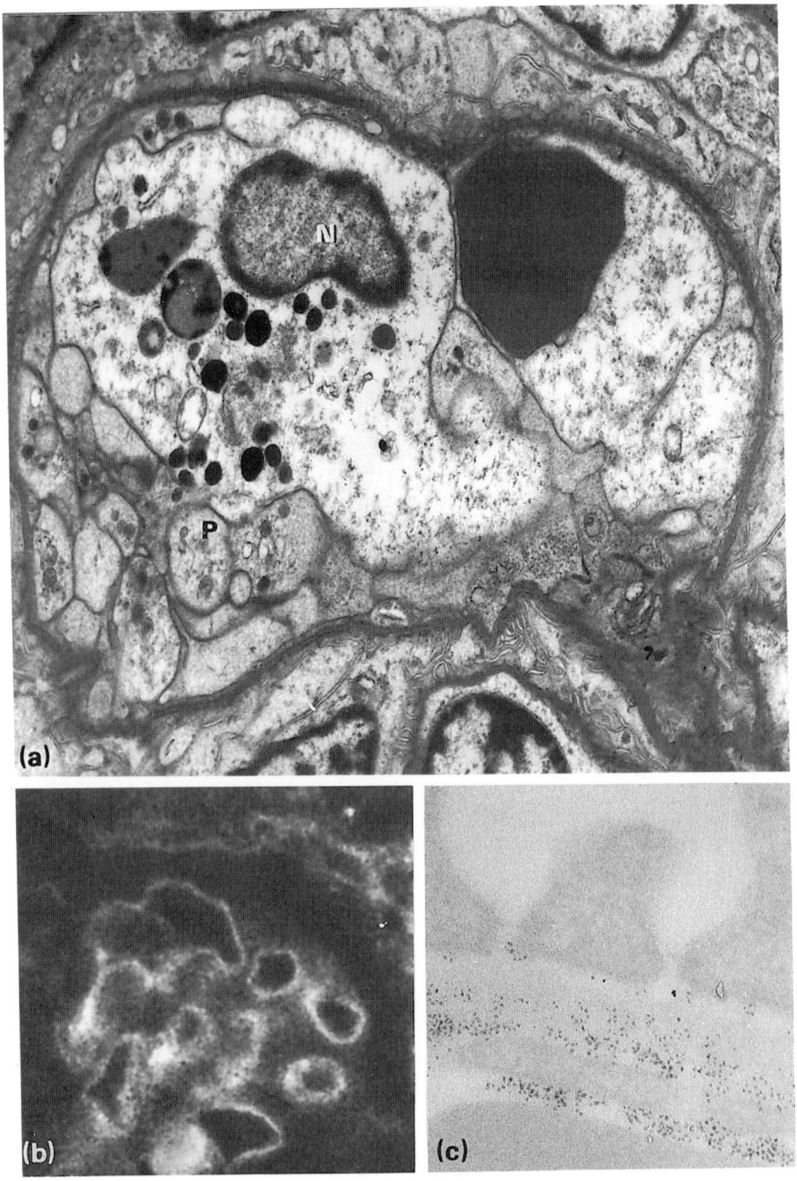

Fig 8.2 (a) Electron micrograph of the kidney of a rabbit injected in the renal artery with 0.6 μg of PAF and sacrificed after 20 min. There is an accumulation of degranulated platelets (P) and polymorphonuclear neutrophils—PMN (N) in the glomerular capillary lumen as well as focal disappearance of foot processes in visceral epithelial cells; (b) Immunofluorescence micrograph showing the localization of platelet-derived cationic proteins in the glomerular capillary walls in a rabbit injected with PAF; and (c) electron micrograph showing the increased penetration of native ferritin particles in the glomerular basement membrane in a rabbit injected with PAF, thus indicating an increase in glomerular permeability. Magnification: (a) × 5000; (b) × 4000; and (c) × 45 000.

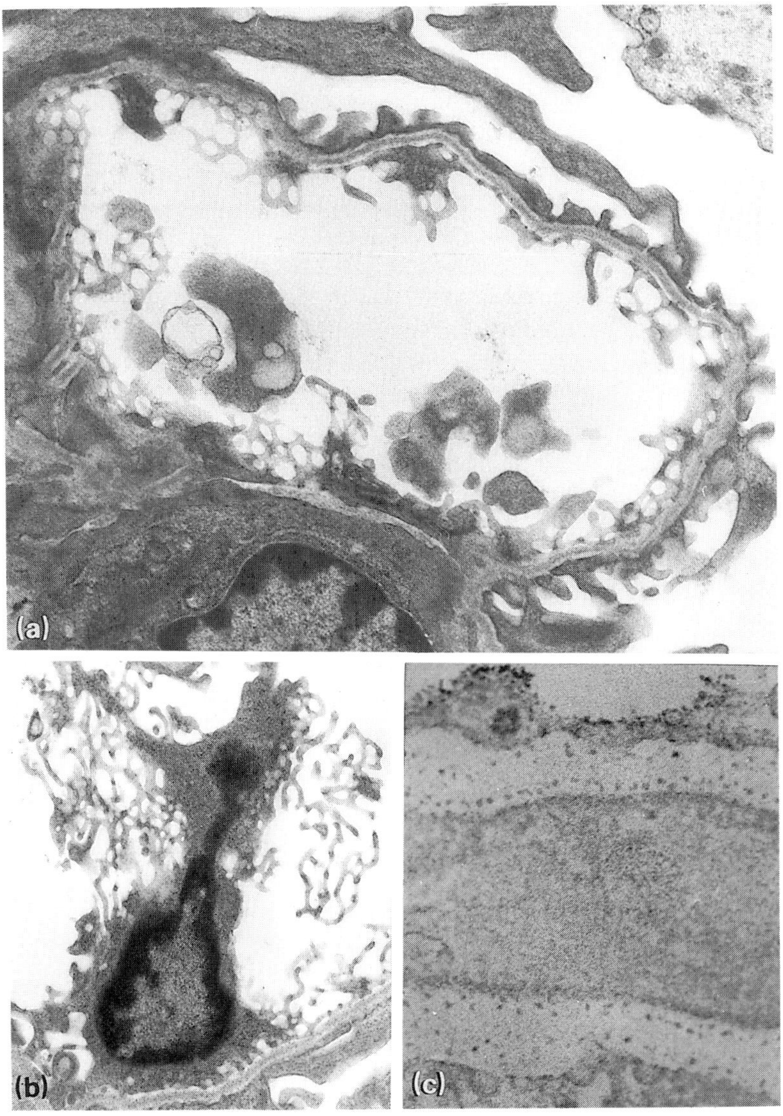

Fig. 8.3 (a) Electron micrograph of a kidney from a PMN- and platelet-depleted rabbit infused with PAF. The rabbit was sacrificed after 20 min. There is an increase in the number and the size of fenestrae of the endothelium in the absence of inflammatory cells; (b) electron micrograph of an endothelial cell protruding into the glomerular capillary lumen with an increased number of microvillus-like projections and morphological changes suggesting contraction; and (c) anionic sites as detected by polyethyleneimine of a normal glomerular basement membrane. Magnification: (a) and (b) × 6000; (c) × 35 000.

Role of PAF in endotoxin-induced acute renal failure

Endotoxaemia is commonly associated with systemic hypotension and acute renal failure. Several lines of evidence suggest that PAF contributes to the alterations observed during endotoxaemia such as systemic hypotension [55], impaired pulmonary haemodynamics and lung injury [56] and acute haemodynamic renal insufficiency [34] in rats.

1 PAF synthesis and release may be triggered in PMN, monocytes and endothelial cells challenged with TNF [25], the main mediator of endotoxin shock [57]; and endotoxin (LPS), a potent inducer of PAF production from cultured mesangial cells [33].

2 Blood concentrations of PAF, as well as the amount of PAF extracted from kidney homogenates are increased in endotoxin shock [55, 58].

3 PAF-receptor antagonists markedly reduce the mortality and reverse hypotension in endotoxin-induced shock [59].

Wang & Dunn [34] have demonstrated that PAF receptor antagonists not only prevent but also reverse the normotensive endotoxin-induced haemodynamic renal insufficiency characterized by a greater reduction in glomerular filtration rate than in renal plasma flow. They have proposed that endogenous PAF produced within the glomerulus during endotoxaemia may mediate to a considerable extent endotoxin-induced acute renal haemodynamic insufficiency [33]. Support for this idea is provided by the protective effect of PAF antagonists in models of bowel necrosis induced by LPS and TNF/cachectin [60,61]. Finally, Stork *et al.* [45] have shown that the local production of PAF may stimulate vascular and glomerular synthesis of vasodilatory prostaglandins that could, in turn, modulate PAF induced renal hemodynamic alterations. These results may suggest potential therapeutic applications for PAF receptor antagonists.

Potential role of PAF in glomerular immunopathology

Several studies have shown that in experimental serum sickness the deposition of immune complexes in vascular and glomerular structures is associated with increased vascular permeability induced by basophil degranulation and release of mediators from platelets [62]. Platelets are directly involved in the pathogenesis of acute serum sickness by a complement-independent, leukocyte-dependent mechanism that has been related to the release of PAF from IgE-sensitized basophils [2]. In acute serum sickness, the release of PAF seems to be generated by an IgE-dependent basophil degranulation and not by the interaction with PMN of circulating immune complexes in antigen excess [63]. In fact, the formation of immune deposits in glomeruli is preceded by intravascular release of PAF, concomitantly with an *in vivo* degranulation of basophils. The role of PAF in the formation of immune deposits in glomeruli is suggested by the following observations: (1) rabbits with high levels of

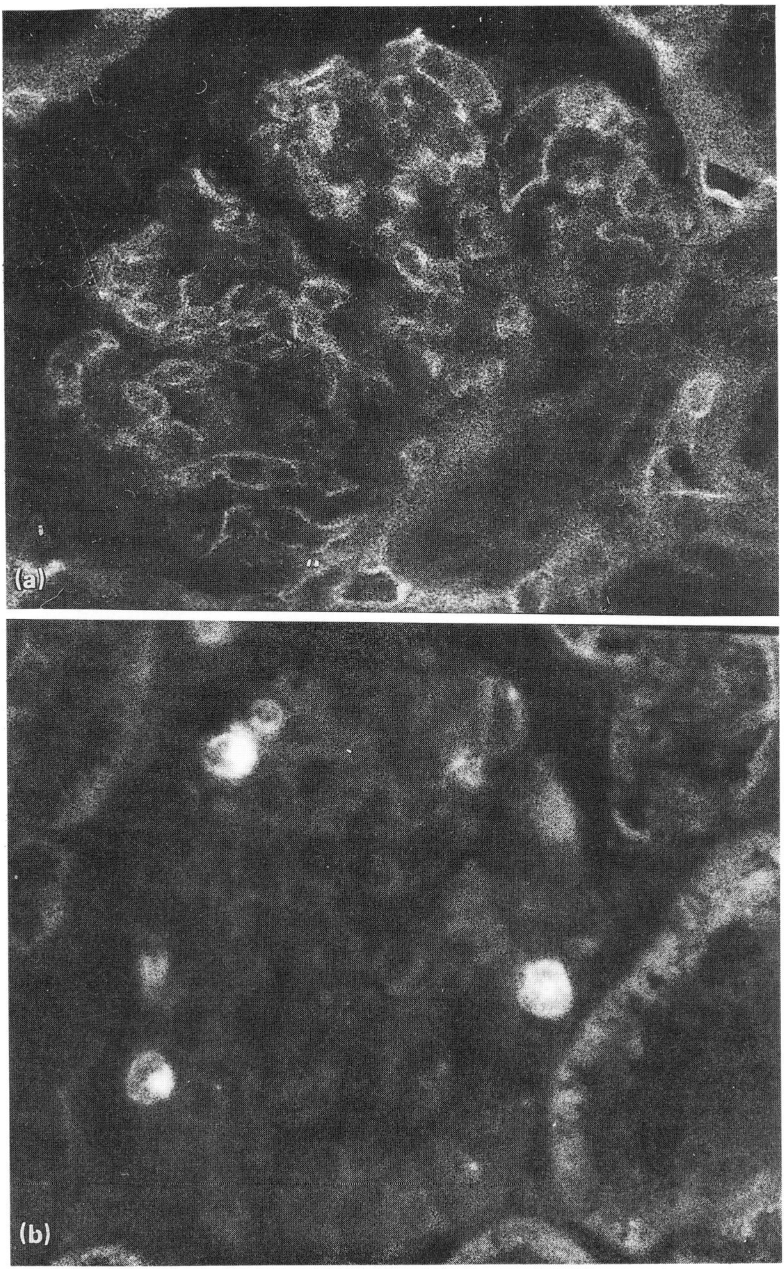

Fig. 8.4 Immunofluorescence micrograph of a glomerulus from a rabbit with acute serum sickness at day 9 showing the binding of platelet-derived cationic proteins (a) to glomerular capillary walls and the intra-cytoplasmic localization of cationic proteins in PMN; and (b) recruited in a glomerulus. Magnification: (a) and (b) × 600.

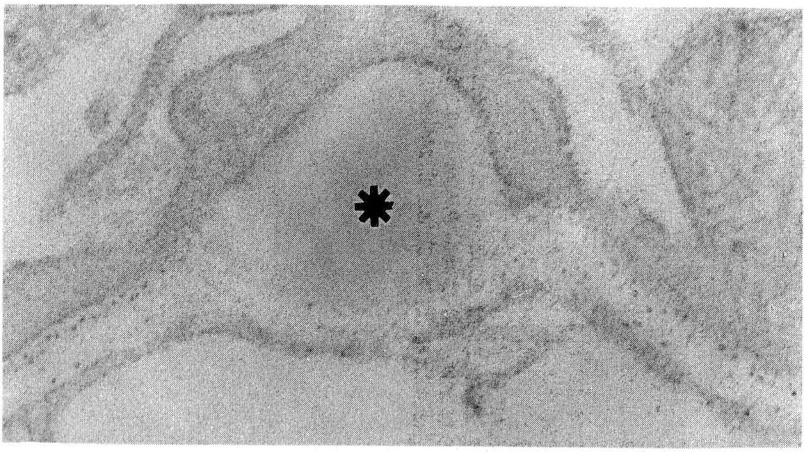

Fig. 8.5 Electron micrograph of a portion of a glomerular capillary of a rabbit with acute serum sickness showing focal loss of anionic sites in correspondence of a sub-epithelial electron-dense deposit (*). Magnification: × 40 000.

immune complexes, but no *in vivo* degranulation of basophils and release of PAF, do not develop glomerulonephritis; (2) in rabbits developing the disease, platelets become specifically desensitized to the action of PAF; (3) as in the experiments of *in vivo* infusion of PAF, intravascular release of PAF is accompanied by platelet activation, glomerular localization of platelet-derived cationic proteins (Fig. 8.4) and focal neutralization of fixed anionic sites [64] (Fig 8.5); and (4) the infusion of PAF increases glomerular permeability [52] and deposition of immune complexes suggesting a role for this mediator in the formation of glomerular immune deposits in acute serum sickness.

The increased glomerular permeability has been associated with the release of vasoactive amines from platelets and of both platelet- and PMN-derived cationic proteins which are capable of neutralizing glomerular anionic charges [52]. In addition, the administration of PAF receptor antagonists in the accelerated form of acute serum sickness markedly reduces proteinuria and glomerular inflammation [65]. The availability of specific PAF-receptor antagonists has allowed the role of PAF in other experimental glomerular inflammatory reactions to be assessed. In nephrotoxic nephritis, a complement- and leukocyte-dependent model of anti-glomerular basement membrane antibody-mediated disease, PAF receptor antagonists prevent the development of severe crescentic glomerulonephritis and renal insufficiency, and reduce proteinuria [66].

Blockade of PAF receptors also inhibits the tissue injury caused by *in situ* formation of immune complexes in the model of unilateral glomerulonephritis produced by implantation of cationic antigen in glomeruli of pre-immunized rats [67] (Fig. 8.6). This model reproduces several of the

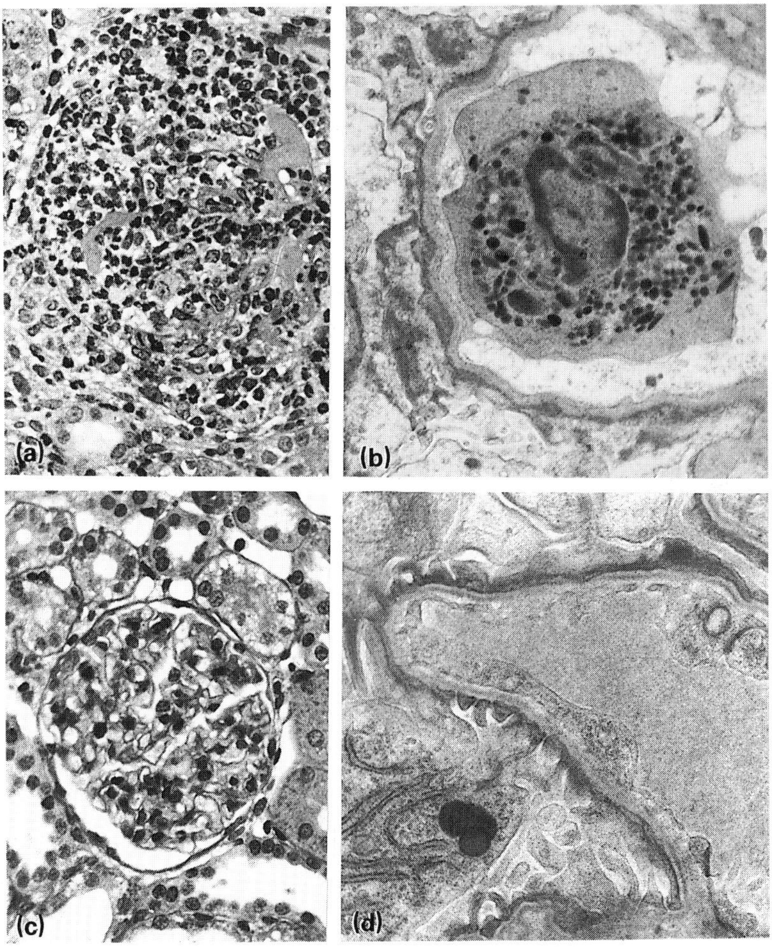

Fig. 8.6 Light microscopy of a glomerulus from a rat with unilateral *in situ* formed immune complex glomerulonephritis induced by implantation of cationic human IgG in pre-immunized animals. The glomerulus is enlarged with proliferation of endocapillary cells and infiltration of PMN; (b) electron micrograph of a glomerular capillary loop of a rat with unilateral *in situ* formed immune complex glomerulonephritis. Electron-dense deposits are present at the epithelial site of a capillary basement membrane. The capillary lumen contains a PMN; (c) light microscopy of a glomerulus; and (d) electron micrograph of a portion of a glomerular capillary of a rat pretreated with SRI 63–072, a PAF-specific antagonist before the induction of unilateral *in situ* formed immune complex glomerulonephritis. The accumulation of inflammatory cells is markedly reduced. Magnification: (a) and (c) × 250; (b) and (d) × 6000.

morphological and immunohistochemical features of human acute immune complex glomerulonephritis. In this model, tissue and proteinuria are complement-, PMN- and monocyte-dependent. The depletion of complement, provided it is initiated before the formation of immune complexes, prevents proteinuria. However, despite complement depletion, PMNs and monocytes accumulate at the sites of immune deposits. Since depletion of leukocytes prevents glomerular injury, it is conceivable that the release of mediators from leukocytes determines tissue injury. While complement has most probably a primary role in activating rather than in recruiting the inflammatory cells, PAF may induce the initial recruitment of these cells in the glomeruli. In fact, PAF receptor antagonists prevent accumulation of inflammatory cells in glomeruli and proteinuria but not the activation of complement.

The initial formation of immune deposits in the sub-endothelial space may cause concomitant activation of complement and generation of PAF from macrophages and endothelial cells (Fig. 8.7). This latter event initiates adherence of leukocytes to the endothelium. The local generation of C3a and C5a anaphylatoxins and phagocytosis of immune complexes

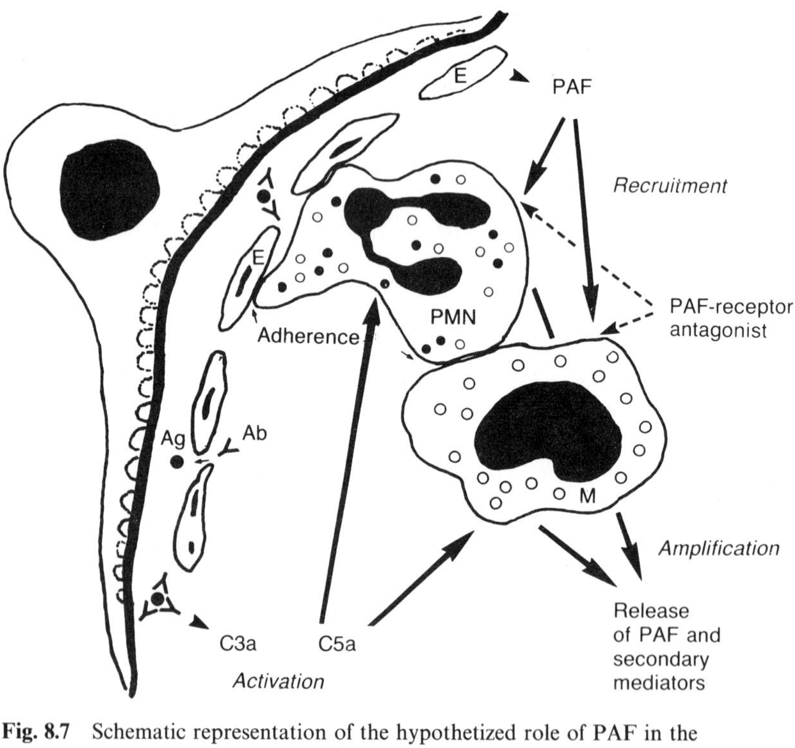

Fig. 8.7 Schematic representation of the hypothetized role of PAF in the recruitment of inflammatory cells and in the amplification of tissue injury in a model of unilateral *in situ* formed immune complex glomerulonephritis. PMN = polymorphonuclear neutrophils; E = endothelial cells; Ag = antigen; Ab = antibody; M = monocyte.

determines the release of inflammatory mediators from the recruited leukocytes and stimulates further release of PAF that may further amplify the inflammatory reaction (Fig. 8.7).

By contrast, PAF receptor antagonists do not prevent proteinuria in passive Heymann nephritis, a disease characterized by formation of sub-epithelial immune deposits due to the *in situ* interaction of circulating antibodies with antigen expressed on the surface of glomerular epithelial cells. Proteinuria in this model is complement-dependent but leukocyte-independent. In fact, proteinuria is caused by the terminal components of complement that determine injury of glomerular epithelial cells [68]. These results suggest that the site of initial antigen–antibody interaction, namely the sub-endothelial space, is of critical importance. In fact, when immune complexes are formed in the sub-epithelial space in Heymann nephritis, they are segregated by the basement membrane and therefore unable to recruit inflammatory cells. In addition, glomerular epithelial cells are unable to synthesize PAF.

These results indicate that PAF acts as a critical mediator of glomerular injury when leukocytes and/or platelets are involved as final effectors of inflammation. Nevertheless, Egido *et al.* [69] recently reported that PAF antagonists prevent proteinuria and morphological alterations of podocytes in the adriamycin model of nephropathy in the rat suggesting that PAF may have a role also in toxic non-inflammatory glomerular pathology.

Role of PAF in renal allograft rejection

The release of PAF has been studied in hyper-acute renal allograft rejection in the rabbit [70,71]. Hyper-acute rejection is actually very rare in humans because of a more accurate selection of compatible donors. This pathological condition is characterized by an acute and dramatic vasoconstriction associated with intravascular aggregates of platelets, leukocytes, erythrocytes and fibrin that occlude small arteries inducing ischaemic necrosis. The pathogenesis of hyper-acute rejection is related to the immediate binding of allo-transplantation antibodies and complement to the endothelium of glomerular and peritubular capillaries, an event that is followed by the appearance of PAF in the venous effluent of the transplanted organ. PAF is probably released by endothelial cells after interaction with allo-transplantation antibodies within 2–10 min after revascularization and during the 60 min of observation. Concomitant with the release of PAF, an influx of platelets and later of PMN is observed. Platelets adhere to the endothelium and are found in intra-vascular thrombi (Fig. 8.8). Platelets are degranulated and by immunofluorescence platelet-derived cationic proteins are localized at the sites of fixed anionic charges in the glomerular capillary wall. The accumulation of PMN

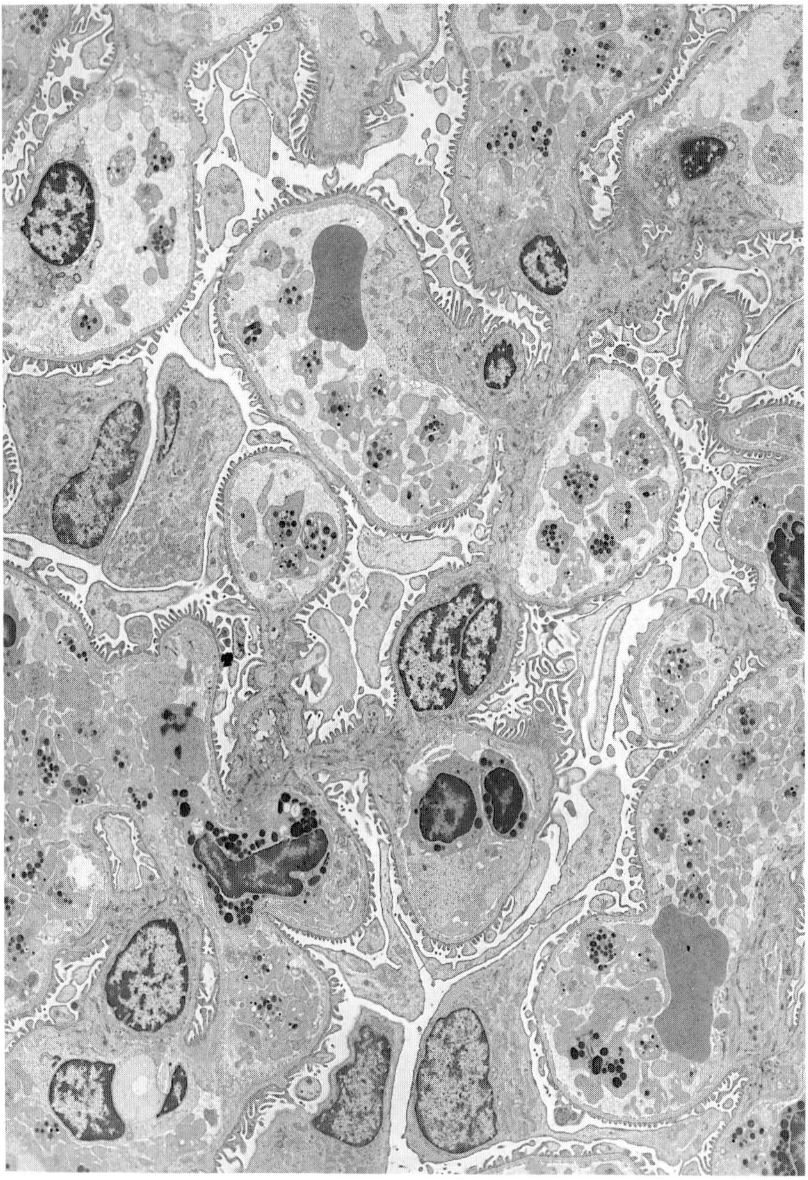

Fig. 8.8 Electron micrograph of a portion of a glomerulus from a graft undergoing hyperacute rejection showing intra-vascular accumulation of partially degranulated platelets, swelling of endothelial cells and accumulation of PMN in glomerular capillaries. Magnification: × 3500.

becomes prominent 1 h after re-vascularization and deposits of PMN-derived cationic proteins are also found in the glomerular capillary wall indicating that PMN undergo degranulation [70].

In spite of the fact that no data currently are available in cell-mediated renal allograft rejection, preliminary evidence obtained in cardiac allografts suggests a potential role of PAF. Treatment of rat cardiac allograft recipients with BN 52021, a PAF receptor antagonist, in combination with azathioprine or cyclosporin A, which by themselves do not prolong graft survival, significantly delays organ rejection [72]. These results are in agreement with the recent evidence that PAF possesses immunomodulatory effects (for review see [6]).

Conclusions

PAF production and release in the renal microvasculature may produce functional and structural changes as result of its direct action on resident renal cells or through the recruitment and activation of inflammatory cells. Thus PAF may contribute to the clinico-pathological expression of renal diseases. The development of specific PAF receptor antagonists or inhibitors of its synthesis may allow a better understanding of the role of this mediator in renal pathophysiology.

References

1 Henson, P. M. Released vasoactive amines from rabbit platelets induced by sensitized mononuclear leukocytes and antigen. *J. Exp. Med.* (1970), **131**, 287–306.

2 Benveniste, J. M., Henson, P. & Cochrane, C. G. Leukocyte-dependent histamine release from rabbit platelets. The role of IgE, basophils and platelet-activating factor. *J. Exp. Med.* (1972). **136**, 1356–1377.

3 Pinckard, R. N., McManus, L. M. & Hanahan, D. J. Chemistry and biology of acetyl glyceryl ether phosphorylcholine (platelet-activating factor). *Adv. Inflam. Res.* (1982), **4**, 147–180.

4 Snyder, F. Chemical and biochemical aspects of platelet-activating factor: a novel class of acetylated ether-linked choline phospholipids. *Med. Res. Rev.* (1985), **5**, 107–140.

5 Vargaftig, B.B., Chignard, M., Benveniste, J., Lefort, J. & Wal, F. Background and present status of research on platelet-activating factor (PAF-acether). *Ann. NY Acad. Sci.* (1981), **370**, 119–137.

6 Braquet, P. & Rola-Pleszczynski, M. Platelet-activating factor and cellular immune responses. *Immunol. Today* (1987), **8**, 345–352.

7 Camussi, G. Potential role of PAF in renal pathophysiology. *Kidney Int.* (1986), **29**, 469–477.

8 Mencia-Huerta, J. M., Hename, S., Sorlin, B., Rola-Pleszczynski, M., Pignol, B. & Braquet, P. Effect of PAF on IL-1 release and synthesis by rat spleen adherent monocytes. In Braquet, P. (ed.) *PAF and Cell Immunology, New Trends in Lipid Mediators Research* (1988), **1**, 1–15. Karger, Basel.

9 Rola-Pleszczynski, M., Pignol, B., Pouliot, C. & Braquet, P. Inhibition of human lymphocyte proliferation and IL-2 production by PAF (PAF-acether): reversal by specific antagonist, BN 55021. *Biophys. Res. Commun.* (1987), **142**, 654–659.

10 Dulioust, A., Vivier, E., Salem, P., Perycelz, S., Benveniste, J. & Thomas, V. Inhibition of human T4 + cell proliferation by PAF-acether (PAF). *Fed. Proc.* (1987), **46**, 784. (Abstract).

11 Rola-Pleszczynski, M., Pouliot, C., Pignol, B. & Braquet, P. PAF induces human suppressor cells activity. *Fed. Proc.* (1987), **46**, 444. (Abstract).

12 Rola-Pleszczynski, M. Immune modulation of PAF: effects on lymphocytes and monocyte function. In Braquet, P. (ed.) *PAF and Cell Immunology, New Trends in Lipid Mediators Research* (1988), **2**, 30–37. Karger, Basel.

13 Chilton, F. H., O'Flaherty, J. T., Walsh, C. E. *et al.* Platelet activating factor stimulation of the lipoxygenase pathway in polymorphonuclear leukocytes by 1-0-alkyl-2-O-acetyl-*sn*-glycero-3-phosphorylcholine. *J. Biol. Chem.* (1982), **257**, 5402–5407.

14 McGivern, D. V. & Basran, G. S. Synergism between PAF (PAF-acether) and prostaglandin E_2 in man. *Eur. J. Pharmacol.* (1984), **102**, 183–185.

15 Camussi, G., Mencia-Huerta, J. & Benveniste, J. Release of platelet activating factor and histamine. I. Effect of immune complexes, complement and neutrophils on human and rabbit mastocytes and basophils. *Immunology* (1977), **33**, 523–534.

16 Camussi, G., Tetta, C., Bussolino, F. *et al.* Mediators of immune complex induced aggregation of polymorphonuclear neutrophils. I. C5a anaphylatoxin, neutrophil cationic proteins and their cleavage fragments. *Int. Arch. Allergy Appl. Immunol.* (1980), **62**, 1–15.

17 Camussi, G., Aglietta, M., Coda, R., Bussolino, F., Piacibello, W. & Tetta, C. Release of platelet-activating factor (PAF) and histamine. II. The cellular origin of human PAF: monocytes, polymorphonuclear neutrophils and basophils. *Immunology* (1981), **42**, 191–199.

18 Betz, S. J., Lotner, G. Z. & Henson, P. M. Generation and release of platelet-activating factor (PAF) from enriched preparations of rabbit basophils: failure of human basophils to release PAF. *J. Immunol.* (1980), **125**, 2749–2755.

19 Lee, T. C., Lenihan, D. J., Malone, B., Roddy, L. L. & Wasserman, S. I. Increased biosynthesis of platelet-activating factor in activated human eosinophils. *J. Biol. Chem.* (1984), **259**, 5526–5530.

20 Mencia-Huerta, J. M., Roubin, R., Morgat, J. L. & Benveniste, J., Biosynthesis of platelet-activating factor (PAF-acether). III. Formation of PAF-acether from synthetic substrates by stimulated murine macrophages. *J. Immunol.* (1982), **129**, 804–808.

21 Camussi, G., Aglietta, M., Malavasi, F. *et al.* The release of platelet-activating factor from human endothelial cells in culture. *J. Immunol.* (1983), **131**, 2397–2403.

22 Prescott, S. M., Zimmerman, G. A. & McIntyre, T. M. Human endothelial cells in culture produce platelet-activating factor (1-alkyl-2-acetyl-*sn*-glyceryl-3-phosphorylcholine) when stimulated with thrombin. *Proc. Nat. Acad. Sci. (USA).* (1984), **81**, 3534–3538.

23 Camussi, G., Pawlowski, I., Bussolino, F. Caldwell, P., Brentjens, J. & Andres, G. Release of platelet-activating factor in rabbits with antibody mediated injury of the lung. The role of polymorphonuclear neutrophils and pulmonary endothelial cells. *J. Immunol.* (1983), **131**, 1802–1806.

24 McIntyre, T., Zimmermann, G., Satoh, K. & Prescott S. Cultured endothelial cells synthesize both platelet-activating factor and prostacyclin in response to histamine, bradykinin and adenosine triphosphate. *J. Clin. Invest.* (1985), **76**, 271–280.

25 Camussi, G., Bussolino, F., Salvidio, G. & Baglioni, C. Tumor necrosis factor/cachectin stimulates peritoneal macrophages, polymorphonuclear neutrophils, and vascular endothelial cells to synthesize and release platelet activating factor. *J. Exp. Med.* (1987), **166**, 1390–1404.

26 Bussolino, F., Breviario, F., Tetta, C., Agliotta, M., Mantovani, A. & Dejana, E. Interleukin-1 stimulates platelet-activating factor (1-O-alkyl-2-acetyl-*sn*-glycero-3-phosphorylcholine) production in cultured human endothelial cells. *J. Clin. Invest.* (1986), **77**, 2027–2033.
27 Malavasi, F., Tetta, C., Funaro, A. *et al.* Fc receptor triggering induces expression of surface activation antigens and release of platelet-activating factor in large granular lymphocytes. *Proc. Nat. Acad. Sci.* (*USA*) (1986), **83**, 2443–2447.
28 Pirotzky, E., Pintos-Morell, G., Burtin, C., Boudet, J., Bidault, J. & Benveniste, J. Renal anaphylaxis. I. Antigen initiated responses from isolated perfused rat kidney. *Kidney Int.* (1987), **32**, 233–237.
29 Pirotzky, E., Ninio, E., Bidault, J., Pfister, A. & Benveniste, J. Biosynthesis of platelet-activating factor (PAF-acether). Precursors of PAF-acether and acetyl transferase activity in isolated rat kidney cells. *Lab. Invest.* (1984), **51**, 567–572.
30 Schlondorff, D., Goldwasser, P. & Satriano, J. A. Synthesis of platelet-activating factor by isolated glomeruli and cultured mesangial cells of the rat kidney. *Clin. Res.* (1985), **33**, 588A. (Abstract).
31 Pintos-Morell, G., Pirotzky, E., Erard, D. *et al.* PAF-acether (platelet-activating factor) and IL-1-like production by lipopolysaccharide-stimulated glomuruli. *Clin. Immunol. Immunopathol.* (1988), **46**, 396–405.
32 Schlondorff, D., Goldwasser, P., Neuwirth, R., Satriano, A. & Clay, K. L. Production of platelet-activating factor in glomeruli and cultured mesangial cells. *Am. J. Physiol.* (1986), **250**, F1123–F1127.
33 Wang, J., Kester, M. & Dunn, M. J. The effects of endotoxin on platelet-activating factor synthesis by cultured mesangial cells. *Biochim. Biophys. Acta* (1988), **969**, 217–224.
34 Wang, J. & Dunn, M. J. Platelet activating factor mediates endotoxin-induced acute renal insufficiency in rats. *Am. J. Physiol.* (1987), **253**, F1–F7.
35 Gemsa, D., Resch, K., Bunsten, S. & Lovett, D. Glomerular mesangial cells secrete interleukin-1 (IL-1) and prostaglandin E in response to bacterial endotoxin (ET). *Kidney Int.* (1987), **31**, 320. (Abstract).
36 Neuwirth, R., Satriano, J. A., De Candido, S. & Schlondorff, D. Angiotensin-II (A-II) causes formation of platelet activating factor (PAF) in cultured rat mesangial cells. *Kidney Int.* (1988), **33**, 278. (Abstract).
37 Lianos, E. A. & Langlis, A. Mesangial cells (MC) synthesis of PAF in response to defined inflammatory mediators. *Kidney Int.* (1988), **33**, 273. (Abstract).
38 Woodward, D. S., Lee, T. C. & Snyder, F. The final step in the *de novo* biosynthesis of PAF. Properties of a unique CDP-choline: 1-alkyl-2-acetyl-*sn*-glycerol-choline-phosphotransferase in microsomes from the renal inner medulla of rats. *J. Biol. Chem.* (1987), **262**, 2520–2527.
39 Sanchez Crespo, M., Inarrea, P., Alvarez, V., Alonso, F. Egido, J. & Hernando, L. Presence in normal human urine of a hypotensive and platelet-activating phospholipid. *Am. J. Physiol.* (1983), **244**, F706–F711.
40 Lee, T. C. & Snyder, F. Function metabolism and regulation of PAF and related ether lipids. In Kuo, J. F. (ed.) *Phospholipids and Cellular Regulation* (1985), **2**, 1–39 CRC, Boco Raton, FA.
41 Schwertschlag, U., Scherf, M., Gerber, J. G. Mathias, M. & Nico, A. G. L-PAF induced changes on renal vascular resistance (RVR), vascular reactivity and renin release (RR) in the isolated perfused rat kidney, *Kidney Int.* (1986), **29**, 388A. (Abstract).
42 Weisman, S. M., Felsen, D. & Vaughan, E. D. Platelet-activating factor is a potent stimulus for renal prostaglandin synthesis: possible significance in unilateral ureteral ligation. *J. Pharmacol. Exp. Ther.* (1985), **235**, 10–15.

43 Schlondorff, D., Satriano, J. A., Hagege, J., Perez, J. & Baud, L. Effect of platelet-activating factor and serum-treated zymosan on prostaglandin E_2 synthesis, arachidonic acid release and contraction of cultured mesangial cells. *J. Clin. Invest.* (1984), **73**, 1227–1231.

44 Ardaillou, N., Hagege, J., Nias, M. P., Ardaillou, P. & Schlondorff, D. Vasoconstriction-evoked prostaglandin synthesis in cultured human mesangial cells. *Am. J. Physiol.* (1985), **248**, F240–F246.

45 Stork, J. E. Sheu, T. Y. & Dunn, M. J. Stimulation of prostaglandin E_2 and thromboxane B_2 production in cultured rat mesangial cells by PAF: inhibition by a specific receptor antagonist. *Kidney Int.* (1985), **27**, 267A. (Abstract).

46 Bussolino, F., Camussi, G. A., Aglietta, M. *et al.* Human endothelial cells are target for platelet-activating factor. I. Platelet activating factor changes in cytoskeleton structures and promotes albumin diffusion across endothelial monolayer. *J. Immunol.* (1987), **139**, 2439–2446.

47 Sedor, J. R. & Abboud, H. E. Platelet-activating factor stimulates oxygen radical release by cultured rat mesangial cells. *Kidney Int.* (1985), **27**, 222A (Abstract).

48 Paller, M. S., Hordal, J. R. & Ferris, F. F. Oxygen free radicals in ischemic acute renal failure in the rat. *J. Clin. Invest.* (1984), **74**, 1156–1164.

49 Lopez-Farre, A., Torralbo, M. & Lopez-Novoa, J. M. Glomeruli from ischemic rat kidneys produce increased amounts of platelet-activating factor. *Biochem. Biophys. Res. Commun.* (1988), **152**, 129–135.

50 Bessin, P., Bonnet, J., Thibaudeon, J., Agier, B., Beand, V. & Gilet, F. Pathophysiology of shock states caused by PAF-acether in dogs and rats. In Benveniste, J. & Arnoux, B. (eds) *PAF, INSERM Symposium No 23* (1983), pp. 343–355. Elsevier, Amsterdam.

51 Scherf, M., Nies, A. S., Schwertschlag, U., Hughes, M. & Gerber, J. G. Hemodynamic effects of PAF in the dog kidney *in vivo. Hypertension* (1986), **8,** 737–741.

52 Camussi, G., Tetta, C., Coda, R., Segeloni, G. & Vercellone, A. Platelet-activating factor-induced loss of glomerular anionic charges. *Kidney Int.* (1984), **25**, 73–81.

53 Perico, N., Delaini, F., Tagliaferri, M. *et al.* Effect of platelet-activating factor (PAF) and its specific receptor antagonist on glomerular permeability in isolated perfused rat kidney. *Lab. Invest.* (1988), **58**, 163–171.

54 Schwertschlag, U., Dennis, V. N. & Camussi, G. Non-immunological alterations of glomerular filtration by L-PAF in the rat kidney. *Current Therapy in Nephrology, (Sorrento)* (1988), 118.

55 Doebber, T. W. Wu, M. S., Robbins, J. C., Choy, P. M., Chang, M. N. & Shen, T. Y. Platelet-activating factor (PAF) involvement in endotoxin-induced hypotension in rats: studies with PAF-receptor antagonist kadsurenone. *Biochem. Biophys. Res. Comm.* (1985), **3,** 799–808.

56 Chang, S. W. Feddersen, C. O., Henson, P. M. & Voelkel, N. F. Platelet-activating factor mediates hemodynamic changes and lung injury in endotoxin-treated rats. *J. Clin. Invest.* (1987), **79**, 1498–1509.

57 Beutler, B., Milsark, I. W. & Cerami, A. C. Passive immunization against cachectin/tumor necrosis factor protects mice from lethal effects of endothoxin. *Science* (1985), **229**, 869.

58 Inarrea, P., Gomez-Cambronero, J., Pascual, J., Ponte M. C., Hernando, L. & Sanchez Crespo, M. Synthesis of platelet-activating factor (PAF-acether) and blood volume changes in gram-negative sepsis. *Immunopharmacology* (1985), **9,** 45–52.

59 Terashita, Z., Imura, Y., Nishikawa, K. & Sumida, S. Is platelet activating factor (PAF) a mediator of endotoxin shock? *Eur. J. Pharmacol.* (1985), **109**, 257–261.

60 Hsueh, W., Gonzalez-Crussi, F. & Arroyave, J. L. Platelet activating factor is an endogenous mediator for bowel necrosis in endotoxemia. *FASEB J.* (1988), **1**, 403–405.

61 Sun, X.-M. & Hsueh, W. Bowel necrosis induced by tumor necrosis factor in rats is mediated by platelet-activating factor. *J. Clin. Invest.* (1988), **5**, 1328–1331.
62 Cochrane, C. G. Mechanisms involved in the deposition of immune complexes in tissues. *J. Exp. Med.* (1971), **134**, 755–795.
63 Camussi, G., Tetta, C., Deregibus, M. C., Bussolino, F., Segoloni, G. & Vercellone, A. Platelet-activating factor (PAF) in experimentally-induced rabbit acute serum sickness: role of basophil-derived PAF in immune complex deposition. *J. Immunol.* (1982), **128**, 86–94.
64 Camussi, G., Tetta, C., Meroni, M. *et al.* Localization of cationic proteins derived from platelets and polymorphonuclear neutrophils and local loss of anionic sites in glomeruli of rabbits with experimentally-induced acute serum sickness. *Lab. Invest.* (1986), **55**, 56–62.
65 Koyama, A., Susuki, S., Kobayashi, N. *et al.* Role of platelet-activating factor in acute serum sickness in rabbits. In *Int. Congr. Nephrol. London July 1987.* Abstracts Book, p. 337.
66 Bertani, T., Livio, M., Macconi, D. *et al.* Platelet-activating factor (PAF) as a mediator of injury in nephrotoxic nephritis. *Kidney Int.* (1987), **31**, 1248–1256.
67 Camussi, G., Pawlowski, I., Saunders, R., Brentjens, J. & Andres, G. Receptor antagonist of platelet activating factor inhibits inflammatory injury induced by *in situ* formation of immune complexes in renal glomeruli and in the skin. *J. Lab. Clin. Med.* (1987), **110**, 196–206.
68 Camussi, G., Salvidio, G., Biesecker, G., Brentjens, J. & Andres, G. Heymann nephritis antibodies induce complement-dependent injury of rat glomerular visceral epithelial cells. *J. Immunol.* (1987), **139**, 2906–2914.
69 Egido, J., Ramirez, F., Rodriguez, M. J. *et al.* The role of platelet-activating factor in glomerular kidney diseases. In *The Role of Platelet-activating Factor in Immune Disorders, New Trends in Lipid Mediators Research* (1988), **2**, 167–180. Basel, Karger.
70 Ito, S., Camussi, G., Tetta, C., Milgrom F. & Andres, G. Hyperacute renal allograft rejection in the rabbit. The role of platelet-activating factor and of cationic proteins derived from polymorphonuclear leukocytes and from platelets. *Lab. Invest.* (1984), **51**, 148–161.
71 Camussi, G. & Salvidio, G. Platelet activating factor in graft rejection. *Prog. Biochem. Pharmacol.* (1987), **22**, 106–117.
72 Foegh, M. L., Khiribadi, B. S., Rowles, J. R., Braquet, P. & Ramwell, P. W. Prolongation of cardiac allograft survival with BN 52021, a specific antagonist of platelet-activating factor. *Transplantation* (1986), **42**, 86–90.

Chapter 9
PAF and the gastro-intestinal tract

Brendan J. R. Whittle and Juan V. Esplugues

Inroduction

Parenteral administration of PAF induces a range of patho-physiological events that resemble the clinical state of shock [1,2]. These actions include an increase in vascular permeability, haemoconcentration, hypotension, neutrophil aggregation and lysosomal enzyme release [2,3,4]. It is well established that shock can induce extensive gastro-intestinal damage, while septic shock is a major risk factor for gastro-intestinal ulceration resulting in mortality [5–7]. Thus, it appears likely that endogenous PAF release could contribute to the pathological events that underlie damage and ulceration to the stomach and intestine. Indeed, parenteral administration of PAF was found to induce gastro-intestinal damage in animal models [8–10]. In the present paper, the actions and role of PAF in the pathogenesis of gastro-intestinal disorders are detailed and the therapeutic potential for the clinical use of inhibitors and antagonists of PAF in gastro-intestinal disease is reviewed.

Action on the gastric mucosa

Effect of intravenous PAF

Intravenous infusion of PAF in low doses induced extensive damage to the rat gastric mucosa. This mucosal damage was macroscopically characterized as extensive hyperaemia and vaso-congestion with areas of haemorrhagic damage [10]. On histological evaluation, microvascular engorgement and congestion was the predominant feature, with extravasation of red-blood cells being apparent as well as epithelial and glandular destruction, with focal areas of necrosis that extended throughout the depth of the mucosal tissues [11]. In addition to the congestion of the mucosal and sub-mucosal microvasculature with red-blood cells, the presence of white-cell aggregates within these vessels was observed, particularly at the base of the mucosal glands and sub-mucosal vessels [11].

Intravenous infuson of picomole doses of PAF, which themselves did not alter systemic arterial blood pressure, substantially augmented the low degree of mucosal damage induced by administration of topical irritants such as dilute ethanol and sodium taurocholate [11]. Intra-peritoneal administration of PAF in the rat likewise enhanced the gastric damage induced by absolute ethanol [12].

Role of endogenous mediators in PAF-induced damage

It is possible that the actions of PAF in the gastro-intestinal tract are exerted via the further release of tissue-destructive mediators. However, histamine, noradrenaline and the cyclooxygenase products of arachidonic acid do not appear to play major roles as mediators of PAF-induced gastric damage since such damage was not prevented by pretreatment with antagonists of histamine-H_1 and -H_2 receptors or α-adrenoceptors [10]. Furthermore, inhibitors of cyclooxygenase (indomethacin, acetylsalicylic acid) or thromboxane synthetase (1-benzylimidazole), failed to reduce the extent of gastric damage [13].

A 2 h pretreatment with the glucocorticoid anti-inflammatory agents, dexamethasone or prednisolone, or administration of the dual lipoxygenase/cyclooxygenase inhibitor, BW 755C, did however, produce a significant reduction of PAF-induced gastric damage. These latter agents also significantly reduced the extent of haemoconcentration induced by PAF administration [13]. These observations could support a contribution of lipoxygenase products of arachidonic acid to PAF-induced gastric damage. Futhermore, the LTD_4-receptor antagonist, FPL 55712 attenuated the macroscopic damage induced by co-administration of intragastric ethanol and intra-peritoneal injection of PAF [12]. However, since this relatively non-specific and weak leukotriene antagonist reduced the damage induced by ethanol alone, the role of leukotrienes in this model is difficult to interpret. In other studies, more chronic pretreatment with dexamethasone over 36 h reduced the stimulated LTB_4 formation in the gastric mucosa following PAF infusion, but had no significant effect on mucosal LTC_4 formation and did not reduce the gastric mucosal damage [14]. Thus, the role of lipoxygenase metabolites in PAF-induced gastric damage remains to be clarified by the use of potent and selective leukotriene-receptor antagonists or 5-lipoxygenase inhibitors.

PAF-induced aggregation of neutrophils or platelets might also contribute to gastro-intestinal mucosal vasocongestion. While there is histological evidence supporting a role for neutrophil aggregation [11], a contribution of platelet aggregation in the ulcerogenic action of PAF in the rat is unlikely, since PAF does not directly aggregate rat platelets, and high doses are required *in vivo* to reduce the platelet count. Furthermore, the ulcerogenic actions of PAF were observed when administered to rats made thrombocytopaenic by prior administration of anti-platelet serum [10].

Since prostaglandins, particularly of the E series, markedly reduce the gastric damage and ulceration induced by a variety of ulcerogens, their actions on PAF-induced mucosal damage were investigated. However, neither PGE_2 nor its 16, 16-dimethyl analogue significantly reduced PAF-induced gastric damage [15]. These studies thus demonstrated that the protective properties of such prostanoids [16] do not extend to this form of damage. Furthermore, the presence of high concentrations of acid in the stomach are not necessary for PAF-induced ulcerogenesis, and pretreatment with anti-secretory doses of cimetidine did not reduce this mucosal damage [10].

Effects of close-arterial administration of PAF

To investigate the actions of local administration of PAF on the integrity of the rat gastric mucosa and to evaluate its effects on the microvasculature using histological criteria, we have utilized a technique for the close-arterial infusion of such mediators through the left gastric artery [17]. Local intra-arterial infusion of PAF resulted in a dose-dependent increase in macroscopically-assessed damage to the gastric mucosa (Fig. 9.1). The macroscopic appearance of this damage was comparable to that described following intravenous infusion and was characterized by extensive hyperaemia and haemorrhage, being located in the corpus region [17].

Local infusion of PAF also induced a dose-related increase in the histological index of damage (Fig. 9.2). Histological examination indicated congestion in the mucosal and sub-mucosal microvasculature throughout the antral and corpus regions, which was accompanied by extensive

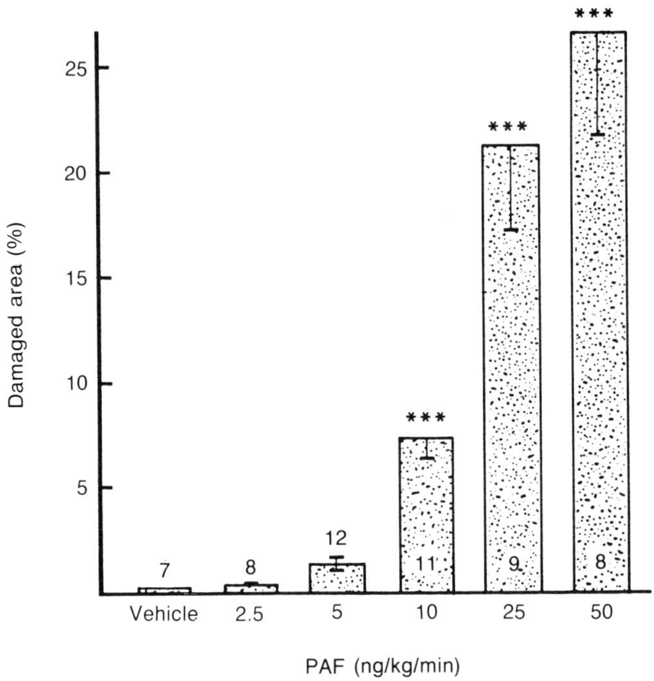

Fig. 9.1 Gastric mucosal damage following local intra-arterial infusion of PAF (2.5–50 ng/kg/min) for 10 min in the rat. The area of macroscopically assessed damage was determined by computerized planimetry and expressed as a percentage of the total mucosal area. Results are shown as mean ± s.e. mean of (*n*) studies, where stastical difference from the vehicle control group is given as ***, $P < 0.001$. Data are adapted from Esplugues & Whittle (1988) [17].

damage to surface epithelium, dilatation of the gastric glands and the presence of sub-epithelial oedema where the epithelium had remained intact.

The threshold doses of PAF for the induction of macroscopic or histological damage in both antral and corpus regions following close-arterial infusion produced minimal systemic hypotension, with the fall in systemic arterial blood pressure (BP) being <20 mmHg. Furthermore, intravenous infusion of PAF (25 ng/kg/min) produced a comparable fall in BP as the same dose infused locally, yet induced minimal damage to the gastric mucosa as assessed both by macroscopical and histological observation [17]. These findings indicate that although systemic hypotension may contribute to the gastric damage induced by high doses of PAF, especially when administered by the intravenous route, PAF can induce extensive disruption of the mucosal tissue and microvasculature by more direct mechanisms.

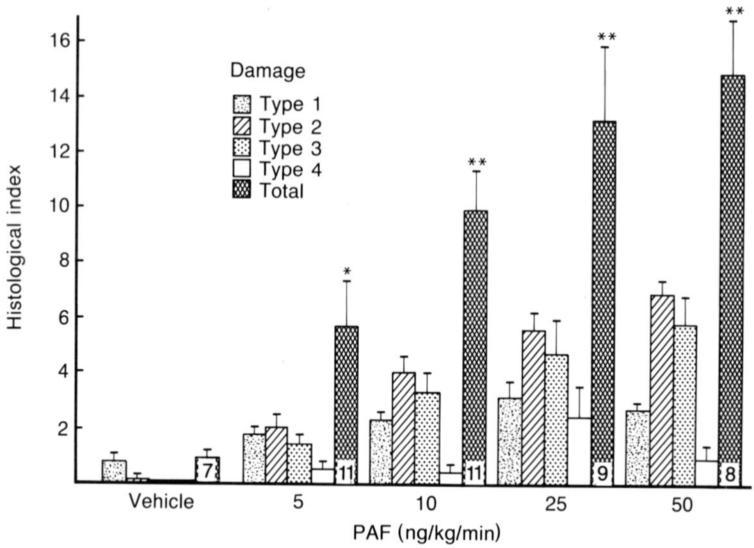

Fig. 9.2 Histological evaluation of the effects of local intra-arterial infusion of PAF (5-50 ng/kg/min) on gastric corpus mucosa of the rat. The data are shown in terms of the histological score for various types of damage (Types 1 to 4). Thus, epithelial cell damage was Type 1, (a score of 1), glandular disruption, vasocongestion or oedema, in the upper mucosa (Type 2), haemorrhagic damage in the mid to lower lucosa (Type 3) and deep necrosis or ulceration (Type 4). Each sub-section was evaluated on a cumulative basis, and the overall mean value of the scores for each of the 5–6 fields was taken as the histological index for that section. Results are shown as mean ± SEM of (*n*) values. For clarity, significant differences from vehicle control is given for total histological index only, where *, $P < 0.05$, and **, $P < 0.01$. Data are adapted from Esplugues & Whittle (1988) [17].

The predominant histological feature of congestion and engorgement of the mucosal microvessels following both local and intravenous administration of PAF suggested that vascular stasis may be an important mechanism underlying the mucosal damage. Such stasis could have been brought about by direct vasoconstrictor effects on the submucosal arterioles and venules resulting in a reduction in mucosal blood flow, or by other microvascular changes. To investigate such possibilities, the effects of PAF on blood flow in the rat gastric mucosa have been determined.

Actions of PAF on gastric microvasculature

To investigate whether the microcirculatory stasis could have resulted from direct vasoconstriction in the sub-mucosal arterioles and venules, an *in vivo* microscopy technique in the rat has been utilized. No change in the diameter of the sub-mucosal vessels could be detected during intravenous administration of PAF in doses that induced mucosal damage [18]. However, slowing of blood flow could clearly be observed during adminis-

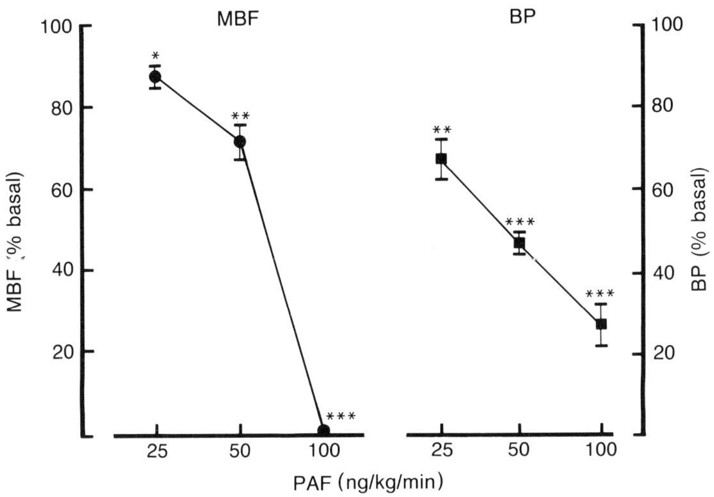

Fig. 9.3 Effect of intravenous infusion of PAF (25–100 ng/kg/min) on gastric mucosal blood flow (MBF), determined by hydrogen-gas clearance and mean systemic arterial blood pressure (BP) in the rat. Results, expressed as a percentage of basal values, are mean ± s.e. mean of 4–7 experiments in each group. MBF was measured 4 min after the start of the PAF infusion. Statistical difference from control data is shown as *, $P < 0.05$, **, $P < 0.01$, and ***, $P < 0.001$. Data are adapted from Whittle *et al.* (1986) [18].

tration of PAF, with stasis of flow being observed in 50% of the arterioles and 58% of the venules with the highest dose investigated [18].

Using hydrogen-gas clearance as a further index of gastric mucosal blood flow, a dose-dependent reduction in blood flow was determined during the intravenous infusion of PAF, accompanied by a corresponding fall in BP (Fig. 9.3). With the highest doses of PAF investigated, clearance reached an abrupt plateau within 4 min, indicating that blood flow had ceased [18].

To investigate whether changes in blood flow could be detected in the mucosal capillaries, red-blood cell velocity was determined, again using *in vivo* microscopy techniques. Intravenous infusion of PAF induced a significant fall in capillary blood flow, within 2–3 min of the start of infusion, with sluggish flow and sludging of blood cells along the capillary walls being observed. At the highest dose of PAF used, capillary blood flow fell to non-detectable levels within 5 min of the start of infusion, and no flow could be detected during the remainder of the infusion period. Stasis of flow in the capillaries could clearly be observed on the video-recordings [18].

Effects on the canine or feline gastric mucosa

The effects of intravenous or local gastric intra-arterial infusion of PAF has also been investigated in the dog, utilizing the chambered gastric

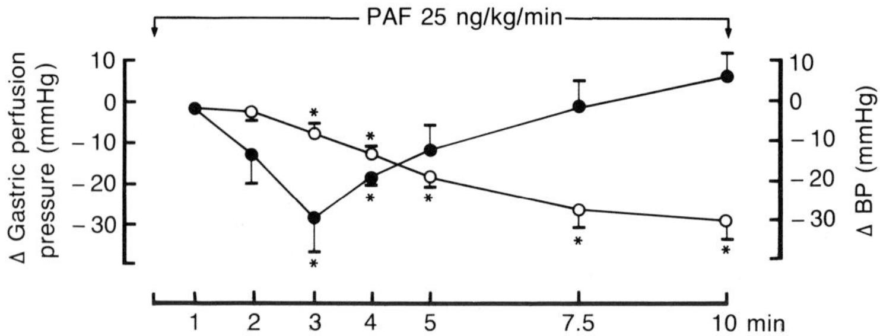

Fig. 9.4 Effect of an intravenous infusion of PAF (25 ng/kg/min for 10 min) on gastric vascular perfusion pressure (●—●) as a measure of vascular resistance and on systemic arterial blood pressure (○—○) in the anaesthetized dog. The initial fall in vascular resistance was followed by a rebound to values greater than the control, while BP gradually fell during the period of PAF infusion. Macroscopically, the intitial flushed appearance of the mucosa was followed by a darkened vasocongested appearance. Results, shown as Δ mmHg, are the mean ± s.e. mean of three experiments, where significant difference from the control is shown as *, $P < 0.05$. Data are adapted from Whittle *et al.* (1987) [19].

mucosa *in situ* [19]. During intravenous infusion of PAF in a dose causing a slow-onset fall in BP, an initial fall in gastric vascular resistance was followed by a rise above the resting value (Fig. 9.4), an effect which was also observed following local intra-arterial infusion. Indeed, following termination of the local PAF infusion, where no change in BP was noted, vascular resistance continued to increase (Fig. 9.5), accompanied by a darkened vaso-congested appearance of the chambered mucosal surface. On histological examination, extensive vascular congestion extended into the sub-mucosa, with extravasation of erythrocytes, prominent sub-epithelial oedema and haemorrhage.

Intravenous bolus administration of PAF in the anaesthetized cat induced a dose-related transient hypotension and increase in haematocrit [20]. Macroscopically, the corpus mucosa appeared blanched with regions of hyperaemia. On histological inspection, extensive vaso-congestion in the mucosal and sub-mucosal microvessels was observed, with substantial sub-epithelial oedema and focal areas where extravasation of erythrocytes could be detected, as well as regions of disrupted epithelium, haemorrhage and fibrin deposition (Fig. 9.6).

Others have likewise found that local intra-arterial infusion of PAF to the canine chambered stomach decreased venous outflow and mucosal blood flow, while enhancing the efflux of sodium and potassium ions, but with no increase in the back-diffusion of hydrogen ions [21].

Mechanisms of gastric mucosal damage

Deposition of blood cells along the walls of the rat gastric microvessels was observed during the periods of sluggish blood flow in the gastric

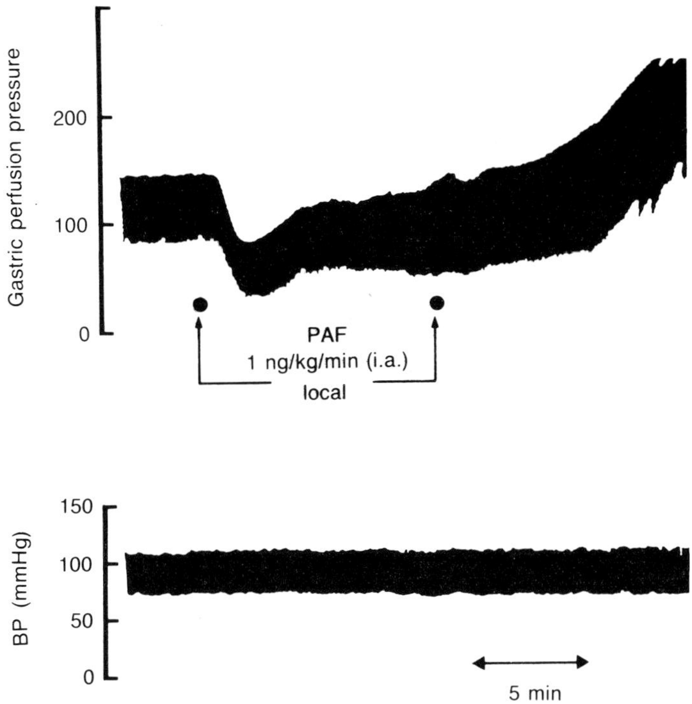

Fig. 9.5 Changes in gastric vascular perfusion pressure (*upper trace*) and systemic arterial blood pressure (BP; *lower trace*) induced by local intra-arterial infusion of PAF (1 ng/kg/min) for 10 min in the anaethetized dog. The trace shows a transient fall in gastric perfusion pressure during local infusion of PAF, followed by a substantial rise in perfusion pressure, but with no change in systemic arterial BP. Results are adapted from Whittle *et al.* (1987) [19].

microcirculation induced by PAF [18]. These cells were not identified as platelets, and indeed despite its name, PAF is only weakly active in stimulating platelet aggregation in the rat. Furthermore, extensive mucosal damage can be induced by PAF in platelet-depleted rats [10].

However, the presence of neutrophil aggregates was observed on histological examination of the rat gastric mucosa and systemic neutropenia has been detected after infusion of ulcerogenic doses of PAF [11]. These aggregates, by initially occluding the smaller capillaries, may thus contribute to the reduction in mucosal blood flow. Such effects would be enhanced by the concurrent marked haemoconcentration resulting from the extensive systemic extravasation of plasma protein that follows administration of PAF in ulcerogenic doses [13]. The changes in the rheological properties of the blood as a consequence of such haemoconcentration, coupled with the presence of aggregated cells, could therefore account for the sluggish flow and eventual stasis observed in the gastric

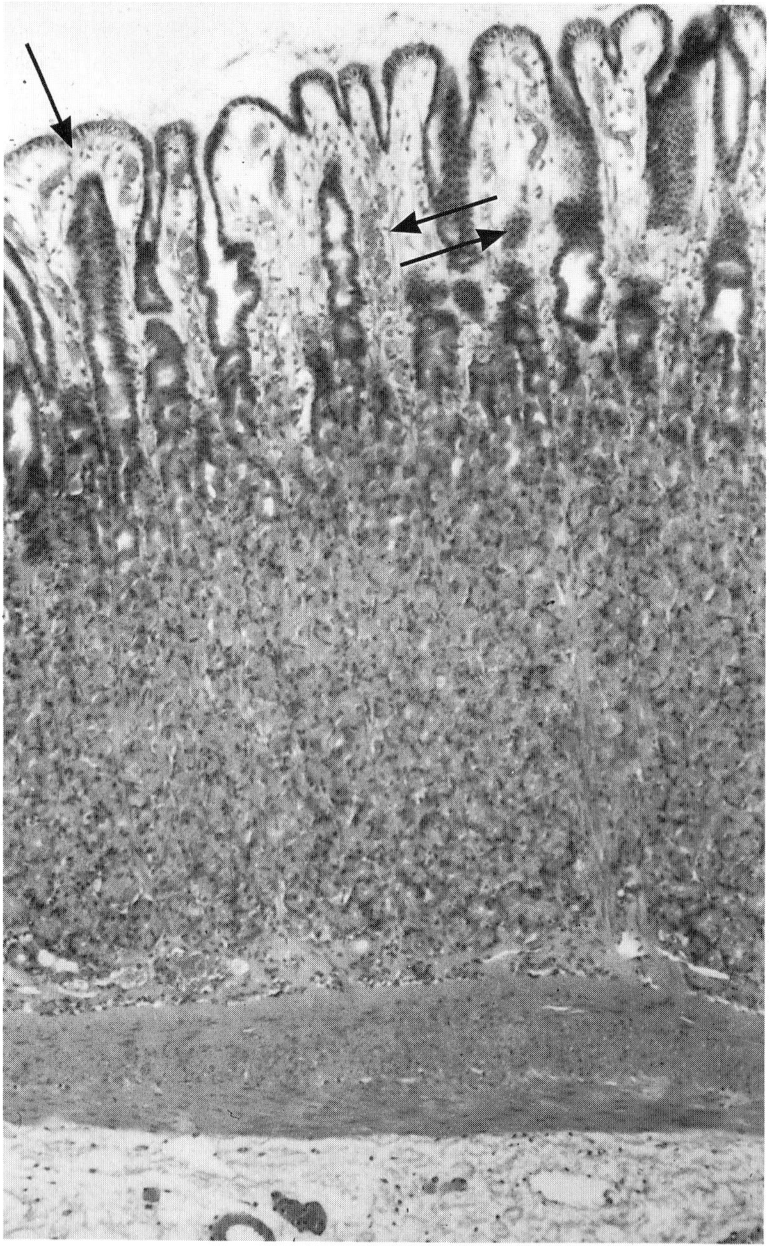

Fig. 9.6 Histological appearance of the gastric mucosa following sequential intravenous bolus administration of PAF (total dose 750 ng/kg) in the anaesthetized cat. Extensive sub-epithelial oedema and vasocongestion, with extravasation of erythrocytes can be seen (arrows). The section, stained with haemotoxylin and eosin, is derived from studies by Lees *et al.* (1986) [20].

microcirculation. In the dog, the pronounced changes in the gastric microcirculatory parameters are also suggestive of direct vascular spasm or the accumulation of macro-aggregates in the mucosal micro-vasculature, reducing blood flow.

Role in gastric ulceration

The gastric ulcerogenic effects of PAF are not simply non-specific actions of a phospholipid since lyso-PAF in doses some 100-fold more than those of PAF failed to induce detectable mucosal damage. Pharmacological evidence that these effects are mediated through activation of specific PAF receptors was provided by the observations that intravenous administration of the structurally dissimilar PAF-receptor antagonists, CV-3988, BN 52021, Ro 19-3704 or L-652731 could inhibit the damage induced by PAF-infusion [17, 22]. Others have also reported that the gastric mucosal damage induced by bolus injections of PAF could be attenuated by the PAF-receptor antagonists, WEB 2086 or BN 52063 and BN 52021 [23, 24].

PAF in endoxin-induced gastric damage

Several early reports indicated that PAF-receptor antagonists could ameliorate the mortality and hypotensive actions of endotoxin administration in rats [25–28]. Since extensive gastro-intestinal damage is observed following endotoxic shock, it was proposed that the release of endogenous PAF may contribute to such gastric ulceration [10]. Indeed, intravenous administration of the PAF-receptor antagonist CV-3988 substantially reduced the damage induced by bolus injection of the lipopolysaccharide (LPS) of *Salmonella typhosa* [29]. In further studies, using LPS from *Escherichia coli* to induce gastric damage, intravenous administration of CV-3988, BN 52021 and Ro 19-3704 reduced both the macroscopic and histological signs of mucosal disruption, as well as the mucosal plasma leakage [22].

In other studies, the gastric damage induced by LPS from *Salmonella enteritidis* was inhibited by oral administration of BN 52021 [24]. These findings thus supports the involvement of PAF, released either locally or systemically, in the pathogenesis of gastric ulceration in endotoxin or septic shock.

PAF in models of gastric ulceration

The involvement of PAF in the mechanisms underlying gastric mucosal damage induced by agents other than endotoxin is not clear. Thus, whereas neither Ro 19-3704 or BN 52021 reduced the haemorrhagic necrotic damage induced by oral administration of ethanol, CV-3988 did exert a protective action, although this is thus likely to reflect a non-specific activity [22]. Others have observed that BN 52021 and kadsurenone exerted inconsistent actions on mucosal damage induced by ethanol, aspirin or restraint stress [24,30].

It is therefore unlikely that PAF release makes a significant contribution to the pathogenesis of these latter models of gastric ulceration.

Actions on gastro-intestinal motility

Spasmogenic effects on isolated smooth muscle

PAF can exert potent spasmogenic actions on segments of gastro-intestinal smooth muscle *in vitro*. Thus, PAF induced long-lasting contractions of isolated strips of guinea pig ileum which were not antagonized by histamine H_1-receptor antagonists, atropine or a leukotriene antagonist and which caused desensitization to subsequent challenge [31,32]. In further studies, high concentrations of PAF were observed to induce only a transient contraction, followed by a relaxation [33]. These contractile actions on guinea pig ileum appear to be receptor-mediated since they were prevented by the PAF antagonists CV-3988 and 48740 RP [34]. Furthermore, specific binding sites for PAF could be detected on purified plasma membranes from ileal smooth muscle [35].

PAF also induced dose-related contractions of isolated segments of rat duodenum, jejunum, ileum and colon, with higher concentrations inducing a biphasic contractile response in the small intestinal tissues [36]. More recent studies on the rat isolated colon indicated that the potent spasmogenic actions of PAF were inhibited by the PAF-receptor antagonists FR 900452 and CV-3988, but not by antagonists of histamine, 5-hydroxytryptamine (5-HT) or leukotriene D_4 [37]. The sustained contractile effect of PAF on the colon was also found in that study to be reversed by washing the tissue with a high concentration of bovine serum albumin.

Effects on gastric contractility

PAF has been demonstrated to induce a spasmogenic effect on isolated strips of rat forestomach muscle [38]. Furthermore, we have observed pronounced increases in motility in the rat stomach *in vivo* following close-arterial infusion of PAF. To quantify this increase in gastric motility, changes in intra-gastric pressure *in vivo* have been determined.

In pentobarbitone-anaesthetized rats, local intra-arterial infusion of PAF induced a maintained rise in intra-gastric pressure followed by a further post-infusion increase (Fig. 9.7). The involvement of the local release of eicosanoids in the initial or secondary phases of the gastric

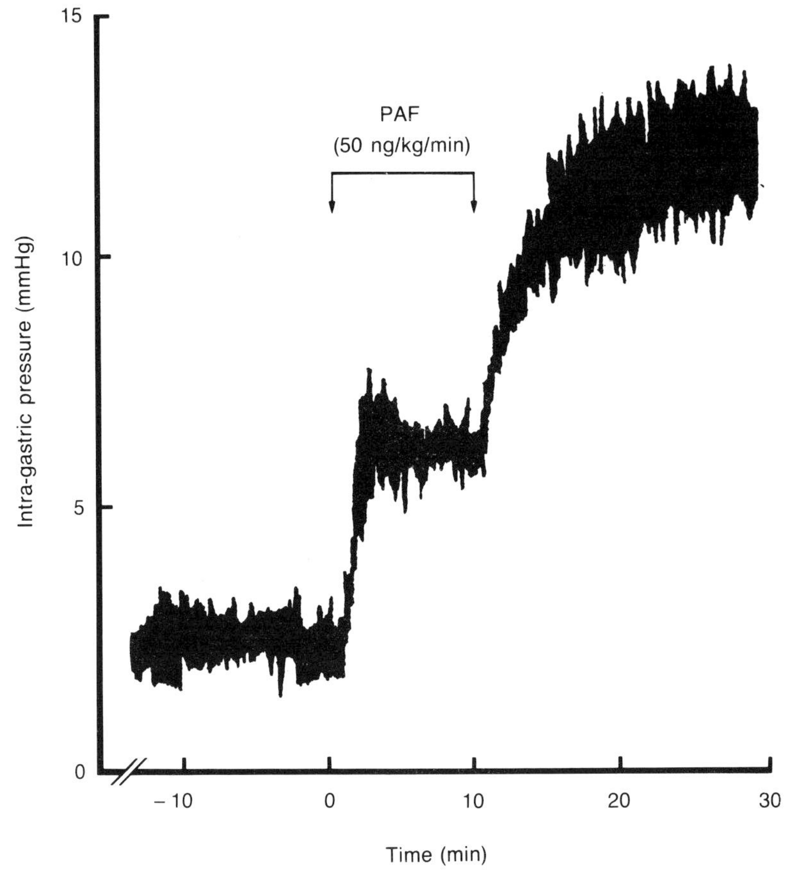

Fig. 9.7 Increase in intra-gastric pressure during the following local intra-arterial infusion of PAF (50 ng/kg/min) for 10 min in the rat. The rapid rise in intra-gastric pressure, as an index of the stomach contractions *in vivo* was maintained during the period of infusion, followed by a substantial further rise in intra-gastric pressure following termination of the infusion. Data are adapted from Esplugues & Whittle (1989) [39].

contraction induced by PAF was excluded since inhibition of cyclooxygenase, thromboxane synthase and lipoxygenase enzymes with potent and selective inhibitors had no effect. The initial contraction was also not dependent on activation of α- or β-adrenoreceptors, since specific antagonists in maximal doses failed to alter this response, nor was it the consequence of activation of cholinergic pathways since atropine, ganglion blockade or vagotomy had no effect [39].

Whereas antagonism of histamine H_1-receptors with maximal doses of mepyramine had no effect on the initial contraction induced by local infusion of PAF, the H_2-antagonist cimetidine and the 5-hydroxytryptamine receptor antagonist, methysergide both exerted a partial inhibitory

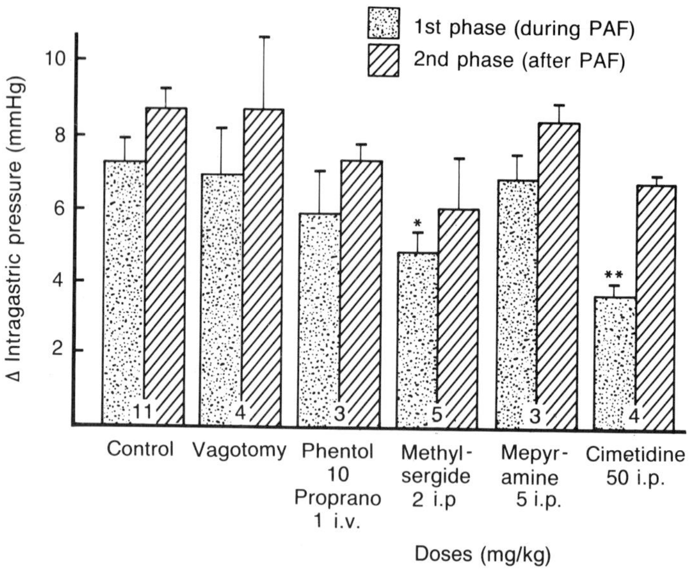

Fig. 9.8 Effects of vagotomy, α and β adrenoceptor antagonism, 5-HT receptor antagonism with methysergide and histamine H_1- and H_2-receptor antagonism on the changes in intra-gastric pressure during (first phase) and following termination (second phase) of a local intra-arterial infusion of PAF (50 ng/kg/min) in the rat. Results are given as mean $\pm$ s.e. mean of (n) experiments. Statistical difference from the control PAF group is shown by *, $P < 0.05$ and **, $P < 0.01$. Data are derived from Esplugues & Whittle (1989) [39].

action (Fig. 9.8). Since both these spasmogenic amines can be released from mast cells, it is possible that this initial response to PAF reflects in part an action on mucosal mast cells or possibly on circulating basophils to liberate such mediators [39]. Likewise, it has been suggested that the effects of PAF on ion transport in the rat jejunum may be secondary to the release of mast-cell mediators [40]. However, PAF itself may in addition, exert a direct contractile effect on gastro-intestinal smooth muscle *in vivo*, although whether both longitudinal or circular smooth-muscle fibres are affected is not yet known.

The second contractile phase that followed the local infusion of PAF was not affected by antagonism of α- or β-adrenoreceptors, 5-HT, histamine H_1- or H_2-receptors, by vagotomy, hexamethonium or by atropine (Fig. 9.8) but was abolished by treatment with the neurotoxin, tetrodotoxin. These findings suggest that PAF may induce gastric motility *in vivo* initially by directly stimulating gastric smooth muscle, and by the release of the mast cell mediators, histamine (acting on H_2-receptors) and 5-HT, and subsequently by non-adrenergic, non-cholinergic, neuronal activity [41]. The involvement of locally-released neuropeptides in this latter response thus warrants investigation.

Role in intestinal damage

PAF-induced intestinal damage

Early studies demonstrated that local intra-aortic administration of high bolus doses of PAF in combination with bacterial lipopolysaccharide (LPS) induced haemorrhagic necrotic lesions in the rat jejunum and ileum, with variable effects on the caecum and with no macroscopic damage to the colon or rectum being detected [8]. The nature of the damage resembled that observed in ischaemic bowel necrosis.

Intravenous infusion of PAF alone also induced damage throughout the rat intestine, as determined by histological techniques and the release of an enzyme marker for tissue damage [42]. Haemorrhagic damage was observed in the duodenum, jejunum and ileum, as was an increase in the release of the lysosomal enzyme, acid phosphatase, whereas the colon was unaffected by this acute administration of PAF. The leakage of radio-labelled plasma albumin in the duodenum, jejunum and ileum was also observed following PAF administration [43]. Both the macroscopically-detected intestinal damage and the plasma albumin leakage induced by infusion of PAF was reduced by intravenous pretreatment with CV-3988, BN 52021 and Ro 19-3704 [22,29,43]. Likewise, oral administration of BN 52021 and BN 52063 reduced the macroscopically-assessed intestinal damage induced by bolus intravenous injection of PAF [24].

Role of leukotrienes and other mediators

In the model of ischaemic bowel necrosis induced by the combination of PAF and endotoxin, administration of the non-specific inhibitors of leukotriene synthesis, diethylcarbamazine and nordihydroguaretic acid, as well as the weak leukotriene antagonist FPL 55712 attenuated the extent of damage in the small intestine [44]. In another investigation, the damage in the small intestine induced by PAF infusion was accompanied by an increase in the LTB_4 tissue formation in the duodenum, jejunum and ileum, but not in the colon, whereas there was a variable effect on LTC_4 synthesis [14]. In that study, dexamethasone pretreatment over 36 h reduced the PAF-induced intestinal damage and LTB_4 formation, yet stimulated LTC_4 formation. Thus, as with the gastric damaging effects of PAF, the role of endogenous leukotriene release in such intestinal damage requires further clarification with selective leukotriene antagonists and 5-lipoxygenase inhibitors.

The release of LTC_4 from the isolated perfused small intestine by PAF has been determined using bioassay techniques, and accounted for the initial vasoconstriction observed [45]. Further studies have suggested that noradrenaline was also released from this *in vitro* preparation after PAF administration, possibly secondary to the LTC_4 release, and accounted for the prolonged vasoconstriction [46]. The involvement of catecholamine release *in vivo* in PAF-induced damage to other gastrointestinal-tissue is not clear since adrenoreceptor blockade did not prevent such gastric mucosal lesions [10,41].

PAF in endotoxin-induced intestinal ulceration

As with the gastric mucosal lesions induced by endotoxin in the rat, the macroscopically assessed damage to the small intestine induced by administration of LPS from *S. typhosa* was substantially inhibited by CV-3988 [29]. Interestingly, like PAF, endotoxin did not induce damage in the distal colon of the rat. In further studies, both the histological and macroscopic damage induced by *E. coli* endotoxin, as well as the leakage of luminal and interstitial plasma albumin in the duodenum, jejunum and ileum, was reduced by CV-3988, BN 52021 and Ro 19-3704 [22,43]. Others have also demonstrated that BN 52021 could reduce the small intestinal disruption induced by *S. enteritidis* [24].

The intestinal damage induced by bolus injections of PAF in combination with LPS damage in the rat was also prevented by pretreatment with the PAF-receptor antagonists, SR1 63-072, SR1 63-119 or ONO-6240 [47].

Release of PAF in endotoxin shock

Early support for the involvement of PAF in the cardiovascular changes induced by endotoxin came from the demonstration of increased blood levels of biologically-assayed PAF [25]. The peak blood levels of PAF (4.7 nM) after endotoxin were calculated as those that could be achieved by intravenous injection of 300 pmol/kg PAF, which is within the range of PAF doses that have been found to induce gastro-intestinal damage [10]. Others have also demonstrated the release of PAF from rat peritoneal cells following endotoxin challenge [48].

If endogenous PAF does play a role in endotoxin-induced gastro-intestinal damage, then elevated levels may be detected in the affected tissues. Indeed, following administration of LPS from *E. coli*, a substantial increase in the formation of PAF in the rat jejunum, following extraction, characterization and bioassay (on rabbit washed platelets) was determined [49]. At 20 min after endotoxin, the jejunal levels of PAF were 20-fold higher than the corresponding control levels, and there was a significant correlation between PAF formation and the severity of the associated jejunal damage (Fig. 9.9). The elevated levels of PAF returned towards control some 2 h following endotoxin challenge [50]. The increased levels of PAF did not appear to reflect a non-specific stimulation

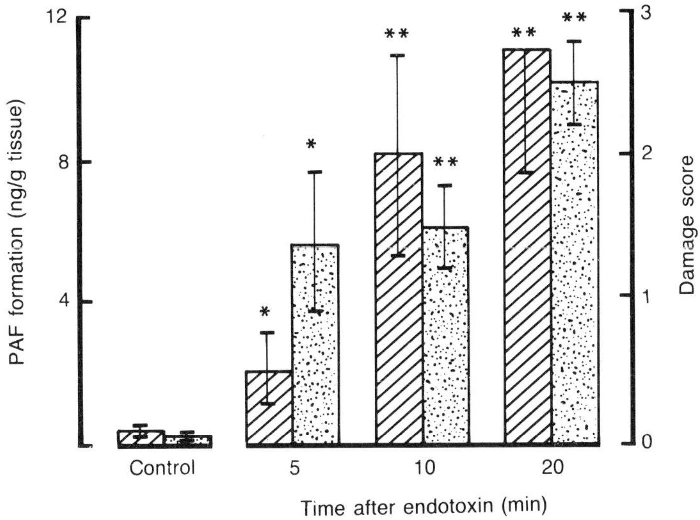

Fig. 9.9 Increase in the formation of PAF by rat jejunum following endotoxin administration and its relationship to intestinal damage. The jejunal damage was scored from 0–3 depending on the severity (speckled columns) and the levels of PAF were measured by bioassay (hatched columns), were assessed at various times after administration of *Escherichia coli* lipopolysaccharide (50 mg/kg i.v.). Results are expressed as mean ± s.e. mean of 9–12 rats in each experimental group where statistical difference from the control is shown as *, $P < 0.05$, and **, $P < 0.01$. Data are derived from Whittle *et al.* (1987) [49].

of phospholipase A_2 and liberation of precursor lipids following damage to the tissue, since the jejunal formation of PGE_2 was not enhanced. However, jejunal thromboxane B_2 levels, as determined by radiommunoassay, were significantly increased following endotoxin challenge, while the intestinal damage could be attenuated by thromboxane synthase inhibitors [51]. In that study, pretreatment with dexamethasone also reduced both endotoxin-induced PAF and thromboxane formation by jejunal tissue, while inhibiting the severity of the tissue damage. These findings indicate a complex interaction or sequential release of these tissue destructive mediators underlying the intestinal damage in this model of endotoxaemia.

PAF and inflammatory bowel disease

In addition to its disruptive actions on the stomach and intestine, PAF may contribute to the pathogenesis of inflammatory conditions throughout the gastro-intestinal tract. Thus, although acute parenteral administration of PAF does not appear to damage the colon [42], its more chronic endogenous release may be involved in the underlying inflammatory processes in the large bowel observed in ulcerative colitis and Crohn's disease.

In an experimental model of colitis in the rat, induced by intra-colonic administration of trinitrobenzene sulphonic acid (TNB), elevated PAF levels were detected in the inflamed colonic tissue 1–3 weeks after challenge [52]. Treatment with BN 52021 during the first or second week after challenge reduced the severity of this colonic damage, although it did not affect the degree of neutrophil infiltration, as assessed by myeloperoxidase activity (MPO). In another study, using the TNB model, an 11-fold increase in colonic PAF levels was detected 24 h after challenge and remained elevated for 1 week, as did the 15-fold increase in MPO activity [53].

Elevated levels of PAF formation were also determined in the guinea pig colon in an immune model of colitis induced by dinitrochlorobenzene and following anaphylactic challenge [53]. In studies of human colonic tissue, increased levels of PAF have also been detected in biopsies from patients with active colitis, following *in vitro* challenge with the ionophore A23187 and anti-IgE, which could be inhibited by *in vitro* incubation with the clinically effective agents, sulphasalazine, 5-amino salicylic acid or prednisolone [54].

Involvement in gastro-intestinal disease: clinical implications

From the studies reviewed above, it is clear that PAF can induce a wide range of deleterious actions on the gastro-intestinal tract. Parenteral administration of PAF has induced vaso-congestion, necrosis and haemorrhagic damage in both the stomach and the small intestine, and is one of the most potent ulcerogens described.

These extremely potent mucosal disruptive actions of PAF throughout the gastro-intestinal tract makes this engodenous mediator of pathological interest. Thus, it has been proposed that the release of PAF makes a major contribution to the associated gastro-intestinal damage in endotoxin or septic shock [10]. The endogenous release of PAF may also contribute to the enhanced gastro-intestinal motility observed in endotoxaemia [41]. Furthermore, an interaction between the endogenous release of both PAF and a further cytotoxic mediator, TXA_2 in the induction of intestinal damage during endotoxin shock has recently been proposed [51]. Experimental studies have demonstrated that such endotoxin-induced gastro-intestinal damage can be substantially ablated by specific antagonists of PAF [22,29]. Studies on the clinical effectiveness of selective PAF-antagonists in attenuating the characteristics of septic shock, including hypotension, haemoconcentration, intra-vascular coagulation and gastro-intestinal disruption are thus anticipated. Furthermore, in combination with endotoxin, PAF can induce disruption in the rat small-bowel comparable to that seen in necrotizing entercolitis, which can be attenuated by PAF-receptor antagonists [8,47]. In patients with diseases of the gastro-intestinal tract, systemic endotoxaemia may be the result of the absorption of endotoxins through the damaged mucosa [55]. Thus, endotoxaemia may both contribute to and be the result of gastro-intestinal damage and the effectiveness of PAF-receptor antagonists as a therapeutic intervention in such situations requires evaluation.

The potent micro-circulatory actions of PAF may underlie the microvascular disturbances and ischaemic episodes that are associated with many gastro-intestinal diseases. Furthermore, local PAF release following activation of phospholipase A_2 release may contribute to mucosal damage resulting from direct ischaemia in the small intestine [56]. Although high systemic doses of PAF may reduce gastro-intestinal motility as a result of profound cardiovascular changes, PAF can exert spasmogenic actions on gastro-intestinal smooth muscle. Thus, its release may be involved in lower bowel motility dysfunction, while enhanced gastric and duodenal motility could affect gastric emptying as well as promote duodenal reflux into the stomach, an action that could aggravate peptic ulcer formation or relapse. These findings point to the potential investigation of PAF-receptor antagonists in such situations.

The local release of PAF may contribute to inflammatory conditions of the gut, and could interact synergistically with the other inflammatory mediators including the eicosanoids, prostanoids, thromboxanes and the leukotrienes. PAF may be involved in gastritis and oesophagitis as well as inflammation of the small intestine and inflammatory bowel diseases. Furthermore, much recent clinical gastro-enterological research has been directed to elucidating the role of the bacterium, *Campylobacter pylori*, in the pathogenesis of peptic ulceration and the events leading to relapse after anti-secretory therapy. The local release of PAF, perhaps following release of a bacterial toxin, may be involved in such actions and indeed a local inflammatory response could make a contribution to the ulcerative process.

PAF may also interact with other pro-inflammatory mediators such as the cytokines. Thus, the local release of PAF has been implicated in vascular permeability changes and leukocyte infiltration induced by interleukin-1 [57]. It has also been suggested that the small bowel necrosis induced by the systemic administration of tumour necrosis factor could result from the release of PAF [58]. The effectiveness of PAF-receptor antagonists may therefore extend to more chronic conditions of inflammation. Thus, the findings of elevated colonic levels of PAF in animal models of colitis [52,53], and the finding that human colonic biopsies from patients with active ulcerative colitis can produce substantially higher levels of PAF on *in vitro* challenge compared with control tissue, further implicate this phospholipid as a pathological mediator of inflammatory bowel diseases [54].

The potential involvement of PAF in pathological conditions of the gastro-intestinal tract thus ranges from endotoxaemic damage, changes in motility and in ischaemic lesions to inflammatory bowel disease. The development of clinically-suitable and selective pharmacological agents that can interfere with the biosynthesis or actions of PAF should offer new therapeutic opportunities for these utilities.

References

1 Bessin, P., Bonnet, J., Apffel, A. *et al.* Acute circulatory collapse caused by platelet-activating factor (PAF-acether) in dogs. *Eur. J. Pharmacol.* (1983), **86**, 403–413.
2 Braquet, P., Shen, T. Y., Touqui, L. & Vargaftig, B. B. Perspectives in platelet-activating factor research. *Pharmacol. Rev.* (1987), **39**, 97–145.
3 McManus, L. M., Hanahan, D. J., Demopoulos, C. A. & Pinckard, R. N. Pathobiology of the intravenous infusion of acetyl glyceryl ether phosphorylcholine (AGEPC), a synthetic platelet-activating factor (PAF), in the rabbit. *J. Immunol.* (1980), **124**, 2919–2924.
4 Doebber, J. W., Wu, M. S., Robbins, Choy, B. M., Chang, M. N. & Shen, T. Y. Platelet activating factor (PAF) involvement in endotoxin induced hypotension in rats; studies with PAF-receptor antagonist kadsurenone. *Biochem. Biophys. Res. Commun.* (1985), **127**, 799–808.
5 Dale, D. C. & Petersdorf, R. G. Septic shock. In Braunwald, E., Isselbacher, K. J., Petersdorf, R. G., Wilson, J. D., Martin, J. B. & Fauci, A. S. (eds) *Harrison's Principles of Internal Medicine* (1983), 11th Ed, pp. 474–478. McGraw-Hill, New York.
6 Robert, A. & Kauffman, G. L. Stress ulcers. In Sleisenger, M. H. & Fordtran, J. S. (eds) *Gastrointestinal Disease* (1983), pp. 612–625. Philadelphia, W. B. Saunders.
7 Shumer, W. Septic shock. *JAMA* (1979), **242**, 1906–1907.
8 Gonzalez-Crussi, F. & Hsueh, W. Experimental model of ischemic bowel necrosis. The role of platelet-activating factor and endotoxin. *Am. J. Pathol.* (1983), **112**, 127–135.
9 Bessin, P., Bonnet, J., Thiboudeau, D., Agie, B., Beaudet, Y. & Gilet, F. Pathophysiology of shock states caused by PAF-acether in dogs and cats. In Benveniste J. & Arnoux, B. (eds) *Platelet-Activating Factor, INSERM Symposium No. 23* (1983), pp. 343–356. Elsevier, Amsterdam.
10 Rosam, A. C., Wallace, J. L. & Whittle, B. J. R. Potent ulcerogenic actions of platelet-activating factor on the stomach. *Nature* (1986), **319**, 54–56.
11 Wallace, J. L. & Whittle, B. J. R. Picomole doses of platelet-activating factor predispose the gastric mucosa to damage by topical irritants. *Prostaglandins* (1986), **31**, 989–998.
12 Konturek, S. J., Brzozowski, T., Drozdowicz, D. & Beck, G. Role of leukotrienes in acute gastric lesions induced by ethanol, taurocholate, aspirin, platelet-activating factor and stress in rats. *Dig. Dis. Sci.* (1988), **33**, 806–813.
13 Wallace, J. L. & Whittle, B. J. R. Effects of inhibition of arachidonic acid metabolism

on PAF-induced gastric mucosal necrosis and haemoconcentration. *Br. J. Pharmacol.* (1986), **89**, 415–422.
14 Wallace, J. L. & MacNaughton, W. K. Gastrointestinal damage induced by platelet-activating factor: Role of leukotrienes. *Eur. J. Pharmacol.* (1988), **151**, 43–50.
15 Steel, G., Wallace, J. L. & Whittle, B. J. R. Failure of prostaglandin E_2 and its 16, 16-dimethyl analogue to prevent the gastric mucosal damage induced by PAF. *Br. J. Pharmacol.* (1987), **90**, 365–327.
16 Whittle, B. J. R. & Vane, J. R. Prostanoids as regulators of gastrointestinal function. In Johnson, L. R. (eds) *Physiology of the Gastrointestinal Tract* (1987), 2nd edn, Vol. 1, pp. 601–638. Raven Press, New York.
17 Esplugues, J. V. & Whittle, B. J. R. Gastric mucosal damage induced by local intra-arterial administration of PAF in the rat. *Br. J. Pharmacol.* (1988), **93**, 222–228.
18 Whittle, B. J. R., Morishita, T., Ohya, Y., Leung, F. W. & Guth, P. H. Microvascular actions of platelet-activating factor on the rat gastric mucosa and submucosa. *Am. J. Physiol.* (1986), **251**, G772–G778.
19 Whittle, B. J. R., Kauffman, G. L. & Wallace, J. L. Gastric vascular and mucosal damaging actions of platelet activating factor in the canine stomach. In Samuelsson, B., Paoletti, R. & Ramwell, P. (eds) *Advances in Prostaglandin, Thromboxane and Leukotriene Research* (1987), pp. 285–292. Raven Press, New York.
20 Lees, I. W., Payne, A. M., Wallace, J. L. & Whittle, B. J. R. (1986), Cardiopulmonary and gastric actions of intravenous PAF in anaesethetized cats. *Br. J. Pharmacol.* **89**, 504p.
21 Soybel, D. I., Ashley, S. W. & Cheung. L. Y. Effects of platelet-activating factor on canine gastric mucosal blood flow and permeability to luminal acid. *Am. J. Surg.* (1988), **155**, 180–185.
22 Wallace, J. L., Steel, G., Whittle, B. J. R. Lagente, V. & Vargaftig, B. Evidence for platelet-activating factor as a mediator of endotoxin-induced gastrointestinal damage in the rat. Effects of three platelet-acting factor antagonists. *Gastroenterology* (1987), **93**, 765–773.
23 Brambilla, A., Ghiozi, A. & Giachetti, A. WEB 2086 a potent PAF antagonist exerts protective effect toward PAF-induced gastric damage. *Pharmacol. Res. Comm.* (1987) **19**, 147–151.
24 Braquet, P., Etienne, A., Mencia-Huerta, J-M. & Clostre, F. Effects of the specific platelet-activating factor antagonists, BN 52021 and BN 52063, on various experimental gastrointestinal ulcerations. *Eur. J. Pharmacol.* (1988), **150**, 269–276.
25 Doebber, J. W., Wu, W. S. & Shen, T. Y. Platelet activating factor intravenous infusion in rats stimulates vascular lysosomal hydrolase secretion independent of blood neutrophils. *Biochem. Biophys. Res. Comm.* (1984), **125**, 980–987.
26 Etienne, A., Hecquet, F., Soulard, C., Spinnewyn, B., Clostre, F. & Braquet P. *In vivo* inhibition of plasma protein and *Salmonella enteritidis*-induced mortality in the rat by a specific PAF-acether antagonist: BN 52021. *Agents & Actions* (1985), **17**, 368–370.
27 Terashita, Z., Imura, Y., Nishikawa, M. K. & Sumida, S. Is platelet activating factor (PAF) a mediator of endotoxin shock? *Eur. J. Pharmacol.* (1985), **109**, 257–261.
28 Casals-Stenzel, J. Protective effect of WEB 2086, a novel antagonist of platelet activating factor, in endotoxin shock. *Eur. J. Pharmacol.* (1987), **135**, 117–122.
29 Wallace, J. L. & Whittle, B. J. R Prevention of endotoxin-induced gastrointestinal damage by CV 3988, an antagonist of platelet-activating factor. *Eur. J. Pharmacol.* (1986), **124**, 209–210.
30 Rainsford, K. D. Relative roles of leukotrienes and platelet activating factor in experimentally-induced gastric ulceration. *Pharmacol. Res. Comm.* (1986), **18**, (Suppl), 209–215.

31 Findlay, S. R., Lichtenstein, L. M., Hanahan, D. J. & Pinckard, R. N. Contraction of guinea pig ileal smooth muscle by acetyl glyceryl ether phosphorylcholine. *Am. J. Physiol.* (1981), **241**, C130–C133.

32 Stimler, N. P., Bloor, C. M., Hugli, T. E., Wykle, R. L., McCall, C. E. & O'Flaherty, J. T. Anaphylactic actions of platelet-activating factor. *Am. J. Pathol.* (1981), **105**, 64–69.

33 Tokumura, A., Harada, K., Fukuzawa, K. & Tsukatani, H. Biphasic action of platelet-activating factor on isolated guinea pig ileum. *Lipids* (1983), **18**, 848–850.

34 Voelkel, N. F., Chang, S., Pfeffer, K. D., Worthen, S. G., McMurtry, I. F. & Henson, P. M. PAF antagonists: different effects on platelets, neutrophils, guinea pig ileum and PAF-induced vasodilation in isolated rat lung. *Prostaglandins* (1986), **32**, 359–372.

35 Hwang, S. B., Lee, C. S., Cheah, M. J. & Shen, T. Y. Specific receptor sites for 1-O-alkyl-2-O-acetyl-*sn*-glycero-3-phosphocholine (platelet activating factor) on rabbit platelet and guinea pig smooth muscle membranes. *Biochemistry* (1983), **22**, 4756–4763.

36 Tokumura, A., Fukuzawa, K. & Tsukatani, H. Contractile effect of 1-O-hexadecyl-2-O-acetyl-*sn*-glycero-3-phosphocholine on strips of isolated rat intestine. *J. Pharm. Pharmacol.* (1984), **36**, 210–212.

37 Tokumura, A., Terao, M., Okamoto, M., Yoshida, K. & Tsukatani, H. Study of platelet activating factor and its antagonists on rat colon strip with a new method avoiding tachyphylaxis. *Eur. J. Pharmacol.* (1988), **148**, 353–360.

38 Levy, J. V. Spasmogenic effect of platelet activating factor (PAF) on isolated rat stomach fundus strip. *Biochem. Biophys. Res. Comm.* (1987), **146**, 855–860.

39 Esplugues, J. V. & Whittle, B. J. R. Mechanisms underlying PAF-induced rat gastric motility *in vivo*. *J. Physiol.* (1988), **398**, 99p.

40 Hanglow, A. C., Bienstock, J., Dyek, N. & Purdue, M. W. Effects of platelet-activating factor (PAF) on rat jejunal mucosa. *Gastroenterology* (1987), **92**, 1424.

41 Esplugues, J. V. & Whittle, B. J. R. The mechanisms contributing to the gastric motility changes induced by PAF-acether and endotoxin in the rat. *Am. J. Physiol.* (1989), **256**, G275–282.

42 Wallace, J. L. & Whittle, B. J. R. Profile of gastrointestinal damage induced by platelet-activating factor. *Prostaglandins* (1986), **32**, 137–141.

43 Wallace, J. L., Steel, G. & Whittle, B. J. R. Gastrointestinal plasma leakage in endotoxic shock. Inhibition by prostaglandin E_2 and by a platelet-activating factor antagonist. *Can. J. Physiol. Pharmacol.* (1987), **65**, 1428–1432.

44 Hsueh, W., Gonzalez-Crussi, F. & Arroyave, J. L. Platelet-activating factor-induced ischemic bowel necrosis. An investigation of secondary mediators in its pathogenesis. *Am. J. Pathol.*(1986), **122**, 231–239.

45 Hsueh, W., Gonzalez-Crussi, F. & Arroyave, J. L. Release of leukotriene C_4 by isolated, perfused rat small intestine in response to platelet-activating factor. *J. Clin. Invest.* (1986), **78**, 108–114.

46 Hsueh, W., Gonzalez-Crussi, F. & Arroyave, J. L. Sequential release of leukotrienes and norepinephrine in rat bowel after platelet-activating factor. *Gastroenterology*, (1988), **94**, 1412–1418.

47 Hsueh, W., Gonzalez-Crussi, F., Arroyave, J. L., Anderson, R. C., Lee, M. L. & Houlihan, W. J. Platelet activating factor-induced ischemic bowel necrosis: the effect of PAF antagonists. *Eur. J. Pharmacol.* (1986), **123**, 79–83.

48 Inarrea, P., Gomez-Cambronero, J., Pascual, J., Carmen Ponte, M., Hernando, L. & Sanchez Crespo, M. Synthesis of PAF-acether and blood volume changes in Gram-negative sepsis. *Immunopharmacology*, **9**, 45–52.

49 Whittle, B. J. R., Boughton-Smith, N. K., Hutcheson, I. R., Esplugues, J. V. & Wallace, J. L. Increased intestinal formation of PAF in endotoxin-induced damage in the rat. *Br. J. Pharmacol.* (1987), **92**, 3–4.
50 Whittle, B. J. R., Boughton-Smith, N. K. Hutcheson, I. & Esplugues, J. V. Intestinal release of eicosanoids and PAF-acether as pathological mediators of endotoxin-induced damage. *Gastroenterology* (1988), **94**, A495.
51 Whittle, B. J. R. & Boughton-Smith, N. K. Interaction between PAF-acether and thromboxane in endotoxin-induced intestinal damage. *Prostaglandins* (1988), **35**, 813.
52 Wallace, J. L. Release of platelet-activating factor (PAF) and accelerated healing induced by a PAF antagonist in an animal model of chronic colitis. *Can. J. Physiol. Pharmacol.* (1988), **66**, 422–425.
53 Boughton-Smith, N. K. & Whittle, B. J. R. Formation of the pro-inflammatory mediator, PAF-acether in different models of colitis. *Gastroenterology* (1988), **94**, A45.
54 Eliakim, R., Karmeli, F., Razin, E. & Rachmilewitz, D. Role of platelet-activating factor in ulcerative colitis. Enhanced production during active disease and inhibition by sulfasalazine and prednisolone. *Gastroenterology* (1988), **95**, 1167–1172.
55 Van Deventer, S. J. H., Ten Gate, J. W. & Tytgat, G. N. J. Intestinal endotoxemia. Clinical significance. *Gastroenterology* (1988), **94**, 825–831.
56 Otamiri, T., Lindahl, M. & Tagesson, C. Phospholipase A_2 inhibition prevents mucosal damage associated with small intestinal ischaemia in rats. *Gut* (1988), **29**, 489–494.
57 Rubin, R. M. & Rosenbaum, J. T. A platelet-activating factor antagonist inhibits interleukin-1-induced inflammation. *Biochem. Biophys. Res. Comm.* (1988), **154**, 429–436.
58 Sun, X. & Hsueh, W. Bowel necrosis induced by tumour necrosis factor in rats is mediated by platelet-activating factor. *J. Clin. Invest.* (1988), **81**, 1328–1331.

Chapter 10
PAF and blood cells: pathophysiological correlates

B. Boris Vargaftig and René Bourgain

Introduction

Platelet activating factor (PAF) is formed by and stimulates monocytes, polymorphonuclear leukocytes, platelets and eosinophils, i.e. cells involved in inflammation. In this Chapter we discuss some of its effects on inflammatory cells and particularly on two important physio-pathological correlates: the ability of PAF to trigger arterial thrombosis in the guinea pig and its role for inflammation-induced perpetuation of asthma. The biochemistry of leukocytes with respect to PAF [1] and more general concepts on the physio-pathology and pharmacology of PAF [2], particularly in asthma [3–5] have been recently reviewed.

Interaction with neutrophils

PAF triggers neutrophil exocytosis, superoxide production and aggregation [6–8] which are enhanced by cytochalasin B [9]. Cyclooxygenase inhibitors do not modify enzyme extrusion, whereas lipoxygenase inhibitors do [10,11]. Small doses of PAF induce neutropenia [12] and formation of thromboxane A_2 [13] when infused intravenously to rabbits, to rats [14] or to guinea pigs; this is accompanied by neutrophil margination in the lungs [15]. Since leukotriene B_4 is formed by neutrophils upon PAF activation, it has been suggested that the effects of PAF are mediated by LTB_4 [11,16]. In view of the contradictory results reported and to species-dependency, it is too early to reach a firm conclusion on whether the effects of PAF on neutrophils are direct or are mediated, at least in part, by lipoxygenase derivatives (reviewed in [1]).

Even though it is now established that activated neutrophils synthesize PAF, it is unclear whether the amounts formed are important for

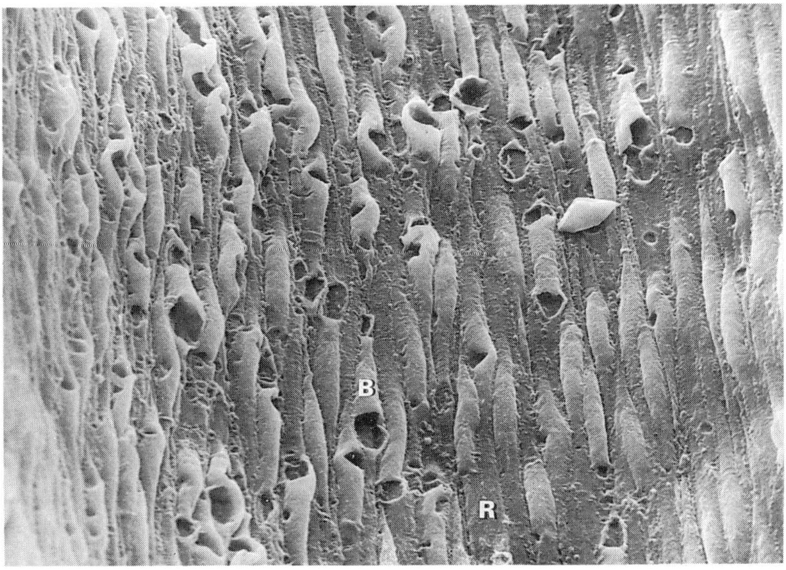

Fig. 10.1 Scanning electron microscopic view of bleb formation (B) in endothelial cells following PAF-acether-mediated challenge of the arterial wall. The endothelial cells involved also demonstrate retraction of the cellular margins (R).

inflammation [17]. The issue is complicated by the fact that: (i) only a small part of the amounts of PAF synthesized by the cell is released and the release varies according to the albumin concentration in the medium [17,18]; (ii) formation of PAF is enhanced by exogenous lyso-PAF provided by nearby activated platelets [19] or serum albumin. Nevertheless, 30 ng of PAF may produce a weal and flare reaction in the human skin [20] and 10^7 human neutrophils stimulated by fMLP release approximately 40 ng PAF into a 4% human serum albumin supernatant [19], suggesting that neutrophil-derived PAF may indeed contribute to inflammation.

It is important to recognize that the effects of PAF on neutrophils may be potentiated by other inflammatory mediators. Thus 5-HETE enhances the degranulation induced by PAF [21]. Conversely, PAF increases the activity of other agonists such as the rate and extent of fMLP-induced superoxide production [22]. The concept of priming is becoming important and refers to aggregation, respiratory burst, degranulation and adhesion of neutrophils to endothelium, which is induced by PAF-primed neutrophils. Mechanisms for the PAF-induced priming are discussed by Braquet *et al.* [23].

Specific PAF antagonists block its actions on neutrophils and may also inhibit the activity of unrelated agonists. BN 52021 and 48740 RP

[24], kadsurenone [25], L-652731 [26] and WEB 2086 [15] inhibit PAF-induced aggregation and exocytosis of azurophilic granules of isolated human neutrophils. By contrast, the protective effect is variable when these antagonists are tested against fMLP-induced neutrophil activation. Thus 48740 RP partly reduces aggregation and lysozyme release but is inactive against β-glucuronidase release and may even enhance it in the absence of cytocholasin B, under conditions in which BN 52021 only inhibits aggregation [24]. These antagonists probably do not interfere with the effects of fMLP, as noted in *in vivo* studies with BN 52021 [28, 29] or CV-3988 [30].

Interaction with eosinophils

Eosinophils are more sensitive to the stimulating effects of PAF, than to histamine, fMLP and eosinophil chemotactic factors of anaphylaxis [31–33]. This effect is blocked by BN 52021 [32]. Leukotriene B_4 is reported not to stimulate the human eosinophil [31,32], but it activates the motility of the guinea pig eosinophil *in vitro* (Coëffier & Joseph, personal communication). PAF-stimulated human eosinophils produce chemoluminescence and LTC_4 [34,35]. The adherence of eosinophils to human vascular endothelial cells is also markedly enhanced by PAF [36]. In addition, PAF synergizes with the calcium ionophore A23187, with arachidonic acid and opsonized zymosan [34,35]. PAF also induces the accumulation of eosinophils in the skin of allergic (but not of non-allergic) patients [37,38] as does allergen. Intravenous injections of PAF or of allergen to guinea pigs leads to platelet and eosinophil margination, diapedesis and migration into the bronchial sub-mucosa and epithelial shedding, a hallmark of asthma (see Chapter 7). Eosinophil migration triggered by PAF and by antigen is blocked by PAF antagonists [27,39], by platelet depletion and PGI_2 administration [39]. PAF is synthesized by human eosinophils stimulated by ionophore A23187 and various chemotactic factors [40,41].

Role of activation of circulating cells for *in vivo* effects

The administration of PAF by the intravenous route [39] or by aerosol [42] induces neutrophil and eosinophil infiltration into the lung parenchyma and PAF antagonists impair cell infiltration following antigen administration. Interestingly, aggregation of leukocytes in the microcirculation as well as a massive infiltration of eosinophils, can be observed when the effects of inhaled PAF and of antigen are compared. Furthermore, 1 h after the administration of PAF, numerous polymorphonuclear leukocyte aggregates are present in the alveolar capillaries and eosinophils are found in the bronchial sub-mucosa [39], suggesting that PAF is implicated in cell recruitment at the site of allergic reactions.

Comparable results have been obtained in human skin when comparing the cell response underlying the cutaneous inflammatory reaction to PAF and to the allergens in atopic and non-atopic subjects. PAF elicits weal and flare responses in both subjects, but these macroscopic effects are accompanied by eosinophil infiltration and by *in situ* activation only in allergic patients [36,37], suggesting that these cells express a qualitative difference in their responsiveness and that PAF might play a key role for augmenting and perpetuating allergic reactions. An enhanced response to PAF of eosinophils from allergic patients has also been demonstrated by Borgeat *et al.* [40]. PAF induced increased production of LTD_4 by eosinophils from asthmatic patients, which was abolished by a PAF antagonist. Furthermore, eosinophils from patients with eosinophilia, including asthmatics, released more PAF as compared with those from control subjects [41].

Using an opto-electronic device to detect platelet–vessel wall interaction and subsequent thrombus formation, Bourgain *et al.* [43] have shown that the topical *in vivo* application of PAF onto a mesenteric arteriole of the guinea pig induces the formation of thrombus, leading to partial or total occlusion of the arterial lumen. The application of an electrical current of 30–40 μA for 1 min to the vessel wall also resulted in the formation of a thrombus comparable to that induced by PAF. When the dose of PAF was reduced to 0.01 μM, no formation of thrombus occurred, but thrombosis was triggered if PAF was added to a sub-threshold electrical challenge (1–5 μA). The ultrastructural findings observed were identical in the three types of challenges and were followed invariably by significant alterations in the structure of the endothelial cells. Retraction of the cell margins and exposure of the underlying sub-intimal structures was observed within the first 2 or 3 min, while the formation of blebs in the cytoplasm of the endothelial cells (Fig. 10.1) was a conspicuous finding. Very rapidly platelets started to adhere onto the sites of exposure of the sub-endothelium and on the retracting endothelial cells. Those platelets then formed small aggregates which increased in size over time, resulting in thrombus formation. Platelet shape change was a constant finding: pseudopodes formed, while the thrombus grew and platelets at different stages of activation were observed (Fig. 10.2). The discoid form of the normal newly arriving platelets was in sharp contrast with the spheroid form of the activated cells. Observations with transmission electron microscopy demonstrated that numerous platelets were completely degranulated at a very early stage, while few if any leukocytes were seen, and then at the site of the retracting endothelial cells. Within minutes, the

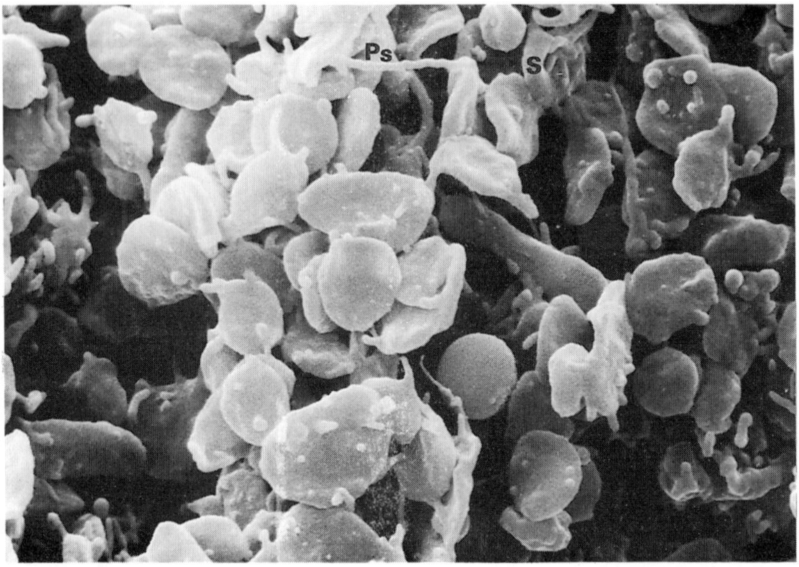

Fig. 10.2 Scanning electron micrscopic view of an early thrombus induced by PAF-acether-mediated challenge. Several states of platelet activation are visible, such as pseudopod formation (Ps) and shape change (S).

platelet thrombus underwent extensive changes, including an increased compactness and invasion by leukocytes, which surrounded the thrombus and rapidly penetrated the thrombotic mass through crevices in its structure. Scanning electron microscopy indicated that the leukocytes were a mixture of lymphocytes, monocytes and eosinophils, with a predominance of neutrophils in an activated state, showing phagosomes, pseudopods, degranulation and phagocytosis images, particularly of platelet debris and fibrin (Fig. 10.3). At this stage of thrombosis, the platelets, particularly those surrounding the leukocytes, showed a marked ballooning and complete degranulation.

The PAF precursor and metabolite lyso-PAF failed to trigger thrombosis, but its addition to a sub-threshold electrical challenge did. In addition, thrombosis was inhibited by a PAF antagonist. Interestingly, the anti-asthma drug ketotifen, which was inactive against PAF itself, was effective both against the combination of lyso-PAF and electrical current and against thrombosis induced by current applied alone. In accordance with the possibility that ketotifen would inhibit PAF generation, it failed to modify thrombosis, once it was established, whereas PAF antagonists were also effective curatively [43,44].

These results do not prove or disprove a role for PAF in thrombosis, even though it is noteworthy that thrombosis induced by the local application of electrical current alone was prevented by PAF antagonists.

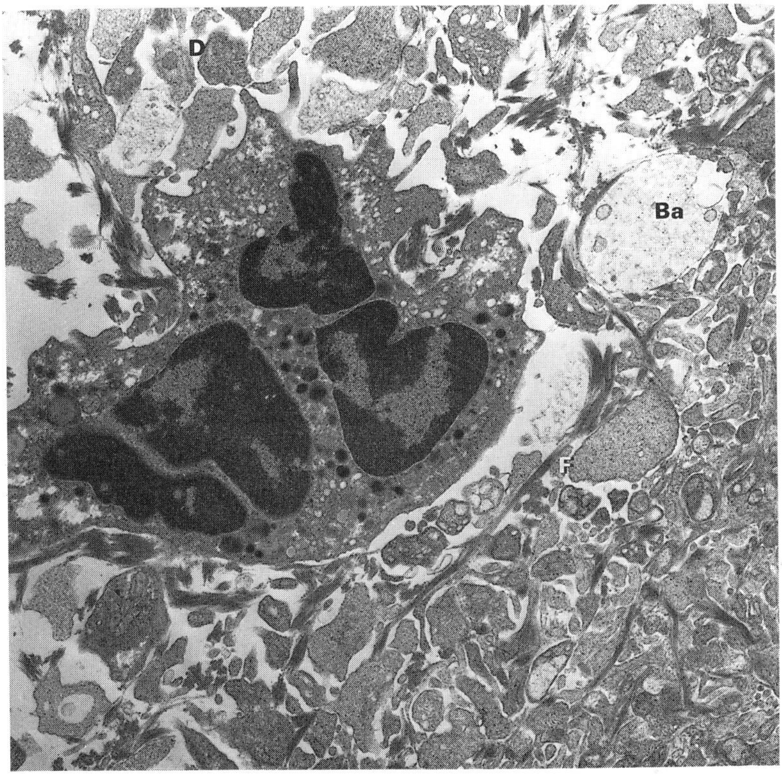

Fig. 10.3 Transmission electron microscopy of a thrombus 15 min following the onset of thromboformation. Leukocyte invasion is present and the platelets are mostly degranulated (D), while some demonstrate marked ballooning (Ba). Fibrin tufts are present (F).

Inflammatory cell recruitment

PAF may play an important role in the development and perpetuation of asthma, since it triggers the recruitment of neutrophils and of eosinophils into the lungs. It is difficult to understand how such a short-lived substance as PAF can display relatively long-lasting effects and promote the recruitment of inflammatory cells after 6 h or even 24 h. In fact, the intra-pleural injection of PAF to the rat is followed by eosinophilia [45] and by the generation of a factor, which induces eosinophilia *in vitro* and *in vivo*, when injected into the pleural cavity of recipient rats. Generation of this factor was suppressed when PAF was co-injected into the donor animals together with dexamethasone, the PAF antagonists BN 52021 or WEB 2086, the anti-allergy drug nedocromil sodium, or the protein synthesis inhibitor cycloheximide. Neither of these inhibitors affected eosinophilia induced by the pre-formed potential mediator, which may be a cytokine. PAF thus appears to favour the migration of eosinophils *in vivo* via a direct as well as an indirect effect. The hypothesized mediator of the indirect effect is either synthesized by a resident cell (such as a mesothelial cell) or by migrating cells, such as neutrophils.

The potential role of PAF as a trigger for the infiltration of eosinophils into the lung in asthma correlates with the observations of Pretolani *et al.* [46–48], showing that the broncho-constrictor response to PAF and the accompanying release of thromboxane B_2 are markedly increased in lungs from actively sensitized guinea pigs boosted with antigen, as compared with those from non-sensitized or sensitized but unboosted animals. In addition, PAF and the tripeptide secretagogue fMLP trigger the release of histamine and LTB_4 which are not released from control PAF-injected non-sensitized lungs. This altered responsiveness to PAF, fMLP (and to LTD_4) strongly suggests that the booster stimulates the recruitment of inflammatory cells, particularly since the enhanced responsiveness to fMLP was suppressed when the animals were treated with the cytotoxic drug vinblastine (Boukili *et al.*, in preparation). The differences between boosted and single-injected animals are probably accounted for by the infiltration of inflammatory cells, and/or by a modification of resident cells, such as alveolar macrophages [49]. Specific hypersensitivity and non-specific hyper-responsiveness start together, but the latter outlasts the former [46], probably because local inflammation persists. Indeed, ovalbumin administration to sensitized animals is followed within 6–24 h by a marked lung infiltration by eosinophils, the appearance of eosinophil-enriched mucous plugs in the bronchial lumen, epithelial desquamation and mucous metaplasia, as induced by PAF. Two PAF antagonists (BN 52021 and WEB 2086) prevent the eosinophil infiltration [39]. There is enough evidence to suggest that allergic asthma is a chronic inflammatory disease of airway, and cell recruitment and mediator release operate as a network for the persistence and aggravation of the disease.

Role in inflammatory pathology

As seen in the past with other potential mediators of inflammation, a role for PAF has been suggested in a large variety of pathological conditions. Future work, particularly the study of PAF antagonists in human disease, will prove or disprove this role. An interesting example is given by asthma, where the hypothesized role of PAF arose from experiments on acute bronchoconstriction [50], whereas now the dominant concept is that PAF is more important in the inflammatory phase of asthma and particularly in the bronchial hyper-responsiveness characterizing this disease. Similarly, the evidence for a role of PAF in thrombosis was provided by its effectiveness as a platelet-aggregating agent and more recently on the guinea pig model discussed above, whereas such a role has not been confirmed in other systems. The natural evolution of these concepts will continue and establish the true role of PAF in human disease.

References

1 Pinckard R. N. Ludwig, J. C. & McManus, M. Platelet-activating factors. In Galin, J. I., Goldstein, I. M. & Snyderman, R. *Inflammation, Basic Principles and Clinical Correlates* (1988), pp 129–167. Raven Press, New York.

2 Braquet, P., Touqui, L., Shen, T. Y. & Vargaftig, B. B. Perspectives in platelet-activating factor research. *Pharmacol. Rev.* (1987), **39**, 97–145.

3 Pretolani, M., Ferrer-Lopez, P. & Vargaftig, B. B. From anti-asthma drugs to PAF-acether antagonsim and back: present status. *Biochem. Pharmacol.* (1989), in press.

4 Barnes, P. J., Chung, K. F. & Page, C. P. Platelet-activating factor as a mediator of allergic disease. *J. Allergy Clin. Immunol.* (1989), **81**, 919–934.

5 Bigby, T. D. & Nadel, J. A. Asthma. In Gallin, J. I. Goldstein, I. M. & Snyderman, R. (eds) *Inflammation, Basic Principles and Clinical Correlates* (1988), pp 679–694. Raven Press, New York.

6 Goetzl, J. J., Derian, C. K., Tauber, A. I. & Valone, F. H. Novel effects of 1-O-alkyl-2-acetyl-*sn*-glyceryl-3-phosphocholine mediators on human leukocyte function: delineation of the specific roles of the acyl substituents. *Biochem. Biophys. Res. Comm.* (1980), **94**, 881–888.

7 O'Flaherty, J. T., Wykle, R. L., Miller, C. H. *et al.* 1-O-alkyl-2-acetyl-*sn*-glyceryl-3-phosphocholine. A novel class of neutrophil stimulants. *Am. J. Pathol.* (1981), **103**, 70–79.

8 Shaw, J. O., Pinckard, R. N., Ferrigni, K. S., McManus, L. M. & Hanahan, D. J. Activation of human neutrophils with 1-O-hexadcyl/octadecyl-2-acetyl-*sn*-glyceryl-3-phosphocholine (platelet-activating factor). *J. Immunol.* (1981), **127**, 1250–1255.

9 Dewald, B. & Baggiolini, M. Platelet-activating factor as a stimulus of exocytosis in human neutrophils. *Biochim. Biophys. Acta* (1986), **888**, 42–48.

10 Smith, R. J. & Bowman, B. J. Stimulation of human neutrophil degranulation with 1-O-octadecyl-2-O-acetyl-*sn*-glyceryl-3-phosphorylcholine: modulation by inhibitors of arachidonic acid metabolism. *Biochem. Biophys. Res. Comm.* (1982), **104**, 1495–1501.

11 Chilton, F. H., O'Flaherty, J. T., Walsh, C. E. *et al.* Platelet activting factor. Stimulation of lipoxygenase pathway in polymorphonuclear leukocytes by 1-O-alkyl-2-O-acetyl-*sn*-glyceryl-3-phosphocholine. *J. Biol. Chem.* (1982), **257**, 5402–5407.

12 McManus, L. M., Hanahan, D. J., Demopoulos, C. A & Pinckard, R. N. Pathobiology of the intravenous infusion of acetyl glyceryl ether phosphorylcholine (AGEPC), a synthetic platelet-activating factor (PAF), in the rabbit. *J. Immunol.* (1980), **124**, 2919–2924.

13 McManus, L. M., Fitzpatrick, F. A., Hanahan, D. J. & Pinckard, R. N. Thromboxane B_2 (TXB_2) release following acetyl glyceryl ether phosphorylcholine (AGEPC) infusion in the rabbit. *Immunopharmacology* (1983), **5**, 197–207.

14 Doebber, T. W., Wu, M. S. & Shen. T. Y. Platelet activating factor intravenous infusion in rats stimulates vascular lysosomal hydrolase secretion independent of blood neutrophils. *Biochem. Biophys. Res. Comm.* (1984), **125**, 980–987.

15 Pretolani, M., Lefort, J., Malanchère E. & Vargaftig, B. B. Interference by the novel PAF-acether antagonist WEB 2086 with the bronchopulmonary responses to PAF-acether and to active and passive anaphylactic shock in guinea pigs *Eur. J. Pharmacol.* (1987), **140**, 311–321.

16 Lin, A. H., Morton, D. R. & Gorman, R. R. Acetyl glyceryl ether phosphorylcholine stimulates leukotriene B_4 synthesis in human polymorphonuclear leukocytes. *J. Clin. Invest.* (1982), **70**, 1058–1065.
17 Ludwig, J. G., Hoppens, C. L., McManus, L. M., Mott, G. E. & Pinckard, R. N. Modulation of platelet-activating factor (PAF). Synthesis and release from human polymorphonuclear leukocytes (PMN): role of extracellular albumin. *Arch. Biochem. Biophys.* (1987), **241**, 337–347.
18 Lynch, J. M. & Henson, P. M. The intracellular retention of newly synthesized platelet-activating factor. *J. Immunol.* (1986), **137**, 2653–2661.
19 Coëffier, E., Chignard, M., Delautier, D. & Benveniste J. Cooperation between platelets and neutrophils of PAF-acether formation. *Fed. Proc.* (1984), **43**, 781. (Abstract).
20 Archer, C. B., Page, C. P., Paul, W., Morley, J. & McDonald, D. M. Inflammatory characteristics of platelet-activating factor (PAF-acether) in human skin. *Br. J. Dermatol.* (1984), **110**, 45–50.
21 O'Flaherty, J. T., Thomas, M. J., Hammett, M. J., Carroll, C., McCall, C. E. & Wykle, R. L. 5-L-hydrosy-6,8,11,14-eicosatetraenoate potentiates the human neutrophil degranulating action of platelet activating factor. *Biochem. Biophys. Res. Comm.* (1983), **111**, 1–7.
22 Dewald, B. & Baggiolini, M. Activation of NADPH oxidase in human neutrophils. Synergism between fMLP and the neutrophil products PAF and LTB_4. *Biochem. Biophys. Res. Comm.* (1985), **128**, 297–304.
23 Braquet, P., Braquet, M., Bussolino, F., Bourgain, R. & Hosford, D. PAF/cytokine auto-generated feed-back networks in microvascular immune injury: consequences in shock, ischemia and graft rejection. *J. Lipid. Med.* (1989), **1**, 75–112.
24 Bureau, M., Joseph, D. & Vargaftig, B. B. Desensitization and antagonism of rat polymorphonuclear leukocytes stimulated with PAF-acether. *Prostaglandins.* (1987), **33**, 37–50.
25 Shen, T. Y., Hwang, S. B., Chang, M. N. *et al.* Characterization of a platelet activating factor receptor antagonist isolated from haifenteng (*Piper futokadsura*): Specific inhibition of *in vitro* and *in vivo* platelet activating factor-induced effects. *Proc. Nat. Acad. Sci. (USA)* (1985), **82**, 672–676.
26 Hwang, S. B., Lam, M. H., Biffu, T., Beattie, T. R. & Shen, T. Y. *Trans*-2, 5-bis-(3, 4, 5, -trimethoxyphenyl)tetrahydrofuran. An orally active specific and competitive receptor antagonist of platelet activating factor. *J. Biol. Chem.* (1985), **260**, 15 639–15 645.
27 Coyle, A. J., Urwin, S. C., Page, C. P., Tonvay, C., Vilain, B. & Braquet, P. The effect of the selective PAF antagonist BN 52021 on PAF and antigen-induced bronchial hyperreactivity and eosinophil infiltration. *Eur. J. Pharmacol.* (1988), **148**, 51–55.
28 Desquand, S., Touvay, C., Randon, J. *et al.* Interference of BN 52021 (ginkgolide B) with the bronchopulmonary effects of PAF-acether in the guinea pig. *Eur. J. Pharmacol.* (1986), **127**, 83–95.
29 Boukili, M. A., Bureau, M., Lagente, V. *et al.* Pharmacological modulation of the effects of N-formyl-L-methionyl-L-leucyl-L-phenylalanine in guinea pigs: involvement of the arachidonic acid cascade. *Br. J. Pharmacol.* (1986), **89**, 349–359.
30 Issekutz, A. C. & Szpejda, M. Evidence that platelet-activating factor may mediate some acute inflammatory response. Studies with platelet-activating factor antagonist, CV 3988. *Lab. Invest.* (1986), **54**, 275–281.
31 Wardlaw, A. J., Moqbel, R., Cromwell, O. & Kay, A. B. Platelet activating factor, a potent chemotactic and chemokinetic factor for human eosinophils. *J. Clin. Invest.* (1986), **78**, 1701–1706.
32 Tamura, N., Agrawal, D., Sumiaman, F. & Townley R. G. Effects of platelet-

activating factor on the chemotaxis of normodense eosinophils from normal subjects. *Biochem. Biophys. Res. Comm.* (1987), **142**, 638–644.

33 Bruijnzeel, P. L. B., Kok, P. M. T., Hamelink, M. L. & Verhagen, J. Platelet activating factor (PAF-acether)-induced leukotriene C_4 formation and luminol-dependent chemoluminescence by human eosinophils. *Pharmacol. Res. Comm.* (Suppl.) (1986), **18**, 61–69.

34 Bruijnzeel, P. L. B., Kok, P. M. T., Hamelink, M. L., Kijne, A. M., & Verhagen J. Platelet activating factor induces leukotriene C_4 synthesis by purified human eosinophils. *Prostaglandins* (1987), **34**, 205–214.

35 Felarca, A. B., & Lowell, F. C. The accumulation of eosinophils and basophils at skin sites as related to intensity of skin reactivity and symptoms in atopic disease. *J. Allergy. Clin. Immunol.* (1971), **48**, 125–133.

36 Kimani, G., Tonnesen, G. & Henson, P. M. Stimulation of eosinophil adherence to human vascular endothelial cells *in vitro* by platelet-activating factor. *J. Immunol.* (1988), **140**, 3161–3166.

37 Hénocq, E. & Vargaftig, B. B. Skin eosinophilia in atopic patients. *J. Allergy. Clin. Immunol.* (1988), **81**, 691–695.

38 Hénocq, E. PAF-acether and eosinophils. *Prog. Biochem. Pharmacol.* (1988), **22**, 141–148.

39 Lellouch-Tubiana, A., Lefort, J., Simon, M. T., Pfister, A. & Vargaftig, B. B. Eosinophil recruitment into guinea-pig lungs after PAF-acether and allergen administration: modulation by prostacyclin, platelet depletion and selective antagonists. *Am. Rev. Resp. Dis.* (1988), **137**, 948–954.

40 Borgeat, P. Fruteau de Laclos, B., Rabinovitch, H. *et al.* Eosinophil-rich human polymorphonuclear leukocyte preparations characteristically release leukotriene C_4 on ionophore A23187 challenge. *J. Allergy. Clin. Immunol.* (1984), **74**, 310–315.

41 Lee, T. C. Lenihan, D. J., Malone, B., Roddy, L. L. & Wasserman, S. Increased biosynthesis of platelet-activating factor in activated human eosinophils. *J. Biol. Chem.* (1984), **259**, 5526–5530.

42 Lellouch-Tubiana, A., Lefort, J., Lagente, V., Cirino, M. & Vargaftig, B. B. Morphological and pharmacological evidences for the participation of PAF-acether in anaphylactic shock in the guinea pig. In Paubert-Braquet, M. (ed.) *Lipid Mediators in the Immunology of Shock* (1987), pp. 209–215. Plenum Press, New York.

43 Bourgain, R., Vermariën, H., Andries, R. *et al.* A standardized '*in vivo*' model for the study of experimental arterial thrombosis. Description of a method. *Adv. Exp. Med. Biol.* (1984), **180**, 653–649.

44 Bourgain, R., Maes, L., Braquet, P., Andries, R., Touqui, L. & Braquet, M. The effect of 1-O-alkyl-2-acetyl-*sn*-glycero-3-phosphocholine (PAF-acether) on the arterial wall. *Prostaglandins* (1985), **30**, 185–197.

45 Martins, M. A., Silva, P. M. S., Faria Lima, H. C. C. *et al.* Pharmacological modulation of PAF-induced rat pleurisy and its role in inflammation by zymosan. *Br. J. Pharmacol.* (1989), **96**, 363–371.

46 Pretolani, M., Lefort, J. & Vargaftig, B. B. Active immunization induces lung hyperresponsiveness in the guinea-pig: pharmacological modulation and triggering role of the booster injection. *Am. Rev. Resp. Dis.* (1988), **138**, 1572–1578.

47 Pretolani, M., Lellouch-Tubiana, A., Lefort, J., Bachelet, M. & Vargaftig, B. B. PAF-acether and experimental anaphylaxis as a model for asthma. *Int. Arch. Allergy Appl. Immunol.* (1989), in press.

48 Pretolani, M., Lefort, J., Dumarey, C. & Vargaftig, B. B. Role of the lipoxygenase metabolites in the hyperresponsiveness to PAF-acether in lungs from actively sensitized guinea pigs. *J. Pharm. Exp. Ther.* (1989), **248**, 353–359.

49 Bachelet, M., Masliah, J., Malanchère, E., Lefort, J., Béréziat, B. & Vargaftig, B. B. Reduced sensitivity of alveolar macrophages from sensitized guinea-pig to the cyclic AMP-stimulating effect of prostaglandin E_2 and β-adrenoceptor agonists. *Pulm. Pharmacol.* (1989), in press.
50 Vargaftig, B. B., Lefort, J., Chignard, M. & Benveniste, J. Platelet-activating factor induces a platelet-dependent bronchoconstriction unrelated to the formation of prostaglandin derivatives. *Eur. J. Pharmacol.* (1980), **65**, 185–192.

Chapter 11
PAF and the skin

Fiona M. Cunningham

Introduction

Amongst the many and diverse biological effects attributed to the phospholipid mediator platelet activating factor (PAF) is the ability to induce vascular and cellular changes in human skin following local administration [1–4]. These properties, together with the more recent identification of PAF in various inflammatory dermatoses [5–11], has led to the suggestion that PAF may be responsible for mediating at least some of the pathological changes associated with such disorders in man. Other mediators, for example, histamine or the eicosanoids, which produce similar effects to PAF in the skin, have also been identified in such conditions [12]. Thus, in order to determine the relative importance of each compound, selective inhibitors of the formation or action of putative mediators must be used in the clinic and any improvement in the disease state correlated with a decrease in the amount of a particular compound, or with inhibition of its effects. The availability of selective PAF receptor antagonists for use in patient studies should provide the information necessary to elucidate more fully the role of PAF in the pathogenesis of human skin disease.

The studies which have established the effects of PAF in skin will be reviewed in this chapter, as will those which have described the presence of PAF in samples from patients with skin disorders, since the rationale for examining the therapeutic effects of PAF receptor antagonists in human skin disease is based upon the results of such studies.

Effects of PAF in the skin of experimental animals

Vascular effects

Intra-dermal injection of PAF into the skin of rats, guinea pigs, rabbits and primates has been shown by a number of groups to result in plasma protein extravasation which is reported, at least in guinea-pig skin, to consist of an early, transient increase in permeability followed, after administration of higher doses, by a more prolonged phase which overlaps with the early response [13–19]. In contrast to the actions of PAF, injection of lyso-PAF, the precursor and breakdown product of PAF, is without effect. The vascular permeability changes induced by intra-dermally injected PAF have been found to be dose dependent, and can persist for up to 1.5 h with the highest doses tested [15]. An initial blanching has also been reported at the site of injection of as little as 1 pmol PAF in guinea pigs, although vasoconstrictor responses were not consistently observed in either rabbit or rat skin [14]. PAF has been reported to be approximately 1000–10 000 times more potent than histamine in eliciting plasma protein extravasation in rabbit, rat and guinea pig skin, the latter species being the most sensitive to the effects of PAF, and 100 times more potent than bradykinin in guinea-pig skin [14,15]. A small difference in the minimum dose of C_{16} and C_{18} PAF molecular species required to induce plasma protein extravasation was also observed in rabbit skin, since 7/11 rabbits responded to a dose of 1 pmol C_{16} PAF as compared to only 2/8 responding to 1 pmol of the C_{18} molecular species [14]. In contrast, octadecyl PAF was more potent at inducing oedema formation in guinea-pig skin [17], although in this study no difference was reported between the potencies of the two molecular species of PAF in the rat. Taira *et al.* [18] have reported, however, that C_{18} at a dose of 200 ng/site induced a greater leakage of Evan's blue dye, and a more persistent response, than an equivalent dose of C_{16} PAF in rat skin.

Co-administration of the vasodilator prostaglandin, PGE_2, was found to enhance responses to PAF in guinea pig, rabbit and rat skin [13,15,19], whilst α- and β-adrenoceptor agonists reduced the increased permeability in guinea-pig skin [15]. PAF-induced plasma protein extra-vasation has been variously reported to be dependent on, or independent of, the formation of cyclooxygenase products since pretreatment with non-steroidal anti-inflammatory drugs such as indomethacin has yielded conflicting results. Oral, but not intra-dermal, administration of indomethacin has been found to inhibit PAF-induced extravasation responses in guinea-pig skin [17,20] yet to be without effect against PAF-induced permeability effects in rat skin if given orally [17,19]. When administered either intra-cutaneously or via the intra-peritoneal route, however, PAF responses were significantly reduced [19]. Leukotrienes are unlikely to be involved in PAF-induced extravasation since responses were not affected by pretreatment with the leukotriene receptor antagonist FPL 55712 or the lipoxygenase inhibitor nordihydroguiaretic acid [19]. The lack of any significant effect of pretreatment with H_1-receptor antagonists [13,14,17,19,20] or compounds which inhibit the release of histamine [19] also suggests that PAF is not acting via release of histamine in rat, rabbit or guinea-pig skin.

The permeability-increasing effects of PAF in rabbit skin were further found to be independent of circulating neutrophils since responses obtained in animals pretreated with intravenously-injected zymosan-activated plasma or with nitrogen mustard were no different to controls [13,21]. A similar neutrophil-independent response was obtained in rats pretreated with nitrogen mustard [21,22]. That platelets are not involved in PAF-induced plasma protein extravasation was also suggested by the finding that increased vascular permeability occurred in the skin of rats pretreated with a combination of mepyramine, methysergide and indomethacin, which prevents platelet accumulation and the platelet release reaction [22]. Plasma protein extravasation in guinea-pig skin was also unaffected by pretreatment with anti-platelet antiserum [23]. In addition, platelet accumulation in guinea-pig skin in response to 200 pmol intra-dermal PAF was reduced by PGE_1, whilst plasma protein extravasation was enhanced [15]. Direct effects of PAF on endothelium have also been demonstrated by transmission electron microscopy which has shown separation of post-capillary endothelial cells associated with extravasation of colloidal carbon occurring 40 min after intra-dermal administration of PAF in guinea-pig skin [24,25].

Cellular effects

In addition to effects on the skin microvasculature, PAF induces cell and platelet accumulation in guinea pig [2,15,26], rat and rabbit skin [21,27–29]. A modest haemorrhage, associated with significant ^{111}Indium-labelled erythrocyte accumulation has been reported to occur within 40 min of PAF injection, and to persist for up to 24 h [15]. Clumps of erythrocytes, together with some neutrophils, have been observed histologically in the dermis at the site of haemorrhage in the guinea pig, although no such haemorrhage was seen in rabbit skin [14]. In addition to early neutrophil accumulation in guinea-pig skin, a mononuclear cell infiltrate was detected at 24 h, consisting of activated macrophages [2,26]. Accumulation of ^{111}Indium-labelled platelets has also been reported in guinea-pig skin following intra-dermal injection of 20–200 pmol PAF/site, the accumulation being complete within 1 h of injection [15].

A dose-dependent increase in ^{51}Cr-labelled neutrophil accumulation occurs in response to intra-cutaneous injection of PAF (10^{-8} to 10^{-5} M) in the rabbit, although the dose–response curves did not plateau at the highest concentration of PAF tested [29]. Maximal responses were observed in 2-h lesions, with only background counts being detected in those which had been established for 4–6 h. Re-stimulation of the same lesion with PAF 6 h after the first challenge resulted in a decreased influx of neutrophils when compared to responses in control sites [28]. A normal response was, however, obtained if sites were re-stimulated with another

Table 11.1 Modulation of PAF-induced plasma protein extravasation (PPE)

Agent/route*	Effect on PPE†	Species	References
PGE_2 (i.d.)	↑	Guinea pig, rat, rabbit, man	[3,13,15,19]
α- and β-agonists (i.d.)	↓	Guinea pig, rat	[15,19]
Indomethacin (p.o.)	↓	Guinea pig	[17]
Indomethacin (i.d.)	–	Guinea pig	[20]
Indomethacin (p.o.)	–	Rat	[17,19]
Indomethacin (i.d., i.p.)	↓	Rat	[19]
Indomethacin (p.o.)	–	Man	[20]
Indomethacin or aspirin (p.o.)	'Slight' enhancement	Man	[1]
FLP 55712 (i.d.)	–	Rat	[19]
NDGA (i.d.)	–	Rat	[19]
Prednisone (p.o.)	–	Man	[1]
Mepyramine (i.d.)	'Modest' reduction	Guinea pig	[20]
Mepyramine (i.d.)	–	Rat	[19]
Chlorpheniramine or brompheniramine (p.o.)	–	Man	[1,20]
Ketotifen (p.o.)	↓	Man	[32]
Methysergide (i.d.)	–	Rat	[19]
Mepyramine + methysergide + indomethacin (i.v.)	–	Rat	[22]
Anti-platelet antiserum	–	Guinea pig	[23]
Neutrophil depletion	–	Rat, rabbit	[13,21,22]
PAF (i.d.)	↓	Rat, rabbit	[28,30]

* i.d. = intra-dermal; i.v. = intravenous; p.o. = oral.
† = No effect.

chemotaxin, illustrating the specific nature of the desensitization response. PAF-induced plasma protein extravasation has also been reported to be inhibited by prior treatment with PAF, but not lyso-PAF, histamine or serotonin in rat skin [30]. Neutrophil accumulation in response to PAF was also observed histologically in rabbit dermis at 3 h, with cell margination and plugging of dermal vessels evident as early as 15 min after injection [21,27]; a decline in cell numbers was apparent by 6 h. Dilated lymphatics were evident after intra-dermal injection of PAF in rat skin, together with leukocyte plugs and intra-mural leukocytes, which were predominantly neutrophils, in the venules [21]. No platelet aggregates were found in rat skin although such aggregates were evident in the rabbit [21]. Intact mast cells were also present at the sites of both PAF and lyso-PAF injection, suggesting that PAF had not induced mast-cell degranulation.

Thus PAF-induced permeability effects in the skin of experimental animals appear to be induced independently of other mediators or circulating blood elements, by a direct effect on endothelial cells (Table 11.1). Following the increased plasma protein extravasation and accumulation of platelets and erythrocytes, PAF induces infiltration of circulating leukocytes into the skin.

Effects of PAF in human skin

Vascular effects

Intra-dermal injection of PAF into the skin of man has been reported to produce an instant blanching followed by vasodilation and an increase in vascular permeability, evident as the characteristic weal-and-flare response [1–3]. Weal responses were found to be maximal within 15 min and had essentially disappeared by 90 min; flare responses were maximal at 5 min and resolved within 30 min. In addition to the acute weal and flare, a late erythematous response was observed at the injection site 3–6 h after injection of the higher doses of PAF used in approximately 50% of subjects [3]. This late-onset response was sometimes associated with hyperalgesia, the hyperalgesia and erythema usually resolving within 1–2 h, although after injection of 800 pmol PAF, a tender indurated papule with surrounding erythema was reported to be evident after 36 h [2,3]. Once again lyso-PAF produced no acute or delayed-onset response in any subject tested. Although it has been suggested that there may be a difference in the vascular response to molecular species of PAFs with differing alkyl side-chain lengths in animal skin [14,17,18], acute weal-and-flare responses in healthy volunteers were not reported to be significantly different after intra-dermal injection of either C_{16} or C_{18} PAFs [31].

As in animal skin, a synergistic interaction between E-type prostaglandins and PAF has been demonstrated in man, both weal volume and flare area being significantly greater in response to a mixture of PAF plus PGE_2 than to either agent alone [3]. Responses have been reported to be unaffected [20] or enhanced by pretreatment with non-steroidal anti-inflammatory drugs and to be unaltered by prior treatment with prednisone [1]. In contrast to the lack of any significant effect of H_1-receptor antagonists on PAF-induced permeability changes in animal skin, chlorpheniramine significantly reduced the flare response to PAF in human skin whilst having no effect on weal volume [20] suggesting that at least some of the effects of PAF in human skin may be mediated by histamine release. Further evidence for histamine involvement in cutaneous responses to PAF in man is provided by the recent finding that whilst the anti-allergic anti-histaminic agent ketotifen reduced weal-and-flare responses to PAF in human skin, responses to histamine were similarly inhibited [32]. The late-phase response to PAF has also been reported to be selectively decreased by disodium cromoglycate [2].

Pruritus has been reported to occur following intra-dermal injection of PAF in 10-μl volumes, the itching being reduced by local administration of H_1-receptor antagonists or prior depletion of histamine from the skin [1,33]. That PAF was not found by others to cause itching has been suggested to be due to inhibition of the pruritic response by the larger injection volumes used in some studies [33,34]. Flare area was also reported by Fjellner & Hagermark [33] to be reduced by antihistamines or histamine depletion, observations which are in agreement with the findings of Archer *et al.* [20]; weal volume was not, however, measured in the study by Fjellner & Hagermark [33].

Cellular effects

Biopsies obtained from normal healthy non-atopic human subjects after administration of 200 pmol PAF demonstrated the presence of intra-vascular erythrocytes with some neutrophils, together with dermal oedema at 30 min [4]. By 4 h, intra-vascular neutrophil accumulation was evident, as well as a mixed peri-vascular cellular infiltrate, composed predominantly of neutrophils, although lymphocytes and histiocytes were also present. At 24 h, the cellular infiltrate, which was less intense, consisted primarily of lymphocytes and histiocytes. Histological examination of sections prepared from a biopsy taken 32 h after intra-dermal injection of 800 pmol PAF in a single volunteer showed some evidence of endothelial swelling and vessel destruction, as well as an intense inflammatory cell infiltrate consisting of lymphocytes, histiocytes and neutrophils. A number of eosinophils, together with some mast cells were also reported to be present in the peri-vascular infiltrate [4].

The effects of PAF on leukocyte accumulation have also been examined in human skin by use of a skin chamber technique [35]. Suction blisters were raised on the skin of healthy non-atopic volunteers, the blister roofs removed and skin chambers placed over the de-nuded dermis. The chambers were then filled with medium alone, or medium plus chemotaxin, and cell accumulation measured with time. In the absence of bovine serum albumin (BSA) PAF induced no dose- or time-dependent cell accumulation. Following addition of BSA to the chambers, however, a significantly greater number of cells accumulated in response to 9×10^{-7} M PAF at 24 h than were found in control chambers which contained BSA alone, with >90% of the cells present being neutrophils. Cell migration was also enhanced by the presence of PGE_2 and was more persistent than with PAF alone. Histological analysis of biopsies taken from the site of application of chambers containing PAF and BSA revealed neutrophils migrating into the superficial dermis at 6 h but accumulating at the base of the fibrin layer covering the skin window and not migrating through. Degranulated basophils and occasional degranulated mast cells were also noted. After 24 h, an intense mononuclear cell infiltrate was evident in the superficial dermis, basophils which were present at 6 h being absent at 24 h. Despite the introduction of fresh PAF into the chamber at 24 h, neutrophil migration was observed to decline. Since the decrease in neutrophils was paralleled by an increase in the number of mononuclear cells, it has been suggested that mediator degradation may take place as a result of the action of enzymes released directly from, or indirectly by, accumulating inflammatory cells [35].

Neutrophil accumulation onto coverslips placed over abraded skin sites that had previously received intra-dermal injections of 200 or 400 ng PAF/site was also observed after 24 h in healthy subjects [36,37]. The nature of the inflammatory-cell infiltrate, however, differed markedly in atopic individuals, despite the weal-and-flare reactions being similar in size to those measured in control subjects. Eosinophils formed up to 33% of the total cells present in atopics, with approximately 33% of the eosinophils showing evidence of degranulation; phagocytosis of the granules by macrophages was also apparent. In contrast, the inflammatory-cell infiltrate in healthy subjects consisted of <1% eosinophils. Antigen challenge, or intra-dermal injection of 5 μg of the chemotactic tripeptide formyl-methionyl-leucyl-phenylalanine in the atopic group also resulted in eosinophil accumulation. Thus the preferential recruitment of these cells to sites of injection of chemoattractants such as PAF which was observed in allergic patients may be of relevance to the onset of the dual response seen after challenge with specific antigen in such subjects, and which is thought to be dependent on cellular accumulation. Interestingly, the macroscopic late-phase reaction to PAF or allergen reported by others [2,4] was not observed by Hénocq & Vargaftig in either control or atopic subjects [37].

In human skin, PAF therefore appears to induce both direct effects on the microvasculature, resulting in plasma protein extravasation, as well as indirect effects, via the release of histamine. Cellular accumulation is also evident after intra-dermal injection of PAF, the nature of the inflammatory cell infiltrate being dependent upon the clinical status of the individual.

Effects of PAF antagonists on cutaneous responses

A number of selective PAF-receptor antagonists have now been described which include, amongst others, CV-3988, kadsurenone, 48740 RP, L-652731, BN 52021 and WEB 2086, and the inhibitory activity of these compounds determined against a range of PAF-induced biological responses (see [38] for review). The increased vascular permeability associated with intra-dermal administration of PAF in guinea pigs and rats has, for example, been shown to be inhibited by kadsurenone [17]. L-652731 and CV-3988 inhibit PAF-induced plasma protein extravasation in rat skin [18,39] and intra-cutaneous injection of SRI 63-072 was found to reduce the permeability increasing effects of PAF in 18/20 tests carried out in 10 rhesus monkeys [40].

Both plasma protein extravasation induced by a combination of PAF and prostaglandin E_2, as well as that associated with a reversed passive Arthus reaction are suppressed by L-652731 in rabbit skin [41]. Oedema responses to local injection of preformed immune complexes were not, however, inhibited by the PAF antagonist. In addition to reducing the extravasation component of the Arthus response, CV-3988 has been found to inhibit the associated platelet accumulation and, to a lesser extent, the leukocyte accumulation in rabbit skin [42]. Platelet accumulation in response to intra-dermal injection of zymosan, zymosan-activated plasma (ZAP) and endotoxin were also reduced by pretreatment with CV-3988 suggesting that PAF may also, at least in part, mediate the platelet response to these agonists. The PAF antagonist, however, had no significant effect on plasma protein extravasation or leukocyte accumulation in response to either ZAP or endotoxin [42]. A reduction in oedema, interstitial haemorrhage and in the numbers of polymorphonuclear leukocytes in the deep dermis was also observed after induction of the Arthus response in rats pretreated with another PAF antagonist, SRI 63-072 [43]. BN 52021, at a dose shown in other animal models to inhibit PAF activity, has now been reported to significantly reduce ear swelling induced by dinitrofluorobenzene, and to a lesser extent that induced by croton oil treatment, suggesting the involvement of PAF in murine allergic contact dermatitis, and perhaps also irritant dermatitis [44]. Since the ear swelling that occurs in this model is thought to result from tissue oedema, followed by cell emigration into the skin, the described ability of BN 52021 to inhibit the response over the entire five days of the experiment would be consistent with PAF affecting both vascular and cellular events. In contrast to a possible role for PAF in allergic contact and irritant dermatitis, as well as the Arthus response, it has recently been reported that neither PAF nor leukotrienes are involved in the 48-h passive cutaneous anaphylaxis reaction, at least in the rat [18].

A single-blind crossover study in man has showed that BN 52063, which comprises a mixture of ginkgolides a, b and c, given as a single oral dose of 80 mg, 90 min before injection of PAF, inhibited both weal and flare responses in the skin of five healthy male volunteers [45]. In a subsequent study [46] the effects of BN 52063 were assessed in a double-blind placebo-controlled crossover trial in six normal subjects. Weal and flare responses were again found to be significantly reduced following ingestion of 80 or 120 mg BN 52063, 2 h prior to intra-dermal administration of PAF. BN 52063 had no effect on histamine-induced responses and was well tolerated by all volunteers [46]. No adverse side effects were reported in either study following the acute administration of this PAF antagonist at doses up to 120 mg. The tolerance of healthy volunteers to intravenous infusion of another PAF antagonist, CV-3988, in amounts sufficient to inhibit platelet aggregation *ex vivo* has also been reported recently [47]. Although no clinically significant adverse effects were documented, a mild local irritation at the injection site was noted which persisted for up to 3 days, as well as small but statistically significant increases in plasma haemoglobin and decreases in serum haptoglobin.

BN 52063 has also been shown to inhibit the late phase of antigen-induced cutaneous responses in atopic subjects [48], inhibition of responses to PAF, but not histamine. Intra-dermal injection of increasing doses of grass pollen or house-dust mite antigens produced an acute weal and flare response followed at the higher doses by a late reaction after 1 h. The early weal response was found to be attenuated in 50% of subjects, but the overall reduction was not significant suggesting that PAF may not be important in allergen-induced cutaneous vascular permeability. That flare responses are unaffected by BN 52063 is in agreement with this response being largely mediated by histamine and the cutaneous axon reflex [49–51]. This study provides further experimental evidence of a role for PAF in the late response to antigen challenge in atopic subjects, although the lack of a significant inhibitory effect of the PAF antagonist on late responses induced by the highest doses of antigen tested suggests that other inflammatory mediators are likely to also be involved.

PAF antagonists, in addition to reducing the vascular effects of PAF and antigen in man have also been reported to inhibit ultraviolet-induced killing of *Candida albicans* by cultured human keratinocytes *in vitro* [38].

Identification of PAF in the skin

Following observations of the pro-inflammatory effects produced by PAF in the skin of experimental animals and man, it was postulated that the actions of this phospholipid, if released into the involved tissues, could contribute to the patho-physiological changes observed in certain skin diseases in man. The recovery of PAF from lesional stratum corneum of three patients with the chronic inflammatory and proliferative skin disorder psoriasis was first reported in 1984, a combination of high-performance liquid chromatographic and bioassay techniques being used to characterize the PAF [5]. Since erythema and cellular infiltration are characteristic features of the psoriatic lesion, the pro-inflammatory effects

Table 11.2 Measurement of PAF in human skin disease

Skin disorder	Sample	References
Psoriasis	Lesional stratum corneum	[6,7,8]
Psoriasis	Skin chambers 30 min after addition of buffer	[8]
Atopics	Skin chambers, hours after addition of antigen or histamine	[9,10]
Cold urticaria	Venous blood after cold challenge	[11]

of PAF, which have been demonstrated in healthy human skin, are consistent with a role for PAF in eliciting certain of the inflammatory changes associated with this disease. The presence of PAF in psoriatic stratum corneum was confirmed in a further study on four psoriatic patients, the biological activity of the PAF being determined in a platelet aggregation assay using washed guinea-pig platelets pretreated with aspirin and an ADP-scavenging system, and its structural identity established by mass spectrometry [6]. The amount of PAF present was estimated to be between 0.5 and 3 ng per 100 mg psoriatic stratum corneum and consisted of more than three times as much $C_{16:0}$ as $C_{18:0}$ PAF. Ramesha *et al.* [7] have now extended these observations to show that other molecular species of PAF are present in lesional psoriatic stratum corneum, in addition to those already described, ranging from $C_{14:0}$ to $C_{19:0}$ PAFs and including several with unsaturated alkyl side chains. The majority of the PAF (51 %) was however found to be the $C_{16:0}$ molecular species (Table 11.2).

Since stratum corneum consists of cornified keratinocytes which are essentially metabolically inert, release of PAF by the more viable layers of the skin was then examined using a skin chamber technique [8,12].

Psoriatic plaques are first abraded with a scalpel blade until a glistening layer with minimal punctate bleeding is obtained, the area of skin abraded typically being 3.5 cm^2. A plastic chamber is then glued over the abrasion and filled with phosphate-buffered saline (PBS) which is left in contact with the skin for 5 min. The PBS is removed, and the chamber filled with a second 1-ml aliquot of the physiological salt solution, which is left in place for a further 30 min to allow mediator release from the lower epidermis and upper dermis into the chamber. The contents are then removed for analysis by bioassay and mass spectrometric techniques. Chambers placed over abraded psoriatic lesions were found to contain between 2 and 9 ng PAF/ ml chamber fluid (mean 6 ± 3 ng/ ml, $n = 4$) and once again, the predominant molecular species identified was $C_{16:0}$ PAF [8]. PAF release into chambers placed over denuded blister base sites has also been reported to occur 5 h after antigen challenge in 6/8 atopic individuals [9]. This work has recently been confirmed by Michel *et al.* [10] who detected significant PAF release into chambers containing either pollen or histamine at 6 and 24 h, but not at 30 min after challenge of atopics. In neither study was PAF released into buffer containing chambers on the skin of these atopic subjects. This finding is in contrast to results obtained using the abrasion technique in healthy subjects since, not only have nanogram quantities of PAF been measured in chambers placed over abraded lesional psoriatic skin after 30 min, but similar amounts have now been recovered from chambers placed over the abraded skin of healthy volunteers (Mallet & Cunningham, unpublished). The denuded blister base may therefore offer an advantage over abrasion as a means of inducing damage to the skin since the trauma of the abrasion may perhaps be sufficient to elicit maximal PAF generation from the injured site, either directly or indirectly via the release of other mediators. The difficulties associated with raising suction blisters on psoriatic plaques unfortunately precludes a comparison of PAF release by lesional and clinically-normal skin in the same psoriatic patients using such a technique.

The cellular origins of the PAF released into these skin chambers has yet to be determined with possibilities including inflammatory cells which may have accumulated in the skin, dermal micro-vascular endothelial cells, or the resident skin cell population. Neutrophils prepared from the venous blood of psoriatic patients were indeed found to produce PAF following challenge with the ionophore A23187 *in vitro* in amounts similar to those reported to be formed by cells prepared from healthy subjects [8]. However, since PAF is released into chambers over abraded normal skin, which, unlike lesional psoriatic skin, would not be expected to contain neutrophils, it is unlikely that these cells are the source of the PAF. In contrast, since the time course of PAF release into allergen containing chambers on the skin of atopic subjects is similar to the time course of eosinophil accumulation, and eosinophils have been shown to produce

PAF *in vitro* [52], PAF may indeed originate from inflammatory cells in this experimental lesion.

Although the capacity of dermal microvascular endothelial cells prepared from human skin to generate PAF has yet to be determined, large-vessel endothelial cells, as well as micro-vascular endothelial cells derived from adipose tissue are known to produce PAF *in vitro* following stimulation with the ionophore A23187 [53,54] and with mediators such as leukotrienes C_4, D_4 or E_4 [55] or interleukin (IL)-1 [56]. Since IL-1 is present in large amounts in normal human skin [57] and release of IL-1 is reported to occur in response to injurious stimuli [58], abrasion with a scalpel blade may be sufficient stimulus to cause IL-1 release from keratinocyte membranes, and this in turn may induce PAF generation from endothelial cells in dermal micro-vessels. However, the time course of the response to IL-1 demonstrated *in vitro* is such that it suggests little PAF would be formed by such a mechanism over the 30 min incubation period used for the *in vivo* chamber studies [56]. Non-specific perturbation of endothelial cell membranes has been reported by Zimmerman *et al.* [53] not to result in PAF generation.

Mixed human epidermal cells have been shown to produce PAF *in vitro* following ionophore challenge [59]. Freshly-trypsinized cell suspensions, consisting of >95% keratinocytes, produced picogram quantities of PAF per 10^7 cells after incubation for 15 min at 37°C with 2 μM A23187. Separate analysis of cell pellet and supernatant fractions indicated that variable amounts of PAF were released into the supernatant. Further studies have now suggested that the amounts of PAF measured after stimulation with the ionophore under the experimental conditions used is not significantly different from those produced by cells in the absence of the ionophore, although PAF was not detectable in cells that were extracted prior to incubation at 37°C (Mallet & Cunningham, unpublished). Lyso-PAF was not, however, measured in these experiments.

Human skin fibroblasts have recently been shown to produce PAF following challenge with the ionophore A23187 *in vitro* [60], at least 50% of the PAF being released into the supernatant. Maximal production was achieved within the first 5 min of the incubation and decreased thereafter. Although no PAF was detected in unstimulated fibroblasts, the precursors lyso-PAF and 1-alkyl-2-acyl-glycero-3-phosphocholine were found to be present, 80% containing a hexadecyl and 20% an octadecyl chain at the first carbon on the glycerol.

Thus PAF release by dermal fibroblasts or epidermal cells could contribute to that measured in chambers placed over abraded lesional psoriatic and normal skin, although the ability of more physiological stimuli than the ionophore to induce PAF formation by these cells has yet to be investigated. That no PAF was detected in buffer containing chambers placed over denuded blister bases in atopic subjects [9,10] may provide a further indication of the possible cellular source of the PAF since the formation of suction blisters results in separation of the epidermis from the dermis and the subsequent removal of the blister roofs would eliminate any contribution to PAF formation by cells in the epidermal layers.

Further evidence for PAF involvement in skin disease comes from studies of an acute inflammatory disorder, urticaria, or hives, which is characterized by local oedema, erythema and pruritus following challenge with an appropriate stimulus. A PAF-like lipid was reported to be released into the blood of three patients with primary acquired cold urticaria and who developed severe responses after immersion of the forearm in cold water at 4–8°C, the release occurring prior to the peak development of oedema [11]. The material co-eluted with PAF on TLC, induced aggregation of, and serotonin release from, rabbit platelets, and was inactivated by acetyl hydrolase. No PAF-like lipid was detected in the blood of normal subjects following cold challenge. Treatment of three patients with doxepin (10 mg twice a day for 1 or 2 weeks), which has antagonist activity at H_1-receptors, abolished (1 subject) or suppressed (2 subjects) the urticarial response and reduced (1 subject) or abolished (2 subjects) the release of the PAF-like lipid into the blood. Histamine and neutrophil chemotactic factor levels, which were also increased in all subjects following cold challenge, were unaffected by doxepin pretreatment. Since, in an earlier study, the degree of suppression of histamine release by prednisone could not be correlated with clinical improvement [61] and since anti-histamines are held to be largely ineffective against any component of the urticarial response other than pruritus, it is likely that doxepin is suppressing cold urticaria by a mechanism other than H_1-receptor antagonism. Although these observations are potentially of great interest, it has been noted by Braquet *et al.* [38] that the inhibitory effects of doxepin could not be repeated by others. Nevertheless, the presence of PAF in the venous blood of patients with cold urticaria following cold challenge, whether it be released directly as a consequence of the challenge or secondarily from cells or tissue stimulated by other mediators released in this condition, together with its demonstrated ability to cause oedema, erythema and pruritus in the skin, suggests that PAF may be worthy of consideration as a potential mediator of this disease.

Injury to the skin has also been shown in experimental animals to result in PAF formation. Thus PAF, identified by mass spectrometry as the hexadecyl molecular species, has been measured in rat skin following moxibustion (ignition of a Chinese therapeutic moxa with an incense stick) [62] and in guinea-pig skin following irradiation with ultraviolet (UV) light [63]. Picogram quantities of PAF were reported to be present per 100 mg tissue in extracts of UV irradiated, but not control skin; lyso-PAF was, in contrast, found in similar amounts in both control and irradiated skin.

Conclusions

PAF has been shown to cause erythema and plasma protein extravasation following injection into the skin of experimental animals or man [1,2,13–26]. These vascular effects could be relevant to the pathology of acute inflammatory skin diseases such as urticaria and the identification of PAF in venous blood draining the site of challenge in patients with primary acquired cold urticaria [11] is further evidence suggestive of a role for PAF in this disorder. Whether the release of this mediator is a primary cause of the disease or occurs as a result of tissue damage remains to be established in further studies.

The effects of PAF may also contribute to cellular events which underlie the late phase of the skin response to allergen challenge since eosinophil accumulation has been demonstrated in atopic subjects, not only after administration of allergen to the skin, but also in response to PAF [10,36,37]. PAF release into skin chambers placed over denuded blister bases has also been shown to occur hours, but not minutes, after allergen challenge in atopic subjects [9,10]; it remains to be established whether or not the PAF is released by infiltrating cells. Furthermore, in view of its cellular effects [4,27–29,35–37] PAF may, at least in part, mediate the inflammatory changes associated with chronic skin diseases such as psoriasis where both vascular changes and an inflammatory cell infiltrate consisting predominantly of neutrophils and T-lymphocytes are characteristic features. Once again PAF has been identified in the involved skin of patients with this disorder, being present in the lesional stratum corneum [5–7] and released into chambers placed over abraded psoriatic plaques [8]. The amounts of PAF released from abraded lesional and clinically-normal skin have yet to be compared in the same patients in the light of the observation that similar quantities can be recovered from chambers placed over the abraded lesional psoriatic skin and that of healthy control subjects. Finally, work in animals has now suggested that damage to the skin caused by UV irradiation [63] or induction of a local inflammatory response by moxibustion [62] results in PAF formation, which may be relevant to the pathology of tissue injury.

In each of the above conditions it must be noted that mediators other than PAF have also been identified and the actions of such compounds may therefore also be relevant to the patho-physiological changes associated with these skin disorders. Thus, in urticaria, mast cell-derived products such as histamine and PGD_2 have been recovered from the venous blood draining the site of cold challenge [64], as have platelet factors such as platelet factor 4 [65]. Leukotriene C_4/D_4 immunoreactivity has, for example, been identified in suction blister fluid in allergic subjects exhibiting late responses 30 min after challenge with anti-IgE or intra-dermal allergen [66]. In one subject, in whom a longitudinal study was performed, elevated levels of the sulfidopeptide leukotrienes persisted for up to 6 h. A second study [67] also showed persistent elevated levels of LTC_4 and D_4, over a 6 h-period, 85% of the immunoreactivity being attributable to LTC_4. Since it has been suggested that mediators responsible for the late cutaneous response in atopic subjects are released soon after intra-dermal allergen challenge, and remain at elevated levels for long periods of time [66], the sulfidopeptide leukotrienes should perhaps also be considered as potential mediators of the delayed-onset response to allergen. Both cyclooxygenase and lipooxygenase products or arachidonic acid metabolism have been identified in UV-B erythema, prostaglandins being considered at least partially responsible for mediating the early response to UV-B [12,68]. The increasing complexity of a disorder such as psoriasis is reflected in the wide range of mediators recovered from the involved tissue and which include eicosanoids, the complement fragment C5a, IL-1, and a number of, so far, uncharacterized chemokinetically-active peptides [12].

In order to ascertain the relative importance of the contribution of another mediator to the pathology of skin disease in man, selective inhibitors of its formation or actions must be now used. Clinical improvement should be correlated with changes in the amounts of the mediator measured in the case of synthesis inhibitors or, when using receptor antagonists, the effects of the mediator must be shown to be inhibited in the appropriate tissue at the doses of antagonist used. It is to be hoped that the availability of PAF antagonists such as BN 52063, which have already been used in volunteer subjects, for use in the clinic, will enable the role of PAF in inflammatory skin diseases to be further elucidated. In this context it is of considerable interest that a recent report [69] has documented the successful use of BN 52063 for the treatment of systemic mastocytosis in a single patient.

References

1 Pinckard, R. N., Kniker, W. T., Lee, L., Hanahan, D. J. & McManus, L. M. Vasoactive effects of 1-O-alkyl-2-acetyl-*sn*-glyceryl-3-phosphorylcholine (AcGEPC) in human skin. *J. Allergy Clin. Immunol.* (1980), **65**, 196.

2 Archer, C. B., Page, C. P., Paul, W., Morley, J. & MacDonald, D. M. Early and late inflammatory effects of PAF-acether in the skin of experimental animals and man. *J. Invest. Dermatol.* (1983), **80**, 346–347.

3 Archer, C. B., Page, C. P., Paul, W., Morley, J. & MacDonald, D. M. Inflammatory characteristics of platelet activating factor (PAF-acether) in human skin. *Br. J. Dermatol.* (1984), **110**, 45–50.

4 Archer, C. B., Page, C. P., Morley, J. & MacDonald, D. M. Accumulation of inflammatory cells in response to intracutaneous platelet activating factor (PAF-acether) in man. *Br. J. Dermatol.* (1985), **112**, 285–290.

5 Mallet, A. I., Cunningham, F. M. & Daniel, R. Rapid isocratic high performance liquid chromatographic purification of platelet activating factor (PAF) and lyso-PAF from human skin. *J. Chromatogr.* (1984), **309**, 160–164.

6 Mallet, A. I. & Cunningham, F. M. Structural identification of platelet activating factor in psoriatic scale. *Biochem. Biophys. Res. Commun.* (1985), **126**, 192–198.

7 Ramesha, C. S., Soter, N. & Pickett, W. C. Identification and quantitation of PAF from psoriatic scales. *Agents & Actions* (1987), **21**, 382–383.

8 Mallet, A. I., Cunningham, F. M., Wong, E. & Greaves, M. W. Platelet activating factor in chronic plaque psoriasis. In Samuelsson, B., Paoletti, R. & Ramwell, P. (eds) *Advances in Prostaglandin, Thromboxane and Leukotriene Research* (1987), 640–642. Raven Press, New York.

9 Valone, F., Shalit, M., Atkins, P., Goetzl, E. & Sireiman, B. Platelet activating factor release in allergic skin sites in humans. *J. Allergy Clin. Immunol.* (1987), **79**, 248.

10 Michel, L., Denizot, Y., Thomas, Y., Benveniste, J. & Dubertret L. Release of PAF-acether and precursors during allergic cutaneous reactions. *Lancet* (1988), **ii**, 404.

11 Grandel, K. E., Farr, R. S., Wanderer, A. A., Eisenstadt, T. C. & Wasserman, S. I. Association of platelet activating factor with primary acquired cold urticaria. *N. Engl. J. Med.* (1985), **313**, 405–409.

12 Camp, R. D. R. & Cunningham, F. M. The role of eicosanoids in inflammatory disorders of the skin. In Church, M. & Robinson, C. (eds) *Advances in Eicosanoid Research: Eicosanoids in Inflammatory Conditions of the Lung, Skin and Joints* (1988), 112–128. MTP Press, Lancaster.

13 Wedmore, C. V. & Williams, T. J. Platelet-activating factor (PAF), a secretory product of polymorphonuclear leukocytes increases vascular permeability in rabbit skin. *Br. J. Pharmacol.* (1981), **74**, 916p.

14 Humphrey, D. M., McManus, L. M., Satouchi, K., Hanahan, D. J. & Pinckard, R. N. Vasoactive properties of acetyl glyceryl ether phosphorylcholine and analogues. *Lab. Invest.* (1982), **46**, 422–427.

15 Morley, J., Page, C. P. & Paul, W. Inflammatory actions of platelet activating factor (PAF-acether) in guinea pig skin. *Br. J. Pharmacol.* (1983), **80**, 503–509.

16 Patterson, R. & Harris, K. E. The activity of aerosolised and intracutaneous synthetic platelet activating factor (AGEPC) in rhesus monkeys with IgE mediated airway responses and in normal monkeys. *J. Lab. Clin. Med.* (1983), **102**, 933–938.

17 Hwang, S. B., Lee, C. S. C., Cheah, M. J. & Shen, T. Y. Characterisation of cutaneous vascular permeability induced by platelet activating factor in guinea pigs and rats and its inhibition by a platelet activating factor antagonist. *Lab. Invest.* (1985), **52**, 617–630.

18 Taira, M., Kohno, S. W., Yamamura, H. & Ohata, K. Lack of involvement of leukotriene and platelet activating factor in passive cutaneous anaphylaxis in rats. *Agents & Actions* (1988), **24**, 189–195.

19 Kusner, E. J., Knee, C. D. & Krell, R. D. Pharmacological analysis of 1-O-alkyl-2-acetyl-*sn*-glycero-3-phosphocholine- induced increases in cutaneous vascular permeability in the rat. *Agents & Actions* (1987), **20**, 61–68.

20 Archer, C. B., Morley, J., MacDonald, D. M., Page, C. P., Paul, W. & Sanjar, S. Effects of serum albumin, indomethacin and histamine H_1-antagonists on PAF-acether-induced inflammatory responses in the skin of experimental animals and man. *Br. J. Pharmacol.* (1985), **85**, 109–113.

21 Humphrey, D. M., McManus, L. M., Hanahan, D. J. & Pinckard, R. N. Morpho-

logic basis of increased vascular permeability induced by acetyl glyceryl ether phosphorylcholine. *Lab. Invest.* (1984), **50**, 16–25.

22 Pirotzky, E., Page, C. P., Roubin, R. *et al.* PAF-acether induced plasma exudation is independent of platelets and neutrophils in rat skin. *Microcirc. Endoth. Lymph.* (1984), **1**, 107–122.

23 Paul, W., Page, C. P., Cunningham, F. M. & Morley, J. The plasma protein response to PAF-acether is independent of platelet accumulation. *Agents & Actions* (1984), **15**, 80–82.

24 Dewar, A., Morley, J., Page, C. P. & Paul, W. Permeability characteristics of platelet activating factor in guinea pig skin. *Br. J. Pharmacol.* (1983), **78**, 180p.

25 Dewar, A., Archer, C. B., Paul, W., Page, C. P., MacDonald, D. M. & Morley, J. Cutaneous and pulmonary histopathological responses to platelet activating factor (PAF-acether) in the guinea-pig. *J. Pathol.* (1984), **144**, 25–34.

26 Archer, C. B., Page, C. P., Paul, W., Morley, J. & MacDonald, D. M. Inflammatory characteristics of PAF-acether in the skin of experimental animals and man. *Int. J. Tiss. Reac.* (1985), **VII**, 363–365.

27 Humphrey, D. M., Hanahan, D. J. & Pinckard, R. N. Induction of leukocytic infiltrates in rabbit skin by acetyl glyceryl ether phosphorylcholine. *Lab. Invest.* (1982), **47**, 227–234.

28 Colditz, I. G. & Movat, H. Z. Desensitisation of acute inflammatory lesions to chemotaxins and endotoxin. *J. Immunol.* (1984), **133**, 2163–2169.

29 Colditz, I. G. & Movat, H. Z. Kinetics of neutrophil accumulation in acute inflammatory lesions induced by chemotaxins and chemotaxinigens. *J. Immunol.* (1984), **133**, 2169–2173.

30 Pirotzky, E., Pfister, A. & Benveniste, J. A role for PAF-acether (platelet activating factor) in acute skin inflammation? *Br. J. Dermatol.* (1985), **113**, (Suppl. 28), 91–94.

31 Archer, C. B., Cunningham, F. M. & Greaves, M. W. Actions of platelet activating factor (PAF) homologues and their combinations on neutrophil chemokinesis and cutaneous inflammatory responses in man. *J. Invest. Dermatol.* (1988), **91**, 82–85.

32 Chung, K. F., Minette, P., McCusker, M. & Barnes, P. J. Ketotifen inhibits cutaneous but not airway responses to platelet-activating factor in man *J. Allergy Clin. Immunol.* (1988), **81**, 1192–1199.

33 Fjellner, B. & Hagermark, O. Experimental pruritus evoked by platelet activating factor (PAF-acether) in human skin. *Acta Derm.-Venereol. (Stockholm)* (1985), **65**, 409–412.

34 Shelley, W. B. & Arthur, R. P. The neurohistology and neurophysiology of the itch sensation in man. *Arch. Dermatol.* (1957), **76**, 296–323.

35 Michel, L., Mencia Huerta, J-M., Benveniste, J. & Dubertret, L. Biological properties of LTB_4 and PAF-acether *in vivo* in human skin. *J. Invest. Dermatol.* (1987), **88**, 675–681.

36 Hénocq, E. & Vargaftig, B. B. Accumulation of eosinophils in response to intracutaneous PAF-acether and allergens in man. *Lancet* (1986), **i**, 1378–1379.

37 Hénocq, E. & Vargaftig, B. B. Skin eosinophilia in atopic patients. *J. Allergy Clin. Immunol.* (1988), **81**, 691–696.

38 Braquet, P., Touqui, L., Shen, T. Y. & Vargaftig, B. B. Perspectives in platelet activating factor research. *Pharmacol. Rev.* (1987), **39**, 97–145.

39 Hwang, S.-B., Lam, M.-Y., Biftu, T., Beattie, T. R. & Shen, T. Y. *Trans*-2,5-bis(3, 4, 5,-trimethoxyphenyl)tetrahydrofuran: an orally active specific and competitive receptor antagonist of platelet activating factor. *J. Biol. Chem.* (1985), **260**, 15 639–15 645.

40 Patterson, R., Harris, K. E., Lee, M. L. & Houlihan, W. J. Inhibition of rhesus monkey airway and cutaneous responses to platelet activating factor (PAF)

(AGEPC) with the anti-PAF agent SRI 63-072. *Int. Arch. Allergy Appl. Immunol.* (1986), **81**, 265–268.
41 Helliwell, P. & Williams, T. J. A specific antagonist of platelet activating factor suppresses oedema formation in an Arthus reaction but not oedema induced by leukocyte chemoattractants in rabbit skin. *J. Immunol.* (1986), **137**, 302–307.
42 Issekutz, A. & Szpejda, M. Evidence that platelet activating factor may mediate some acute inflammatory responses. Studies with the platelet-activating factor antagonist CV 3988. *Lab. Invest.* (1986), **54**, 275–281.
43 Camussi, G., Pawlowski, I., Saunders, R., Brentjens, J. & Andres, G. Receptor antagonist of platelet activating factor inhibits inflammatory injury induced by *in situ* formation of immune complexes in renal glomeruli and in the skin. *J. Lab. Clin. Med.* (1987), **110**, 196–207.
44 Csato, M. & Czarnetzki, B. M. Effect of BN 52021, a platelet activating factor antagonist, on experimental murine contact dermatitis. *Br. J. Dermatol.* (1988), **118**, 475–480.
45 Guinot, Ph., Braquet, P., Duchier, J. & Cournot, A. Inhibition of PAF-acether induced weal and flare reactions in man by a specific PAF antagonist. *Prostaglandins* (1986), **32**, 160–163.
46 Chung, K. F., Dent, G., McCusker, M., Guinot, Ph., Page, C. P. & Barnes, P. J. Effect of a ginkgolide mixture (BN 52063) in antagonising skin and platelet responses to platelet activating factor in man. *Lancet* (1987), **i**, 248–250.
47 Arnout, J., Van Hecken, A., deLepeleire, I. *et al.* Effectiveness and tolerability of CV-3988, a selective PAF antagonist, after intravenous administration to man. *Br. J. Clin. Pharmacol.* (1988), **25**, 445–451.
48 Roberts, N. M., Page, C. P., Chung, K. F. & Barnes, P. J. Effect of a PAF antagonist BN 52063 on antigen induced acute and late-onset cutaneous responses in atopic subjects. *J. Allergy Clin. Immunol.* (1988), **82**, 236–241.
49 Smith, J. A., Mansfield, L. E., DeShazo, R. D. & Nelson, H. S. An evaluation of the pharmacological inhibition of the immediate and late cutaneous reactions to allergen. *J. Allergy Clin. Immunol.* (1980), **65**, 118–121.
50 Bedard, P., Atkins, P. C. & Zweiman, B. Antigen induced local mediator release and cellular inflammatory responses in atopic subjects. *J. Allergy Clin. Immunol.* (1983), **71**, 394–398.
51 Phillips, M. J., Meyrick Thomas, R. H., Moodley, I. & Davis, R. J. A comparison of the *in vivo* effects of ketotifen, clemastine, chlorpheniramine and sodium cromoglycate on histamine and allergen induced weals in human skin. *Br. J. Clin. Pharmacol.* (1983), **15**, 277–286.
52 Lee, T.-C., Lenihan, D. J., Malone, B., Roddy, L. L. & Wasserman, S. I. Increased synthesis of platelet-activating factor in activated human eosinophils. *J. Biol. Chem.* (1984), **259**, 5526–5530.
53 Zimmerman, G. A., McIntyre, T. M. & Prescott, S. M. Production of platelet activating factor by human vascular endothelial cells: evidence for a requirement for specific agonists and modulation by prostacyclin. *Circulation* (1985), **72**, 718–727.
54 Lynch, J. M. & Henson, P. M. The intracellular retention of newly synthesised platelet activating factor. *J. Immunol.* (1986), **137**, 2653–2661.
55 McIntyre, T. M., Zimmerman, G. A. & Prescott, S. M. Leukotrienes C_4 and D_4 stimulate human endothelial cells to synthesise platelet activating factor and bind neutrophils. *Proc. Nat. Acad. Sci. (USA)* (1986), **83**, 2204–2208.
56 Bussolino, F., Breviario, F., Tetta, C., Aglietta, M., Mantovani, A. & Dejana, E. Interleukin-1 stimulates platelet-activating factor production in cultured human

endothelial cells. *J. Clin. Invest.* (1986), **77**, 2027–2033.
57 Gahring, L., Buckley, A. & Daynes, R. A. Presence of epidermal-derived thymocyte activating factor/interleukin-1 in normal human stratum corneum. *J. Clin. Invest.* (1985), **76**, 1585–1591.
58 Luger, T. A. Possible relevance to dermatology of epidermal cell thymocyte-activating factor (ETAF). *Am. J. Dermatopathol.* (1983), **5**, 97–102.
50 Cunningham, F. M., Leigh, I. & Mallet, A. I. The production of platelet activating factor (PAF) by human epidermal cells. *Br. J. Pharmacol.* (1987), **91**, 117p.
60 Michel, L., Denizot, Y., Thomas, Y. *et al.* Biosynthesis of PAF-acether by human skin fibroblasts *in vitro. J. Immunol.* (1988), **141**, 948–953.
61 Kobza Black, A., Keahey, T. M., Eady, R. A. J. & Greaves, M. W. Dissociation of histamine release and clinical improvement following treatment of acquired cold urticaria by prednisone. *Br. J. Clin. Pharmacol.* (1981), **12**, 327–331.
62 Nakayama, R., Oda, M., Satouchi, K. & Saito, K. Generation of acetyl glyceryl ether phosphorylcholine from the rat skin and muscle tissues stimulated with moxibustion. *Biochem. Biophys. Res. Commun.* (1985), **127**, 629–634.
63 Calignano, A., Cirino, G., Meli, R. & Persico, P. Isolation and identification of platelet activating factor in UV-irradiated guinea pig skin. *J. Pharmacol. Meth.* (1988), **19**, 89–91.
64 Heavy, D. J., Kobza Black, A., Barrow, S. E., Chappell, C. G., Greaves, M. W. & Dollery, C. T. Prostaglandin D_2 and histamine release in cold urticaria. *J. Allergy Clin. Immunol.* (1986), **78**, 458–461.
65 Wasserman, S. I. & Ginsberg, M. H. Release of platelet factor 4 into the blood after cold challenge of patients with cold urticaria. *J. Allergy Clin. Immunol.* (1984), **74**, 275–279.
66 Dorsch, W., Ring, J., Weber, P.-C. & Strausser, T. Detection of immunoreactive leukotrienes C_4/D_4 in skin blister fluid after allergen testing in patients with late cutaneous reactions. *Acta Dermatol. Res.* (1985), **277**, 400–401.
67 Talbot, S. F., Atkins, P. C., Goetzl, E. J. & Zweiman, B. Accumulation of leukotriene C_4 and histamine in human allergic skin reactions. *J. Clin. Invest.* (1985), **76**, 650–656.
68 Kobza Black, A., Barr, R. M., Wong, E. *et al.* Lipoxygenase products of arachidonic acid in human inflamed skin. *Br. J. Clin. Pharmacol.* (1985), **20**, 185–190.
69 Guinot, Ph., Summerhayes, C., Berdah, L., Duchier, J. & Revillaud, R. J. Treatment of adult systemic mastocytosis with a PAF-acether antagonist BN 52063. *Lancet*, (1988), **ii**, 114.

Chapter 12
PAF and the nervous system

Elizabeth Kornecki and Yigal H. Ehrlich

Introduction

Although platelet activating factor (PAF) has effects on several cell types [1,2], until recently there were no reports of studies on direct interactions of PAF with cells in the nervous system. A potential role for PAF in neuronal function was first suggested by the discovery that certain neuroactive drugs, the triazolobenzodiazepines alprazolam [3] and triazolam [4], are specific, competitive antagonists of shape change, aggregation and secretion induced in human platelets by PAF. The specificity of alprazolam and triazolam in exerting these effects was expressed in two ways: (i) PAF (but not ADP, epinephrine, collagen, thrombin, arachidonic acid, or the ionophore A23187) was the only platelet agonist whose action was antagonized by these drugs; and (ii) benzodiazepines lacking the triazole moiety were not effective in inhibiting PAF-mediated cellular responses. This pharmacological specificity was demonstrated when we compared the IC_{50} values of various benzodiazepines for the inhibition of aggregation of washed human platelets [5,6]. The IC_{50} values for triazolam and alprazolam, two triazolobenziodiazepines, were 0.3 μM and 0.5 μM, respectively. In contrast, chlordiazepoxide ($IC_{50} = 67$ μM) and diazepam ($IC_{50} = 130$ μM), two clinically-used benzodiazepines without a triazole component, were far less potent. Furthermore, the experimental drug Ro 5-4864, a preferred ligand for peripheral benzodiazepine receptors, had an IC_{50} value of 45 μM. Ro 5-4864 also failed to block, or interfere with the inhibition by alprazolam and triazolam of PAF-induced platelet responses. We therefore concluded that the platelet benzodiazepine receptor is not involved in this activity and that the triazolobenzodiazepines interact directly with PAF receptors. Similar findings were reported by Casals-Stenzel [7,8] who found, in addition, that the triazolothienodiazepine brotizolam is a potent antagonist of PAF action both *in vitro* and *in vivo*.

The finding that neuroactive drugs can act as potent antagonists of PAF-elicited cellular responses have suggested that PAF and PAF-like ether phospholipids may play a role in the regulation of neuronal function [4–6]. Recently, Casals-Stenzel & Weber [9] reported that the PAF antagonistic activity of triazolodiazepines is not mediated by classical central or peripheral benzodiazepine receptors. This finding led to the development of a novel generation of thienotriazolodiazepine antagonists of PAF [10]. In this context, it is important to emphazise that alprazolam, triazolam and brotizolam have psychotherapeutic effects which are not exerted by benzodiazepines without a triazole ring. It was thus hypothesized [4] that the specialized clinical uses of these drugs in the treatment of psychiatric disorders may be related to their unique ability, among the benzodiazepines, to interact directly with PAF receptors. This hypothesis, and the reports on the interactions of triazolobenzodiazepines with PAF receptors, served to focus the attention on the importance of investigating directly the interaction of PAF with cells in the nervous system, and on the need to study the effectiveness of PAF antagonists in the treatment and/or prevention of neuropathological disorders.

Interactions with excitable cells

PAF exerts potent effects on the cardiovascular system, with the main influences being hypotension, decreased coronary flow, lowered cardiac output, depressed cardiac contractility and enhanced vascular permeability. PAF was also shown to induce contraction in isolated preparations of smooth-muscle containing tissues. These studies have been extensively reviewed recently [11–14]. None the less, since the elucidation of mechanisms underlying neuronal responsiveness to agonist stimulation has been enhanced by studies of mechanisms operating in the activation of non-neuronal excitable cells, we summarize here recent progress in studies on the interactions of PAF with the myocardium and smooth-muscle cells.

The hypotension produced by PAF administration *in vivo* is associated with reduced cardiac output [15,16]. Indeed, studies of isolated guinea-pig heart preparations revealed that PAF directly induces a decrease in myocardial contractility [17,18]. This effect does not require the presence of platelets and is inhibited by PAF antagonists in a manner suggesting mediation by specific PAF receptors [17]. The mechanism of this negative inotropic effect of PAF was studied in detail by Robertson *et al.* [18], using isolated guinea-pig right-ventricular papillary muscles. These preparations responded to concentrations of PAF from 1 nM to 1 μM with shortening of the action potential duration, accompanied by a decrease in intracellular Na^+ activity. The authors suggested that the decreased contractility induced by PAF was brought about by a fall in the intracellular levels of

Ca^{2+}, caused by enhanced $Na^{+}Ca^{2+}$ exchange occurring as a result of decreased intra-cellular Na^{+} activity. Different effects were observed in similar preparations by Tamargo *et al.* [19] who reported results consistent with PAF-induced increase in Ca^{2+} influx via slow channels. The reasons for these conflicting findings are yet to be resolved, and may be related to the possibility that PAF stimulates cells by interacting with two receptor sub-types that activate different pathways of signal transduction. This possibility is supported also by a study which found that the early effects of PAF on guinea-pig papillary muscles were expressed as positive inotropism and in increased action potential [20]. These early effects of PAF could be inhibited by propranolol, an adrenergic antagonist [20]. A 'cross-talk' between PAF and adrenergic systems was also observed in studies where synthetic PAF (1-alkyl-2-acetyl-GPC) produced over two-fold increase in plasma norepinephrine levels when administered to spontaneously hypertensive rats [21].

PAF-induced contraction of smooth muscles has been shown in guinea-pig ileum [22] and in rabbit iris [23]. This latter study, by Yousofzai & Abdel-Latif [23], had investigated the biochemical pathways involved in the response of iris smooth muscle to physiological concentrations (10^{-12} to 10^{-8}M) of PAF. It was found that PAF, in a dose and time-dependent manner, stimulated the release of arachidonic acid and consequently the biosynthesis of prostaglandins in iris smooth muscle. This effect, which required Ca^{2+} in the extracellular environment, was inhibited by the calcium-channel blockers nifedipine, verapamil and diltiazem, but was not affected by cyclooxygenase and lipooxygenase inhibitors. In contrast to the mechanisms operating in platelets, in iris smooth muscle, PAF did not stimulate the generation of phospholipase C products, but appeared to exert its biological effects by stimulating Ca^{2+} influx with subsequent activation of phospholipase A_2 [23]. As discussed below, similar mechanisms appear to operate in the activation of neuronal cells by PAF.

Effects on calcium-ion flux

The influx and efflux of Ca^{2+} through the plasma membrane and the delicately balanced control of the intracellular level of free calcium ions ($[Ca^{2+}]_i$) plays a crucial role in the maintenance of neuronal physiological activity. In addition, Ca^{2+} fluxes control the communication between neurons by regulating the critical process of neurotransmitter release (for many recent reviews, see [24]). Thus, the evidence obtained from studies of platelets that the action of PAF involves interaction with Ca^{2+}-mobilizing systems had a significant impact on subsequent investigations of the role of PAF in neuronal function. The activation of platelets by PAF is dependent on extracellular Ca^{2+}. In 1981, Lee *et al.* [25] reported that PAF promotes Ca^{2+} uptake in rabbit platelets, and later investigated some of the mechanisms involved by measuring net ^{45}Ca uptake [26]. The limitations of this technique are that much of the ^{45}Ca taken up by platelets is bound to the external surface of the plasma membrane [27], and that this method cannot quantify the mobilization of Ca^{2+} from intracellular stores. These limitations have been overcome by using the fluorescent calcium probe, Quin-2. Using this probe, Hallam *et al*, [28] demonstrated that PAF induces an increase in intra-platelet free Ca^{2+} levels which involves mainly an influx of Ca^{2+} from the extracellular environment and partly the mobilization of Ca^{2+} from intracellular stores. Subsequent studies measuring Mn^{2+} influx into Quin-2 loaded platelets provided experimental evidence that the PAF-induced Ca^{2+} influx is mediated by the action of selective channels [29]. These findings were confirmed and expanded by Valone & Johnson [30]. They reported that low concentrations of PAF (4.5 ± 2.4 nM), which are sufficient to induce 100% platelet aggregation, cause only about half of the maximal increase induced in $[Ca^{2+}]_i$ by higher PAF concentrations. At these low PAF levels about 85–90% of the increase in $[Ca^{2+}]_i$ was dependent on extracellular calcium, namely, mediated by Ca^{2+} influx. Repeated exposure to low concentrations of PAF desensitized the $[Ca^{2+}]_i$ responses of platelets to this agonist, again indicating involvement of PAF receptors. Similar results were also obtained with other cells, such as macrophages [31] and endothelial cells [32]. Recently, PAF-induced rise in intracellular Ca^{2+} was studied in a continuous line of human cells of committed monocytic origin using the advanced Ca^{2+} probe, Fura-2 [33]. The involvement of PAF receptors in this process was supported by the demonstration that specific PAF antagonists of five different structural classes, all inhibited the PAF-induced increase in $[Ca_{2+}]_i$ in these cells.

Another experimental approach which implicated Ca^{2+} influx in the action of PAF was based on the use of calcium channel blockers. Verapamil and diltiazem were found to inhibit PAF-induced aggregation of rabbit platelets [34]. Verapamil also inhibited the PAF-induced Ca^{2+} uptake in rabbit platelets [26]. In human platelets, PAF-induced platelet aggregation was inhibited by verapamil but not by dihydropyridine [35]. The order of potency of different classes of Ca^{2+}-channel blockers towards the action of PAF in platelets, and the need for high concentrations of the active blockers to exert these effects, are in agreement with the evidence that platelets lack voltage-gated Ca^{2+} channels [36]. Taken together, all the above findings suggest that in platelets, and perhaps also in other cells, PAF stimulates Ca^{2+} influx by interacting with receptor-operated Ca^{2+} channels. The finding that at high concentrations (IC_{50} of 47 and 64 μM, respectively), diltiazem and verapamil can inhibit the binding of PAF to platelets [37], may suggest that the binding sites for PAF and for calcium blockers are situated in very close proximity within a tightly-linked receptor-channel complex.

The increase in Ca^{2+} influx by stimulation of PAF receptors coupled to agonist-gated channels in the plasma membrane could activate phospholipase A_2, with ensuing release of arachidonate and accumulation of free fatty acids. On the other hand, the mobilization of Ca^{2+} from intracellular stores would be secondary to PAF-receptor mediated stimulation of phospholipase C and increased turnover of polyphosphoinositides [38,39]. PAF action and its influence on cellular Ca^{2+} homeostasis can thus be mediated by at least two different biochemical pathways triggered by receptor-linked signal-transduction systems. The products of these pathways can interact and produce synergistic responses, as well as feedback signals that regulate subsequent responsiveness to PAF, such as protein kinase C-mediated receptor desensitization [40]. All these possibilities should be considered when studying the mechanisms of action of PAF in various tissues, including the nervous system, since the relative contribution of each of these pathways to the induction of specific responses may not be the same in different cell types.

Metabolism in the nervous system

The consideration of a role for PAF in neuronal function requires demonstration of the presence of PAF in nervous tissue. PAF originating from cells in the circulation may interact with peripheral neurons. However, in order to act in the central nervous system (CNS), PAF must cross the blood–brain barrier, or be synthesized endogenously within cells in the brain. Using isolated perfused rat brain, Kumar *et al.* [41] found that infused 1-O-[^{3}H]alkyl-2-acetyl-*sn*-glycero-3-phosphorylcholine is cleaved even more rapidly than infused [^{14}C] inulin, indicating that PAF does not readily cross the blood–brain barrier. While PAF from the circulation may enter the CNS in some pathological processes in which the blood–brain barrier is compromised, it is clear that involvement of PAF in physiological regulation of CNS functions is dependent on the biosynthesis of PAF within brain tissue.

Brain tissue contains high levels of phospholipids, among which $> 4\%$ are ether-lipids and about half of these contain phosphatidylcholine. About 5% of the total phosphatidylcholine content of rat brain is alkylacylphosphatidylcholine which can serve as precursor for PAF synthesis [42]. Indeed, Tokumura *et al.* [43] identified, in lipid extracts of bovine brain, a bioactive PAF fraction which was analysed by gas–liquid chromatography/mass spectrometry and found to contain four species of PAF and ten acyl analogues of PAF. Total PAF content in bovine brain was about 25 μg/g tissue of which approximately 75% was $PAF_{18:0}$ [43].

Two pathways operate in PAF biosynthesis, a remodelling route and a *de novo* route (for details see Chapter 1). In the remodelling route, which is involved mainly in inflammatory reactions, the enzyme 1-O-alkyl-2-lyso-*sn*-glycero-3-phosphocholine:acetyl-CoA acetyltransferase, transfers acetate from acetyl-CoA to the *sn*-2 position of 1-alkyl-2-lyso-*sn*-glycero-3- phosphocholine (GPC). This enzyme is not present in brain tissue (see table 2 in [44]). Two of the main enzymes in the *de novo* biosynthetic pathway of PAF—alkyl lyso-GP:acetyl-CoA acetyl transferase and alkyl-acetyl-GP phosphohydrolase—are present in relatively high levels in brain [45,46]. The implication is that PAF can be formed for physiological function in nervous tissue through the *de novo* pathway. A well-balanced biological regulatory process also requires the presence of an inactivating enzymatic system. Indeed, substantial amounts of specific PAF-acetyl-hydrolase were also found in the brain [47].

The first direct demonstration of PAF biosynthesis in tissue derived from the CNS was reported by Bussolino *et al.* [48], using preparations of chick retina. Extracted PAF was analysed by TLC, HPLC, by chemical and lipase treatments, and by assays of bioactivity using rabbit platelets. Basal levels of extractable PAF in retina was found to be 1.12 $\pm$ 0.3 ng/mg protein. This level increased 5–6 fold after stimulation with 50 μM acetyl-choline or dopamine. Other neurotransmitters tested (L-glycine, GABA and epinephrine) had no effect. The acetylcholine- and dopamine-stimulated production of PAF was found to be carried out by the *de novo* pathway. The calcium ionophore A23187 also stimulated PAF production in retina, but this biosynthesis was mediated by acetyltransferase activity of the remodelling pathway. The PAF produced in response to these stimulations was not released, but accumulated within retinal cells. Thus, it cannot yet be stated whether PAF serves as an extracellular mediator in the CNS or whether it only acts intracellularly. Dopamine receptors are present in the retina on neurons whereas acetylcholine receptors are present in neurons as well as in glia, suggesting that the stimulated PAF productions occurs in neurons only, or in both neurons and glial cells. These questions will have to be resolved in future studies. Bussolino *et al.* [49] have demonstrated production of PAF in embryonic chick retina and have related the findings to a potential role in neuro-development.

The biosynthesis of PAF in rat brain tissue was recently studied by Kumar *et al* [41]. They found that in the isolated, fluorocarbon perfused rat brain there was a detectable low basal level of extractable PAF (0.25 $\pm$ 0.15 pmol/g tissue). PAF was identified by bioassays and HPLC analysis. Intra-peritoneal injection of the convulsant drugs, bicuculline or picrotoxin, increased brain PAF levels considerably, to 4.97 $\pm$ 0.75 and 10.6 $\pm$ 2.18 pmol/g tissue, respectively. Since quantitatively similar results were obtained with isolated perfused rat brain, the authors concluded that PAF biosynthesis in brain tissue was independent of systemic metabolism.

Neuroregulatory actions

Only a few reports have appeared to date of studies which have directly examined the interaction of PAF with neuronal cells and have demonstrated the physiological consequences of this stimulation. The results of these studies, however, clearly point out that this line of investigation can provide important new information on the regulation of neuronal function and, in addition, can shed light on the mechanisms underlying the interaction of the immune system with cells in the nervous system. The first indication of such a possibility came from the studies of Stimler-Gerard [50] who obtained pharmacological evidence that the PAF-induced contraction of isolated lung parenchymal tissue is mediated by parasympathetic stimulation. In this study [50], PAF was applied at nanomolar concentrations to parenchymal strips isolated from guinea-pig lung. The PAF-induced contraction was significantly inhibited by tetrodotoxin, which specifically blocks fast Na^+ channels in axons and thus isolates pharmacologically the neuronal component of smooth-muscle responses to agonist stimulation. In addition, the PAF-induced contraction was inhibited by atropine, a cholinergic antagonist, and moderately enhanced by physostigmine, an inhibitor of acetylcholinesterase. These findings suggested that the PAF action observed here is mediated by endogenously-released acetylcholine. Since hexamethonium, a selective blocker of pre-ganglionic sites, had no effect on this response, it was concluded that the site of action of PAF was at a point distal to the parasympathetic ganglion and proximal to the neuromuscular junction [50]. A subsequent study of PAF-induced contraction in canine trachealis *in vivo* has confirmed that PAF induces tracheal smooth-muscle contraction at least in part by post-ganglionic activation of parasympathetic nerves [51]. Using a very different experimental system, our studies have also implicated PAF action as an inducer of acetylcholine release by demonstrating enhancement of minature end-plate potential production when PAF was applied to *in situ* preparations of the snake neuromuscular junction [52].

The effects of PAF on electrophysiological activity also were demonstrated in isolated retina preparations, where it was found that PAF inhibits the electro-retinogram elicited by a brief light flash, and that this effect is blocked by PAF antagonists [53,54]. It was hypothesized that a PAF-induced increase in the levels of intracellular free Ca^{2+} interferes with the response of the retina to light. Direct evidence for the interactions of PAF with neuronal cells and elucidation of the mechanisms underlying these interactions are very difficult to obtain in complex preparations consisting of heterogeneous cell populations such as those studied above. Some of these difficulties have been overcome by investigating simplified model systems of cloned neural cells.

The availability of homogeneous populations of cloned cell lines of neuronal origin enabled detailed investigation of the mechanisms operating in stimulus–response coupling processes of neurons, and elucidation of the biochemical pathways involved in the regulations of neuronal development and differentiation by hormones and trophic factors. One such extensively studied model is the hybrid clone designated NG108-15 [55,56]. We reported that addition of nanomolar concentrations of PAF to cultures of NG108-15 cells maintained in a chemically-defined, serum-free medium [57] caused growth arrest and induced morphological differentiation in neural cells [6,58]. The possibility raised by these findings, that PAF may play a role in neuronal development, also emerged from the demonstration of PAF production in immature cells of chick embryonic retina: Bussolino *et al.* [49] found that acetylcholine stimulated PAF synthesis via the *de novo* pathway even at day 8 of embryonic development, when the retinal cells are still immature. In older stages, dopamine stimulated this pathway. A sharp increase in dopamine stimulation of PAF synthesis occurred after day 16, when D_2-dopamine receptors become detectable. This differential regulation of PAF biosynthesis by neurotransmitters suggests a significant role for PAF in the physiological processes regulating neuronal differentiation and maturation.

The differentiation induced by PAF in cultured NG108-15 cells was expressed in the extension of short and thick neurites [58], distinctly different from the morphology of neurites extended when the same cells are induced to differentiate by agents that increase the levels of intracellular cyclic AMP in these cells [57]. The mechanism underlying the responsiveness of NG108-15 cells to PAF appears to involve an increase in the intracellular levels of free Ca^{2+}. This was determined in experiments using cells pre-loaded with a chemiluminescent probe of Ca^{2+}, the photoprotein aequorin. Using this probe, we found in NG108-15 cells a PAF-induced transient increase in intracellular levels of free Ca^{2+} which was dependent on the presence of Ca^{2+} in the extracellular medium, inhibited by the PAF-antagonist CV-3988, and by the Ca^{2+}-uptake blockers prenylamine and diltiazem [58]. The blocker nitrendipine had no effects, indicating that voltage-dependent Ca^{2+} channels are not involved in the stimulation of Ca^{2+} influx which was observed here. Similar results were also obtained with an adrenergic neuronal cell line, the PC12 cells, in which the PAF-induced rise in $[Ca^{2+}]_i$ was found to be associated with vesicular exocytosis, measured as a Ca^{2+}-dependent release of ATP that is stored in PC12 cells within secretory vesicles together with dopamine and norepinephrine [58].

Taken together, the results described above have suggested that in neural cells, PAF stimulates the activity of receptor-operated Ca^{2+} channels. This conclusion remains tentative due to the relatively high concentrations of PAF required to demonstrate aequorin signals, which measure free Ca^{2+} levels in the micromolar range. We emphasized [58] the need to use fluorescent probes with sensitivity to free Ca^{2+} in the physiological range (100–900 nM) for demonstrating neuronal responsiveness to very low concentrations of PAF. Such results were obtained in our laboratory using the probe Fura-2 in conjunction with a fluorescent cell-imaging system (Kornecki & Ehrlich, in preparation). Convincing evidence that PAF regulates Ca^{2+} homeostasis in neural cells was reported recently by Bussolino *et al.* [59]. Using cultured PC12 cells, it was shown that nanomolar concentrations of PAF stimulated influx and efflux, measured with $[^{45}Ca]$. PAF also induced a rise in $[Ca^{2+}]_i$ in PC12 cells, measured with the fluorescent probes Quin-2 and Fura-2 [59]. These effects of PAF were obtained when the autocoid was presented in its biologically-active steric configuration, the *R*-form, but not in its *S*-form nor when presented as the 2-lyso derivative. The physiological consequences of the PAF-induced increase in $[Ca^{2+}]_i$ in neural cells was evaluated by measuring dopamine release. This measure was more sensitive than Fura-2 responses, responding significantly to 0.1 nM PAF. The absence of extracellular Ca^{2+} inhibited the release of dopamine induced by 30 nM PAF, although about one-third of the rise in $[Ca^{2+}]_i$ measured with Fura-2 was still in evidence when extracellular Ca^{2+} was chelated [59]. These results indicate that PAF can induce release of Ca^{2+} from intracellular Ca^{2+} stores as well as stimulate Ca^{2+} influx into neural cells, and that the PAF-induced dopamine release is dependent on Ca^{2+} influx from the extracellular environment [59]. Since the PAF-induced dopamine release was inhibited by two structurally different antagonists of PAF receptors, CV-3988 and BN 52021 [59], it may be concluded that in neural cells, PAF can stimulate vesicular exocytosis by activating receptor-operated Ca^{2+} channels.

Consistent with the conclusion that PAF can stimulate vesicular release from neurosecretary cells [58,59] are the findings that PAF can stimulate the secretion of ACTH [60], prolactin and growth hormone [61] from primary cultures of rat anterior pituitary tissue and from halves of rat anterior pituitary incubated *in vitro*. Furthermore, PAF-induced release has been demonstrated in brain tissue itself. Bernardini *et al.* [60,62] measured the release of immunoreactive corticotropin-releasing hormone (iCRH) from explants of rat hypothalamus *in vitro*. PAF at 10 nM induced a 300% increase of iCRH release above baseline values and this effect could be blocked by 1 μM alprazolam but not by diazepam, a benzodiazepine without PAF-antagonistic activity [62]. Subsequent studies [60] provided evidence that PAF-induced iCRH release can also be observed *in vivo* and that this effect was inhibited by several classes of PAF antagonists, thus suggesting the presence of PAF receptors in the brain.

Biochemical pathways in neuronal cells

The effectiveness of PAF antagonists in inhibiting several neuroregulatory actions of PAF (discussed above) have suggested the existence of PAF receptors in neural cells in general, and in the CNS in particular. Recently, specific binding sites for [^{3}H]PAF were detected in gerbil brain membranes [63]. Binding of [^{3}H]PAF was measured in a preparation containing synaptic membranes, myelin, mitochondria and microsomes (a lysed P2 fraction). Non-specific binding was rather high and represented about 80% of total binding. The results should thus be interpreted with caution and it may be expected that future studies with radiolabelled antagonists will provide considerable improvements. Radiolabelled PAF displayed specific, saturable, reversible and time-dependent binding to brain membranes. However, the specific binding of [^{3}H]PAF was only partially inhibited by the antagonist BN 52021 [63]. Computer modelling analysis of Scatchard plots of the binding data revealed a good fit with a two-site model; a high-affinity site with $K_d = 3.66 \pm 0.92$ nM and $B_{max} = 0.83 \pm 0.23$ pmol/mg protein, and another with $K_d = 20.4 \pm 0.56$ nM and $B_{max} = 1.1 \pm 0.32$ pmol/mg protein. Brain regional analysis indicated highest specific binding in the mid-brain and hippocampus and lowest in the cerebellum [63].

Separate sub-populations of specific PAF receptors in brain may be linked to different signal-transduction systems. The present knowledge suggests that two parallel pathways can be activated by PAF in neural cells. In one biochemical pathway, PAF receptors appear to be linked directly to agonist-gated Ca^{2+} channels [58,59]. The studies on the properties and mechanism of PAF-stimulated arachidonate release in iris smooth-muscle cells [23] indicated the operation of a pathway in which increased influx of Ca^{2+}, induced by PAF, stimulates phospholipase A_2 activity. That a similar pathway is operating in brain is suggested by a recent study using PAF antagonists. Birkle *et al.* [64] reported that the PAF antagonist BN 52021 decreased the ischaemia and electroconvulsive shock (ECS)-induced accumulation of free polyunsaturated fatty acids in mouse brain. Specifically, BN 52021 pretreatment decreased the ischaemia-associated accumulation of free palmitic (16:0), 18:0, 20:4 and docosahexaenoic (22:6) acids with no effect on the fatty acids in diacylglycerol or the loss of phosphatidylinositol-4,5-diphosphate (PIP_2), in a manner consistent with interference by the PAF antagonist with the pathway involving phospholipase A_2/phospholipase A_1/lysophospholipase action, but not with the ECS-induced activation of the phospholipase C/diacylglycerol lipase pathway [64]. Unless BN 52021 directly inhibits phospholipase A_2 activity, a possibility that has not been tested yet, these results can be interpreted to mean that agonist occupation of PAF receptors in brain cells stimulates Ca^+ influx which, in turn, increases phospholipase A_2 activity.

As discussed above, in addition to stimulating Ca^{2+} influx, PAF can also increase neuronal Ca^{2+} mobilization from intracellular stores. The signal transduction system operating to bring about this response is known to involve receptor-linked phospholipase C activation and accelerated turnover of polyphosphoinositides, a system which is very prevalent in brain tissue [65]. Using preparations enriched in pinched-off nerve endings (synaptosomes) pre-labelled with ^{32}P, Kumar *et al.* [41] demonstrated a PAF-stimulated turnover of polyphosphoinositides in a manner expected from the activity of receptor-linked phospholipase C. Since these effects were dependent on the presence of Ca^{2+} in the extracellular medium [41], future studies should examine the relationships between PAF-stimulated Ca^{2+} influx and PAF-induced acceleration of polyphosphoinositide metabolism in molecular mechanisms underlying the regulation of neuronal function by PAF.

Involvement in neuropathological processes

Every available review of research on PAF reveals that while numerous reports implicate PAF in various pathobiological processes, only a few studies assign to PAF a role as a physiological regulator in the maintenance of normal homeostasis. It is not surprising, therefore, that evidence has begun to accumulate implicating PAF in several neuropathological disorders. The neuronal dysfunctions associated with the inherited developmental disorder Zellweger syndrome may be directly related to the known lack of PAF synthesis in individuals with this disorder [66,67], as suggested by the findings implicating PAF in neuronal development and differentiation [49,58]. The ability of PAF to stimulate Ca^{2+} influx into neural cells and to induce an increase in intra-neuronal Ca^{2+} levels [58,59] suggests that PAF may also play a role in processes that induce neuro-degeneration in the mature nervous system. Extensive studies in another field of investigation lead to this assumption. The over-activity of excitatory amino acid neurotransmitters has been associated in recent years with the pathophysiological processes operating in several types of neuro-degenerative disorders, including epilepsy, stroke, hypoxia- and hypoglycaemia-induced brain damage, spinal-cord injury and possibly Huntington's, Alzheimer's and Parkinson's diseases [68,69]. The mechanisms underlying the neuro-degeneration induced by excessive stimulation of excitatory amino acid receptors involves activation of agonist-gated Ca^{2+} channels, an exaggerated increase in Ca^{2+} influx and sustained abnormal elevation of intracellular free Ca^{2+} levels [70]. The blockade of receptor-gated ion channels can prevent excitotoxinmediated neuro-degeneration in experimental systems [71]. Analogously, PAF may cause damage to neuronal cells by operating through similar mechanisms. Indeed, when PAF was added to the medium used for the maintenance of neural NG108-15 cells in culture, it caused a concentration- and time-dependent cell death [58]. The neurotoxic effects were not immediate but developed with time. Only PAF concentrations which were found to induce an exaggerated increase in intracellular levels of free Ca^{2+}, well above the physiological range, caused neuronal degeneration [6,58]. Such programmed cell death is consistent with a pathway of agonist-induced, Ca^{2+}-dependent activation of phospholipase A_2, accumulation of free polyunsaturated fatty acids [64], and ensuing production of cytotoxic superoxide and hydroxyl radicals, that can cause neuronal cell death [72]. Studies using cultured CNS neurons currently underway in our laboratory are specifically designed to examine these possibilities. At present, only indirect evidence is available concerning the role of PAF as a mediator in the patho-physiological processes that cause brain injury, as discussed below.

A body of evidence, based primarily on documenting the protective effects of PAF antagonists, demonstrates the involvement of PAF in cerebral ischaemia. Several extensive reviews of these investigations were published recently [73–75] and therefore, these studies are summarized here only in brief. Spinnewyn *et al.* [76] reported that PAF antagonists administered to Mongolian gerbils improved cerebral metabolism and protected the brain in the post-ischaemic phase induced by bilateral carotid ligature. The PAF antagonists BN 52021 and several of its analogues, when given in this study as a prophylactic (for 1 week prior to clamping) antagonized morbidity as assessed by the stroke index and improved mitochondrial respiration as evaluated by the respiratory control ratio. When given 1 h after declamping, BN 52021, kadsurenone, and brotizolam were able to reverse a cerebral impairment trend [76]. Panneta *et al.* [77] showed that BN 52021 inhibits the late deterioration of regional blood flow elicited by ischaemia–reperfusion injury in the gerbil brain. Thus, PAF antagonists can enhance post-ischaemic recovery and increase cerebral perfusion after ligation. These effects are associated with decreased accumulation of free polyunsaturated fatty acids involved in ischaemic brain injury [64]. Similar results were obtained with another model, post-decapitation ischaemia in the mouse brain. There it was found that BN 52021 attenuated the decapitation-induced accumulation of free 20:4 and 22:6 in diacylglycerol but had no effect on the loss of phosphatidylinositol diphosphate [64], again implicating PAF in the activation of phospholipase A_2 (but not of phospholipase C) in injured brain tissue.

Studies using specific antagonists have implicated PAF in biological processes underlying behavioural disorders. Alprazolam, the first triazolobenzodiazepine described as a competitive antagonist of PAF receptors [3,4], is used clinically in the treatment of panic–anxiety disorders and depression (reviewed in [5,6]). Recently, Clostre *et al.* [78] reported that alprazolam inhibited the behavioural despair induced in mice by forced swimming. Moreover, the same study also demonstrated that the specific PAF antagonist BN 52063, which does not interact with central benzodiazepine receptors, has reversed the behavioural inhibition produced by inescapable stress [78]. Such behavioural inhibition is considered one of the best available models of depression [79] and the results thus suggest a role of PAF in the biological processes underlying this behaviour. In view of the data indicating a role for corticotropin-releasing hormone (CRH) in major depression [80], and the finding that PAF can stimulate the release of hypothalamic CRH [60,62], it is possible that PAF plays an important role in the regulation of the hypothalamic–pituitary–adrenal axis and contributes significantly to the behavioural manifestations of the activity of this hormonal loop.

The beneficial and protecting effects of PAF antagonists in the various models of brain injury described above are assumed to be mediated by the blockade of PAF receptors in brain tissue. However, it is not known yet whether the PAF that participates in such neuropathological processes is synthesized in brain tissue or originates from the circulation. Although it has been shown that PAF cannot significantly penetrate the blood–brain barrier [41], there is some evidence that PAF itself can cause an increase in the permeability of the blood–brain barrier. This effect may play a role in the enhancing effect that PAF showed in the development of experimental allergic encephalomyelitis in rats [81] and other brain dysfunctions. Moreover, in many neuropathological situations, the blood–brain barrier is compromised. Under such circumstances relatively high levels of PAF originating from circulating cells may come into contact with cells in the CNS, and induce the exaggerated increase in intracellular free Ca^{2+} levels that can trigger the chain of biochemical events leading to irreversible neuronal degeneration [58]. It may be expected, therefore, that continued studies on the interaction of PAF and its specific antagonists with cells in the nervous system will lead to the development of new therapeutic approaches in the treatment and prevention of neuronal degeneration associated with ischaemia, trauma, stroke and spinal-cord injury, as well as shedding light on the role of PAF in developmental disabilities associated with impaired neuronal development, and on neuronal dysfunctions underlying certain behavioural disorders.

References

1 Benveniste, J., Henson, P. M. & Cochrane, C. G. Leukocyte-dependent histamine release from rabbit platelets. The role of IgE, basophils and a platelet-activating factor. *J. Exp. Med.* (1972), **136**, 1356–1377.

2 Braquet, P., Touqui, L., Shen, T. Y. & Vargaftig, B. B. Perspectives in platelet-activating factor research. *Pharmacol. Rev.* (1987), **39**, 97–145.

3 Kornecki, E., Ehrlich, Y. H. & Lenox, R. H. The antipanic/antiphobic drug, alprazolam, inhibits the aggregation of human platelets by platelet activating factor. *Society for Neuroscience* (1984), **10**, 18.

4 Kornecki, E., Ehrlich, Y. H. & Lenox, R. H. Platelet-activating factor induced aggregation of human platelets specifically inhibited by triazolobenzodiazepines. *Science* (1984), **226**, 1454–1456.

5 Kornecki, E., Lenox, R. H., Hardwick, D. H. & Ehrlich, Y. H. A role for platelet activating factor in neuronal function: specific inhibition of platelet activation by triazolobenzodiazepines and interactions of PAF with cultured neural cells. In Winslow, C. M. & Lee, M. L. (eds) *New Horizons in Platelet Activating Factor Research* (1987), pp 285–292. John Wiley, New York.

6 Kornecki, E., Lenox, R. H., Hardwick, D. H., Bergdahl, J. A., & Ehrlich, Y. H. Interactions of the alkyl-ether-phospholipid, platelet activating factor (PAF) with platelets, neural cells, and the psychotropic drugs triazolobenzodiazepines. In Ehrlich, Y. H., Lenox, R. H., Kornecki, E. & Berry, W. O. (eds) *Molecular Mechanisms of Neuronal Responsiveness. Advances in Experimental Medicine and Biology* (1987), **221**, pp 477–488. Plenum Press, New York.

7 Casals-Stenzel, J. Inhibition of PAF-induced effects by brotizolam and related compounds. *Naunyn-Schmiedeberg's Arch. Exp. Pathol. Pharmakol.* (1985), **332**, (Supplement), R71.

8 Casals-Stenzel, J. Triazolodiazepines are potent antagonists of platelet activating factor (PAF) *in vitro* and *in vivo*. *Naunyn-Schmiedeberg's Arch. Exp. Pathol. Pharmakol.* (1987), **335**, 351–335.

9 Casals-Stenzel, J. & Weber, K. H. Triazolodiazapines: dissociation of their PAF (platelet activating factor) antagonistic and CNS activity. *Br. J. Pharmacol.* (1987), **90**, 139–146.

10 Casals-Stenzel, J., Muacevic, G. & Weber, K. H. Pharmacological actions of WEB 2086, a new specific antagonist of platelet activating factor. *J. Pharmacol. Exp. Ther.* (1987), **241**, 974–981.

11 Levi, R., Burke, J. A., Guo, Z. G. *et al.* Acetylglyceryletherphosphorylcholine (AGEPC), A putative mediator of cardiac anaphylaxis in the guinea pig. *Circ. Res.* (1984), **54**, 117–124.

12 Levi, R., Shen, T. Y., Yee, S. J. *et al.* Platelet activating factor: Effects on human and guinea-pig heart preparations. In Winslow, C. M. & Lee, M. L. (eds) *New Horizons in Platelet Activating Factor Research* (1987), pp. 255–267. John Wiley, New York.

13 Stimler-Gerard, N. P. Parasympathetic action of platelet activating factor in lung. In Winslow, C. M. & Lee, M. L. (eds) *New Horizons in Platelet Activating Factor Research* (1987), pp. 269–275. John Wiley, New York.

14 Feuerstein, G. & Siren, A. L. Platelet-activating factor and shock. *Progr. Biochem. Pharmacol.* (1988), **22**, 181–190.

15 Bessin, P., Bonnet, J., Apful, D. *et al.* Acute circulatory collapse caused by platelet activating factor (PAF-acether) in dogs. *Eur. J. Pharmacol.* (1983), **86**, 403–413.

16 Feuerstein, G. & Hallenbeck, J. M. Prostaglandins, leukotrienes, and platelet-activating factor in shock. *Ann. Rev. Pharmacol. Toxicol.* (1987), **27**, 301–313.

17 Robertson, D. A., Genovese, A. & Levi, R. Negative inotropic effect of platelet-activating factor on human myocardium: A pharmacological study. *J. Pharmacol. Exp. Ther.* (1987), **243**, 834–839.

18 Robertson, D. A., Wang, D. Y., Lee, C. O. & Levi, R. Negative inotropic effect of platelet-activating factor: association with a decrease in intracellular sodium activity. *J. Pharmacol. Exp. Ther.* (1988), **245**, 124–128.

19 Tamargo, J., Tajerina, T., Delgado, C. & Barrigon, S. Electrophysiological effects of platelet-activating factor (PAF-acether) in guinea-pig papillary muscles. *Eur. J. Pharmacol.* (1985), **109**, 219–227.
20 Camussi, G., Alloatti, G., Montrucchio, G., Moda, M. & Emanuelli, G. Effect of platelet activating factor on guinea-pig papillary muscle. *Experentia (Basel)* (1984), **40**, 697–699.
21 Hubbard, J. W., Cox, R. H., Lawler, J. E., Blank, M. L. & Snyder F. Antihypertensive effects of 1-hexadecyl-2-acetyl-*sn*-glycero-3-phosphocholine on plasma renin activity and catecholamine responses in spontaneously hypertensive rats. *Life Sci.* (1983), **32**, 221–232.
22 Findlay, S. R., Lichtenstein, L. M., Hanahan, D. J. & Pinckard, R. N. Contraction of guinea pig ileum smooth muscle by acetyl glyceryl ether phosphorylcholine. *Am. J. Physiol.* (Cell Physiol). (1981), **10**, C130–133.
23 Yousufzai, S. Y. K. & Abdel-Latif, A. A. Effects of platelet-activating factor on the release of arachidonic acid and prostaglandins by rabbit iris smooth muscle. Inhibition by calcium channel antagonists. *Biochem. J.* (1985), **228**, 697–706.
24 Ehrlich, Y. H., Lenox, R. H., Kornecki, E. & Berry, W. O. (eds) Molecular mechanisms of neuronal responsiveness. In *Advances in Experimental Medicine and Biology* (1987), p. 221. Plenum Press, New York.
25 Lee, T. C., Malone, B., Blank, M. L. & Snyder, F. 1-Alkyl-2-acetyl-*sn*-glycero-3-phosphocholine (platelet-activating factor) stimulates calcium influx in rabbit platelets. *Biochem. Biophys. Res. Commun.* (1985), **102**, 1262–1268.
26 Lee, T.C., Malone, B. & Snyder, F. Stimulation of calcium uptake by 1-alkyl-2-acetyl-*sn*-glycero-3-phosphocholine (platelet-activating factor) in rabbit platelets: possible involvement of the lipoxygenase pathway. *Arch. Biochem. Biophys.* (1983), **223**, 33–39.
27 Brass, L. F. & Shattil, S. J. Changes in surface-bound and exchangeable calcium during platelet activation. *J. Biol. Chem.* (1982), **257**, 14 000–14 005.
28 Hallam, T. J., Sanchez, A. & Rink, T. J. Stimulus–response coupling in human platelets. Changes evoked by platelet-activating factor in cytoplasmic free calcium monitored with the fluorescent calcium indicator Quin-2. *Biochem. J.* (1984), **218**, 819–827.
29 Hallam, T. J. & Rink, T. J. Agonists stimulate divalent cation channels in the plasma membrane of human platelets. *FEBS Lett.* (1985), **186**, 175–179.
30 Valone, F. H. & Johnson, B. Modulation of cytoplasmic calcium in human platelets by the phospholipid platelet-activating factor 1-O-alkyl-2-acetyl-*sn*-glycero-3-phosphorylcholine. *J. Immunol.* (1985), **134**, 1120–1124.
31 Conrad, G. W. & Rink, T. J. Platelet activating factor raises intracellular calcium ion concentration in macrophages. *J. Cell Biol.* (1986), **103**, 439–450.
32 Bussolino, F., Aglietta, M., Sanavio, F., Stacchini, A., Lauri, D. & Camussi C. Alkyl-ether phosphoglycerides influence calcium fluxes into human endothelial cells. *J. Immunol.* (1985), **135**, 2748–2753.
33 Ward, S. G. & Westwick, J. Antagonism of the platelet activating factor-induced rise of the intracellular calcium ion concentration of U937 cells. *Br. J. Pharmacol.* (1988), **93**, 769–774.
34 Coeffier, E., Cerrina, J., Jouvin-Marche, E. & Benveniste, J. Inhibition of rabbit platelet aggregation by the Ca^{2+}-antagonists verapamil and diltiazem and by trifluroperazine. *Thromb. Res.* (1983), **31**, 565–576.
35 MacIntyre, D. E. & Shaw, A. M. Phospholipid-induced human platelet activation: effects of calcium channel blockers and calcium chelators. *Thromb. Res.* (1983), **31**, 833–844.

36 Doyle, V. M. & Ruegg, A. T. Lack of evidence for voltage dependent calcium channels in platelets. *Biochem. Biophys. Res. Commun.* (1985), **113**, 598–604.

37 Valone, F. H. Inhibition of platelet activating factor binding to human platelets by calcium channel blockers. In Winslow, C. M. & Lee, M. L. (eds) *New Horizons in Platelet Activating Factor Research.* (1987), pp.215–221. John Wiley, New York.

38 Billah, M. M. & Lapetina, E. G. Platelet activating factor stimulates metabolism of phosphoinositides in horse platelets: possible relationship to Ca^{2+} mobilization during stimulation. *Proc. Nat. Acad. Sci. (USA)* (1983), **80**, 965–968.

39 Lapetina, E. G. & Siegel, F. L. Shape change induced in human platelets by platelet-activating factor. Correlation with the formation of phosphatidic acid and phosphorylation of a 40 000-dalton protein. *J. Biol. Chem.* (1983), **258**, 7241–7244.

40 Lapetina, E. G. The role of GTP-binding proteins in receptor activation of phospholipase C. In Ehrlich, Y. H., Lenox, R. H., Kornecki, E. & Berry, W. O. (eds) *Molecular Mechanisms of Neuronal Responsiveness. Advances in Experimental Medicine and Biology* (1987), **221**, pp.95–100. Plenum Press, New York.

41 Kumar, R., Harvey, S. A. K., Kester, M., Hanahan, D. J. & Olson, M. S. Production and effects of platelet-activating factor in the rat brain. *Biochem. Biophys. Acta* (1988), **963**, (2), 375–383.

42 Rabinowitz, J. L. & Hercker, E. S. Total plasmalogens and O-(acylalkylglycerophosphoryl)ethanolamine from labelled hexadecanol and palmitate during hypoxia and anoxia in rat heart. *Biochem. J.* (1976), **160**, 463–466.

43 Tokumura, A., Kamiyasu, K., Takauchi, K. & Tsukatani, H. Evidence for existence of various homologues and analogues of platelet activating factor in a lipid extract of bovine brain. *Biochem. Biophys. Res. Commun.* (1987), **145**, 415–425.

44 Wykle, R. L., Malone, B. & Snyder, F. Enzymatic synthesis of 1-alkyl-2-acetyl-*sn*-glycero-3-phosphocholine, a hypotensive and platelet-aggregating lipid. *J. Biol. Chem.* (1980), **255**, 10 256–10 280.

45 Lee, T. C., Malone, B. & Snyder, F. A new *de novo* pathway for the formation of 1-alkyl-2-acetyl-*sn*-glycerols, precursors of platelet activating factor. Biochemical characterization of 1-alkyl-2-lyso-*sn*-glycero-3-P:acetyl-CoA acetyltransferase in rat spleen. *J. Biol. Chem.* (1986), **261**, 5373–5377.

46 Lee, T. C., Malone, B. & Snyder, F. Formation of 1-alkyl-2-acetyl-*sn*-glycerols via the *de novo* biosynthetic pathway for platelet-activating factor. Characterization of 1-alkyl-2-acetyl-*sn*-glycero-3-phosphate phosphohydrolase in rat spleens. *J. Biol. Chem.* (1988), **263**, 1755–1760.

47 Blank, M. L., Lee, T. C., Fitzgerald, V. & Snyder, F. A specific acetyl-hydrolase for 1-alkyl-2-acetyl-*sn*-glycero-3-phosphocholine (a hypotensive and platelet-activating lipid). *J. Biol. Chem.* (1981), **256**, 175–178.

48 Bussolino, F., Gremo, F., Tetta, C., Pescarmona, G. P. & Camussi, G. Production of platelet-activating factor by chick retina. *J. Biol. Chem.* (1986), **261**, 16 502–16 508.

49 Bussolino, F., Pescarmona, G., Camussi, G. & Gremo, F. Acetylcholine and dopamine promote the production of platelet activating factor in immature cells of chick embryonic retina. *J. Neurochem.* (1988). **9,** 1755–1759.

50 Stimler-Gerrard, N. P. Parasympathetic stimulation as a mechanism for platelet-activating factor-induced contractile responses in the lung. *J. Pharmacol. Exp. Ther.* (1986), **237**, 209–213.

51 Leff, A. R., White, S. R., Munoz, N. M. *et al.* Parasympathetic involvement in PAF-induced contraction in canine trachealis *in vivo*. *J. Appl. Physiol.* (1987), **62**, 599–605.

52 Kornecki, E., Neel, D., Parsons, R. & Ehrlich, Y. H. Neuronal stimulation by the alkyl-ether phospholipid, platelet activating factor (PAF-acether). *J. Neurochem.* (1987), **48**, (Supplement), 5113.

53 Doly, M., Braquet, P., Bonhomme, B. & Meyniel, G. Effects of PAF-acether on electrophysiological response of isolated retina. *Int. J. Tiss. Reac.* (1987), **IX**, 33–37.
54 Doly, M., Bonhomme, B., Braquet, P., Chabrier, P. E. & Meyniel, G. Effects of platelet-activating factor on electrophysiology of isolated retinas and their inhibition by BN 52021, a specific PAF-acether receptor antagonist. *Immunopharmacol.* (1987), **13**, 189–1194.
55 Nirenberg, M., Wilson, S., Higashida, H. *et al.* Modulation of synapse formation by cyclic adenosine monophosphate. *Science* (1983), **222**, 793–799.
56 Hamprecht, B., Glaser, T., Reiser, G., Bayer, E. & Propst, F. Culture and characteristics of hormone-responsive neuroblastoma X glioma hybrid cells. *Methods Enzymol.* (95), **109,** 316–341.
57 Ehrlich, Y. H., Davis, T., Bock, D., Kornecki, E. & Lenox, R. H. Ecto-protein kinase activity on the external surface of intact neural cells. *Nature* (1986), **320**, 67–70.
58 Kornecki, E. & Ehrlich, Y. H Neuroregulatory and neuropathological actions of the ether-phospholipid platelet-activating factor. *Science* (1988), **240**, 1792–1794.
59 Bussolino, F., Tessari, F., Turrini, F. *et al.* Platelet activating factor induces dopamine release in PC-12 cell line. *Am. J. Physiol.* (1988), **255**, C559–C565.
60 Bernardini, R., Calogero, A. E., Ehrlich, Y. H., Brucke, T., Chrousos, G. P. & Gold, P. W. The alkyl ether-phospholipid platelet activating factor is a stimulator of the hypothalamic–pituitary–adrenal axis in the rat. *Endocrinology*, in press.
61 Grandison, L. & Camoratto, A. M. PAF stimulates prolactin and growth hormone secretion from rat anterior pituitary tissue *in vitro*. In *Second International Conference on Platelet-Activating Factor and Structurally Related Alkyl Ether Lipids* (1986) p. 71. (Abstract).
62 Bernardini, R., Calogero, A. E. & Chrousos, G. P. Platelet activating factor stimulates hypothalamic corticotropin releasing hormone secretion *in vitro*. *Neuroscience Abstracts* (1987), **13**, (No. 450.9), 1622.
63 Domingo, M. T., Spinnewyn, B., Chabrier, P. E. & Braquet P. Presence of specific binding sites for platelet-activating factor (PAF) in brain. *Biochem. Biophys. Res. Commun.* (1988), **151**, 730–736.
64 Birkle, D. L., Kurian, P., Braquet, P. & Bazan, N. G. Platelet-activating factor antagonist BN 52021 decreases accumulation of free polyunsaturated fatty acid in mouse brain during ischemia and electroconvulsive shock. *J. Neurochem.* (1988), **51**, 1900–1905.
65 Agranoff, B. W. Receptor-mediated phosphoinositide metabolism. In Ehrlich, Y. H., Lenox, R. H., Kornecki, E. & Berry, W. O. (eds) *Molecular Mechanisms of Neuronal Responsiveness. Advances in Experimental Medicine and Biology.* (1987), pp. 69–79. Plenum Press, New York.
66 Datta, N. S., Wilson, G. N. & Hajra, A. K. Deficiency of enzymes catalyzing the biosynthesis of glycerol-ether lipids in Zellweger syndrome. *New Engl. J. Med.* (1984), **311**, 1080–1083.
67 Sturk, A., Schaap, M. C. L., Prins, A. *et al.* Age-related deficiency of the synthesis of platelet activating factor by leucocytes from Zellweger patients. *Blood* (1987), **70**, 460–463.
68 Fuxe, K., Roberts, P. & Schwarcz, R. (eds) *Excitotoxins* (1983). Macmillan, London.
69 Jenner, P. (ed.) *Neurotoxins and their Pharmacological Implications* (1987). Raven Press, New York.
70 MacDermott, A. B., Mayer, M. L., Westbrook, G. L. & Smith, J. L. B. NMDA-receptor activation increases cytoplasmic calcium concentration in cultured spinal cord neurones. *Nature* (1986), **324**, 519–522.

71 Olney, J., Price, L., Salles, K. S., Labruyere, J. & Frierdich, G. MK-801 powerfully protects against N-methyl aspartate neurotoxicity. *Eur. J. Pharmacol.* (1987), **141**, 357–361.

72 Dykens, J. A., Stern, A., & Trenkner, E. Mechanism of kainate toxicity to cerebellar neurons *in vitro* is analogous to reperfusion tissue injury. *J. Neurochem.* (1987), **49**, 1222–1228.

73 Braquet, P., Paubert-Braquet, M., Koltai, M., Bourgain, R., Bussolino, F. & Hosford, D. PAF antagonists and the treatment of ischemic diseases: proposed mechanism of action and therapeutic applications. *Trends Pharmacol. Sci.* (1989), **101**, 23–30.

74 Braquet, P., Spinnewyn, B., Blavet, N., Marcheselli, V., Rossawska, M. & Bazan, N. G. Platelet activating factor as a mediator in cerebral ischemia and related disorders. *Biomed. Biochim. Acta* (1988), **47**, S175–218.

75 Braquet, P., Spinnewyn, B., Demerle, C., Hosford, D., Marcheselli, V., Rossawska, M. & Bazan, N. G. The role of platelet activating factor in cerebral ischemia and related disorders. In Barkai, V. & Bazan, N. G. (eds) *New York Academy of Science.* (1989), 559, 296–312.

76 Spinnewyn, B., Blavet, N., Clostre, F., Bazan, N. & Braquet, P. Involvement of platelet-activating factor (PAF) in cerebral post-ischemic phase in Mongolian gerbils. *Prostaglandins* (1987), **34**, 337–346.

77 Panetta, T., Marcheselli, V., Braquet, P., Spinnewyn, B. & Bazan N. G. Effects of a platelet activating factor antagonist (BN 52021) on free fatty acids, diacylglycerols, polyphosphoinositdes and blood flow in the gerbil brain: inhibition of ischemia–reperfusion induced cerebral injury. *Biochem. Biophys. Res. Commun.* (1987), **149**, 580–587.

78 Clostre, F., Millerin, M., Betin, C., Bazan, N. & Braquet, P. Effects of two platelet-activating factor antagonists, BN 52063 and alprazolam, on forced swimming-induced behavioral despair in mice. In Braquet, P. & Prous, J. R. (eds) *Ginkgolides —Chemistry, Biology, Pharmacology and Clinical Perspectives* (1988), pp. 649–664. J. R. Prous Science Publishers, Barcelona.

79 Porsolt, R. D., LePichon, M. & Jalfre, M. Depression: a new model sensitive to antidepressant treatment. *Nature* (1977), **266**, 730–732.

80 Gold, P. W., Goodwin, F. K. & Chrousos, G. P. Clinical and biochemical manifestations of depression: Relation to the neurobiology of stress. *New Eng. J. Med.* (1988), **319**, 413–420.

81 Howat, D. W., Chand, N., Moore, A. R., Braquet, P. & Willoughby, D. A. The effects of platelet-activating factor and its specific antagonists BN 52021 on the development of experimental allergic encephalomyelitis in rats. *Int. J. Immunopathol. Pharmacol.* (1988), **1**, 11–15.

Chapter 13
PAF and the immune system

Marek Rola-Pleszczynski and Pierre Braquet

Introduction

In most instances when the host is asked to mount a specific immune response, the initial event or the subsequent response, or both, are associated with non-specific inflammation. In recent years, with the identification of numerous molecular and cellular components of the inflammatory response, many laboratories have undertaken studies of potential interactions between the latter and the protagonists of more specific immunological reactions. In particular, soluble mediators of inflammation, produced by phagocytes, endothelial cells, skin or nerves have been studied with regard to the possibility that they modulate lymphocyte and monocyte-macrophage functions. Among them, histamine [1], prostaglandins [2], leukotrienes [3] and neuropeptides [4] have been shown to exert varied immunoregulatory effects.

Platelet-activating factor (PAF) is also a potent mediator of inflammation, being released during numerous and varied inflammatory, allergic or immune reactions, and participating in their development. The discovery of selective PAF receptor antagonists has contributed immensely to the definition of a role for PAF in many disease processes. In this Chapter PAF will be discussed as a potentially powerful immunoregulatory agent (Fig. 13.1). Because both PAF and leukotrienes can be derived from the same membrane phospholipid, alkyl-arachidonyl-glycero-phosphorylcholine [5], they may be produced simultaneously, or in sequence, and some of the effects of PAF appear to be mediated by subsequent leukotriene (LT) production.

Cellular sources of PAF are numerous and include various leukocyte populations, endothelial cells and probably other cell types [6]. Resting lymphocytes are unable to produce PAF, possibly due to a lack of acetyl transferase [7]. However, several T- and B- cell lines [8] and large

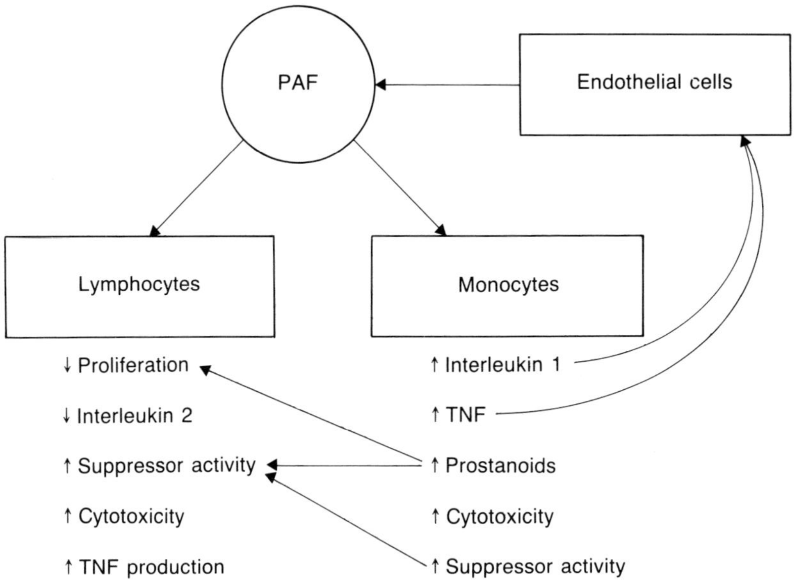

Fig. 13.1 Interactions of PAF with lymphocytes, monocytes and endothelial cells as related to immune functions. TNF = tumour necrosis factor.

granular lymphocytes [9] can be activated to produce PAF under certain circumstances. Many of the cells or tissues which produce PAF are themselves targets of PAF-induced bioactions, with the potential for amplification processes to occur.

Effects on lymphocytes

Proliferation

When PAF was added to cultures of human peripheral blood mononuclear leukocytes (PBML) stimulated with phytohemagglutinin (PHA) or concanavalin A (Con A), we observed a concentration-dependent inhibition of PBML proliferation [10]. The IC_{50} was between 10^{-12} and 10^{-10} M and PAF needed to be present during the first 3 h of the 72-h culture for suppression to be observed. Lyso-PAF or (*S*)-PAF were inactive, while a similar effect was seen with the non-hydrolysable PAF analogue, ethoxy-PAF [11]. PAF-induced inhibition of PBML proliferation was prevented by the use of the PAF-receptor antagonists BN 52020 and BN 52021 indicating that PAF mediated this effect via a class of receptors analogous to that found on platelets. Suppression was also reversed by the cyclooxygenase inhibitor indomethacin, suggesting that prostaglandins were involved as second messengers in the PAF-induced inhibition of lymphocyte proliferation. Some of these initial findings were confirmed by Dulioust *et al.* [12] who reported that PAF suppressed CD4 + T-cell proliferation; the effect occurred at high concentrations of PAF and could be seen when PAF was added late during culture. Similarly, Gebhardt *et al.* [13] reported inhibition by PAF of lymphocyte proliferation in response to allogeneic stimuli in primary or secondary mixed-lymphocyte cultures. BN 52021 not only blocked the effects of PAF but had by itself a stimulatory effect on MLC. In contrast, Behrens & Goodwin [14] reported augmented CD4 + T-cell proliferation in response to PAF, which could be blocked by BN 52021.

In a different system, PAF and two non-hydrolysable PAF analogues increased the proliferation of IL-2-stimulated human lymphoblasts, while some PAF receptor antagonists (CV-3988 and L-652731 but not WEB 2086 or BN 52021) inhibited such proliferation [15]. This inhibition was observed even when the drugs were added 48 h after initiation of the 72-h culture, suggesting an interference by the antagonists with later events in proliferation of pre-activated T-cells. Furthermore, the possibility that endogenously-produced PAF could be involved in some step of IL-2-induced proliferation of human T-lymphoblasts was suggested by the inhibition of such proliferation by the PAF synthesis inhibitor, L-648611 [15].

Interleukin-2 production

Because lymphocyte proliferation involves, in its early stages, the production of IL-2, we measured the production of this lymphokine by PBML at 24 h of stimulation with PHA, in the presence or absence of PAF. Again, a concentration-dependent inhibition of IL-2 production was observed with an IC_{50} of 10^{-11} M and reversal by the PAF antagonist BN 52021 [10]. It was necessary for PAF to be present during the first hour of the 24-h culture for the effect to be measurable. In contrast, Dulioust *et al.* [12] reported that PAF suppressed CD4 + T-cell proliferation, but the inhibition was not associated with inhibition of IL-2 production.

In vivo infusion of PAF into rats via osmotic mini-pumps has allowed the study of PAF effects in whole animals. After 7 days of infusion, splenocytes from PAF-treated rats showed enhanced IL-2 production in response to Con A [16], indicating that contrary to its direct effects *in vitro*, PAF could exert a positive effect on T-cells *in vivo*, potentially via interactions with selected lymphocyte sub-populations or with non-lymphoid cells (macrophages, endothelial cells, etc.).

As will be indicated below, both inhibition of lymphocyte proliferation, on the one hand, and augmentation of lymphoblast responses to IL-2, on the other, in the presence of PAF, could be explained by the simultaneous actions of this lipid mediator on separate T-cell sub-populations with divergent immunoregulatory properties.

Induction of suppressor and helper cell activity

Inhibition of lymphocyte functions may be due to interference with one or more stages of activation. It can also be due to induction or activation of suppressor cells. To test the latter hypothesis in relation to PAF-induced effects, we pre-incubated human lymphocytes with PAF for 3–18 h. The cells were then washed and added to fresh autologous lymphocytes stimulated with mitogens. Using this co-culture system, we found that PAF-pretreated PBML exerted a significant suppressor effect on proliferation of indicator PBML [17,18]. When PBML were fractionated into selected sub-sets and purified as monocytes, T-cells or selected T-cell sub-populations before pre-incubation with PAF, a remarkable spectrum of activities emerged: PAF-preincubated monocytes were induced to express indomethacin-sensitive suppressor cell function. Monocyte-depleted lymphocytes showed slight helper effect, while CD8 + T-cells were induced to become indomethacin-resistant suppressor cells. CD8 + T-cells required 10–100-fold lower concentrations of PAF to exert suppression. CD4 + T-cells, in contrast, were activated to exert a very marked helper effect.

During inflammation, blood lymphocytes cross the wall of blood vessels to infiltrate the tissues. Endothelial cells, which line the vessels, can thus modulate lymphocyte functions; in particular, some products of endothelial cells, such as PAF, can inhibit the proliferation of lymphocytes. We have therefore exposed human endothelial cells (HEC), isolated from the umbilical cord vein, for 1 h to PAF, the PAF antagonist BN 52021 (10^{-4} M), interleukin-1 (IL-1) or to the cyclooxygenase inhibitor indomethacin (10^{-6} M), alone or in combination. The HEC were then treated with mitomycin C, and washed and incubated for 72 h with lymphocytes and Con A. We observed that the pre-incubation of HEC with IL-1 alone or with indomethacin induced a significant suppression of lymphocyte proliferation of 20 and 25%, respectively [19]. Concomitant use of BN 52021 completely prevented this suppressor activity exerted by HEC, suggesting that endogenous PAF from HEC was mediating the suppressive effect. Pre-incubation of HEC with exogenous PAF (10^{-12} to 10^{-8} M) also induced suppressor cell activity and this was blocked by BN 52021. These results suggest that IL-1 and indomethacin together stimulate the production of PAF by HEC, which in turn suppresses lymphocyte proliferation. This effect of PAF is blocked by BN 52021 which can thus restore normal lymphocyte proliferation. Immunoregulation by endothelial cell-derived PAF and its prevention by a PAF antagonist may have important bearings in the numerous disease states where vascular inflammation is a prominent component.

Membrane antigen expression

The induction of suppressor lymphocytes was accompanied, in our studies, by an increase in CD8 + T-cell numbers and a slight decrease in CD4 + T-cells [18], as assessed by indirect immunofluorescence and flow cytometry. CD2 + (sheep erythrocyte receptor-positive) T-cells were also increased in number, but the most striking increase was seen in T-cells bearing DR antigens. No effect was seen on the number of IL-2 receptor (Tac)-positive T-cells. In contrast, Vivier *et al.* [20] reported partial down-regulation of CD2 and CD3 antigen expression by PAF following incubation with PAF in a time- and concentration-dependent manner. HLA class-I antigen expression was not affected. The very high (0.2–1×10^{-5} M) concentrations of PAF used in the latter study, in contrast to those (10^{-12} to 10^{-8}M) used in ours, may account for the differences observed.

Cytotoxic cell functions

Cytotoxic cells and their various effector mechanisms are thought to play an important role in host defences against a whole array of foreign invaders, including parasites, viruses, neoplastic and grafted cells. Many effector cell types (T-cells, NK cells and other natural cytotoxic lymphocytes, macrophages, polymorphonuclear leukocytes, etc.) participate in these functions and most of the effector mechanisms involved appear distinct but are still largely undefined.

Preliminary data from several laboratories suggest that PAF may play a role during certain cytotoxic activities, as PAF receptor antagonists have been shown to inhibit them. For example, BN 52021 can inhibit rat splenic lymphocyte-mediated lysis of Langerhans islet cells [21]. In other non-lymphocyte systems, keratinocyte killing of *Candida albicans* [22] and eosinophil-mediated cytotoxicity against *Schistosoma mansoni* [23] were also found to be blocked by the PAF antagonist.

Several lines of evidence indicate that NK-cell activation involves membrane phospholipid metabolism and we have previously described modulation of NK function by the arachidonic acid metabolites, leukotriene B_4 [24,25] and thromboxane A_2 [26]. When human monocyte-depleted lymphocytes were cultured with the NK-sensitive K562 target cells in a standard 4-h ^{51}Cr release assay, in the presence of graded concentrations of PAF, we found NK activity to be significantly enhanced (32–110%) at all effector target cell ratios, but predominantly so at lower ratios [27,28]. Maximum activity was found at PAF concentrations of

10^{-13} to 10^{-11} M, and this was not blocked by the PAF antagonists BN 52021 and WEB 2086. In contrast, PAF concentrations of $\geqslant 10^{-7}$ were often associated with inhibition of NK activity, an effect which could be reversed by PAF antagonists. While optimal enhancement was observed when PAF was added at the initiation of the cytotoxicity coculture, or within the first 30 min, significant enhancement was also seen when PAF was added as late as 1 h into the culture. Lymphocytes could also be pre-incubated for 1–18 h with PAF, followed by washing to avoid interaction of PAF with target cells, and significant enhancement of NK activity still ensued. Both binding of lymphocytes to K562 cells and post-binding single cell lytic efficiency were augmented by PAF [28].

Although it is impossible to verify at present, the above findings could be explained by the presence of two PAF receptors on NK cells, one with a lower affinity, which could be linked with inhibition of cell function, and another with high affinity, linked with augmentation of cell function. Mandi *et al.* [29] reported a marked inhibition of both rat and human NK-cell function by BN 52021 and other structurally non-related PAF antagonists such as BN 52111 and BN 52115. Conversely, data concerning allo-specific cytotoxic T-lymphocytes (CTL) suggest that PAF may have inhibitory effects, since BN 52021 enhances the generation of CTL when included in the mixed-lymphocyte culture [13].

In several transplantation models, however, PAF appears to act as a pro-rejection mediator [30]. BN 52021 increases cardiac allograft survival in rats, acting synergistically with azathioprine and cyclosporine A [31]. Analogous findings have also been reported with skin [32], liver [33] and kidney [34] grafts. The mechanism(s) and cells involved in these phenomena in relation to PAF are essentially unknown at present.

Additional studies were undertaken to evaluate the possibility that PAF could modulate NK activity by enhancing the production of cytotoxic cytokines. In these investigations, large granular lymphocytes (LGL) were incubated with various target cell lines (K562, Clone I, MA-160, SK-MEL 109), in the presence or absence of PAF. Supernatants were collected and assayed for cytotoxicity in a 20-h ^{51}Cr-release assay against WEHI 164 and U-937 target cells which are sensitive to cytotoxic cytokines. The results showed that LGL incubated with several types of target cells, in the presence of PAF released significantly increased amounts of cytotoxic factors [35]. The maximal release was obtained after 8–10 h of incubation. Mannose 6-phosphate (10 mM) which inhibits natural killer cytotoxic factor (NKCF) was not able to block supernatant cytotoxicity against U-937 target cells, while anti-tumour necrosis factor-α (TNF) antibody completely abolished supernatant activity. These findings suggest that picomolar concentrations of PAF enhance the release of cytotoxic factor(s), mainly TNF, by LGL following interaction with target cells.

Effects on monocytes–macrophages

That PAF can activate monocyte or macrophage functions has been known for some time, as shown by Hartung [36]. More recently, Ho *et al.* [37] observed that PAF could modulate the expression of c-*fos* and c-*myc* oncogenes in human monocytes, indicating that PAF can initiate activation or differentiation of monocytes at the gene level. Studies on the early PAF-induced events of GTPase stimulation, adenylate cyclase inhibition, phosphoinositide metabolism, calcium mobilization and protein phosphorylation [38–43] have led to suggestions that there is more than one class of PAF receptor and that PAF interacts with a GTP-binding (guanine nucleotide regulatory) protein which differs from the classical N_s and N_i proteins by its insensitivity to cholera and pertussis toxins. Elucidation of the molecular events leading to modulation of the various monocyte–macrophage functions is presently the object of numerous studies, in particular as it relates to cytokine synthesis and release.

Interleukin-1 production

When exogenous PAF is added to monocytes or macrophages, several patterns of responsiveness in terms of IL-1 production can be seen, as reported from different laboratories. Mouse peritoneal macrophages, elicited either with thioglycollate or starch, respond in a varied and irregular manner to PAF (unpublished). In contrast, rat splenic macrophages present a biphasic response [44]: low concentrations of PAF (10^{-12} to 10^{-10} M) significantly enhance IL-1 production while higher concentrations are inhibitory. Continuous low-rate administration of PAF *in vivo*, in rats, via osmotic mini-pumps also revealed a biphasic effect on subsequent *ex vivo* IL-1 production by rat splenic monocytes [16]: cells from rats having received 28 μg of PAF during 7 days showed impaired IL-1 (both released and cell-associated) production in response to LPS stimulation. In contrast, cells from rats having received 1–9 μg of PAF showed augmented IL-1 production. These effects were abolished in animals having received a concomitant treatment with BN 52021, given orally.

IL-1 production by human monocytes is also modulated by PAF. Barret *et al.* [45] initially reported an enhanced production of IL-1 when human monocytes were cultured in the presence of graded concentrations of PAF. Even in the absence of any other stimulus, such as lipopolysaccharide (LPS), (*R*)PAF and PAF analogues PR 1501 and PR 1502, but not (*S*) PAF, were capable of inducing IL-1 production. Salem *et al.* [46] also showed that PAF could increase IL-1 production by human monocytes stimulated with muramyl dipeptide, with higher concentrations of PAF inducing the maximum responses.

Studies in our laboratory also indicate a positive effect of PAF on IL-1 production by human monocytes stimulated with muramyl dipeptide (MDP) or LPS [47]. Using platelet-free, elutriated human monocytes, we found that PAF augmented IL-1 production in a concentration-dependent manner characterized by 2 peaks, one at high (10^{-8} to 10^{-6} M) and another at low (10^{-15} to 10^{-14} M) concentrations. Failure to remove platelets following isolation of monocytes by adherence resulted in varied responses to PAF, with predominant inhibition of IL-1 production at higher concentrations. BN 52021 abrogated the PAF effects, mainly in the higher concentration range.

PAF can also synergize with interferon-γ (IFN) and TNF to induce higher levels of IL-1 production by human monocytes [48]. This may be part of an amplification loop since cytokines (IL-1, TNF, IFN) stimulate a biphasic synthesis of PAF by human monocytes [49]. Thus, in addition to directly modulating monocyte activity, at very low concentrations, PAF can also 'prime' the cells to respond in an enhanced manner to subsequent stimuli that would otherwise be ineffectual. We have recently shown that PAF can prime (following an 18-h pre-incubation) monocytes to produce augmented quantities of IL-1. This may be analogous to the observations in polymorphonuclear (PMN) leukocytes where priming with PAF augments their superoxide generation, elastase release and lysis of endothelial cells in response to phorbol ester or formyl-methionyl-phenylalanine (fMLP) [50]. TNF can also prime PMN for enhanced PAF-induced superoxide production [51]. When human PMN were incubated for 3 h at 37°C with various concentrations of TNF (1–1000 ng/ml), a significant dose-dependent generation of superoxide was observed. The response was maximal with 10 ng/ ml TNF and after 60–90 min of incubation, $O_2^{\cdot -}$ production declining after this time. PAF alone (0.1 fM–0.1 nM) failed to elicit any superoxide production, however, when PAF was added for 10 min to cells previously incubated for 80 min with 10 ng/ml TNF, superoxide production was enhanced relative to that induced by TNF alone. Maximum amplification (+30%) was obtained with 10 fM PAF and the enhancing effect of the mediator was completely abolished by four structurally-unrelated PAF antagonists (BN 52021, kadsurenone, BN 52111 and WEB 2086), added either simultaneously with TNF or PAF [51]. In addition, the PAF antagonists also decreased by 50% the superoxide production elicited solely by TNF, indicating that TNF-induced superoxide generation is partially mediated by a mechanism involving endogenous PAF (M. Braquet, unpublished). LPS can also prime PMN for enhanced PAF production [52].

Tumour necrosis factor production

Another major cytokine produced by monocytes and macrophages is TNF, which has been found to mediate not only cytotoxic activities against various target cells but also inflammatory and immunoregulatory functions.

When rat alveolar macrophages (AM) were cultured with PAF alone, no change in TNF production was observed. However, the concomitant addition of PAF and muramyl dipeptide (MDP) to AM cultures markedly enhanced (2–3 fold) TNF production in a concentration-dependent fashion with a maximum effect at 10^{-10}M PAF [53,54]. This enhancement occurred when MDP and PAF were present together at the initiation of the 24-h culture. Stimulation of TNF production by PAF was blocked by specific PAF receptor antagonists, BN 52020, BN 52021 and WEB 2086 with IC_{50} of respectively, 1×10^{-6} M, 2.0×10^{-7} M and 8.0×10^{-8} M. Additionally, the stereoisomer of PAF, (*S*) PAF, used at 10^{-10} to 10^{-12} M failed to induce significant enhancement in TNF production. In parallel, addition of PAF to AM triggered leukotriene B_4 (LTB_4) release in a concentration-dependent manner. Inhibition of 5-lipoxygenase by NDGA or AA-861 blocked the PAF-induced augmentation of both TNF and LTB_4 production. These findings suggest that PAF stimulates TNF production by interaction with a specific putative receptor and by subsequent induction of endogenous leukotriene production.

The ability of lipoxygenase products, mainly leukotriene B_4, to participate in immunoregulatory processes and to modulate cytokine production has been previously documented [3]. Exogenous and endogenous LTB_4 was found to enhance IL-1, IL-2 and IFN production [55,56]. Recently, we observed that exogenous and endogenous LTB_4 can up-regulate TNF production by rat alveolar macrophages [57] and human monocytes [58]. Thus, the findings of a concentration-dependent LTB_4 production by AM stimulated with PAF and the concomitant inhibition of PAF-induced TNF production as well as LTB_4 generation by lipoxygenase inhibitors are consistent with the possibility that the action of PAF on AM can be mediated by the generation of endogenous lipoxygenase metabolites, probably LTB_4, which will further act as second messengers to induce TNF production. Human monocytes–macrophages can also be stimulated by PAF to produce augmented quantities of TNF [47,53,59]. We have observed that TNF production is enhanced at two concentration ranges of PAF, 10^{-15} to 10^{-13} M and 10^{-9} to 10^{-7} M in LPS-treated monocytes. BN 52021 blocks both effects, while pertussis toxin partially inhibits the effect of higher PAF concentrations, suggesting mediation through a N_i-type guanine nucleotide regulatory protein.

Furthermore, PAF or IL-1 can prime monocytes to respond to LPS with enhanced production of TNF during a subsequent culture with IL-1 or PAF, respectively. These findings suggest again that a cascade of inflammatory signals may have much greater effects than simultaneous or individual activities.

Cytotoxic activity

Although several studies are in progress to assess the effects of PAF in monocyte-macrophage-mediated cytotoxicity, relatively little is known at present. Bonavida *et al.* [59] reported that the presence of TNF inhibitors may be responsible for lack of cytotoxicity when TNF production by human monocytes was enhanced in response to PAF. In our studies, PAF-treated rat alveolar macrophages show augmented killing of P815 (TNF-resistant) target cells while killing of WEHI-164 (TNF-sensitive) targets is only moderately enhanced.

Conclusions and perspectives

As shown by the results of numerous current studies, PAF appears to exert several potent immunoregulatory functions at various levels of the immune response. Some studies, such as those on NK-cell activity and macrophage production of TNF suggest that these cells may bear more than one class of receptors for PAF, with different patterns of inhibition by PAF antagonists and distinct coupling to GTP-binding proteins. Further studies on the binding and molecular definition of PAF receptors on cells of the immune system will be needed to determine this potentially important mechanism for modulating the immune function.

Acknowledgements

Studies by the authors presented in this chapter were supported by grants from the National Cancer Institute and the Medical Research Council of Canada, and by the Institut Henri Beaufour, France, M. R.-P. is a Research Scholar of the Fonds de la Recherche en Santé du Québec.

References

1 Rocklin, R. E. & Haberek-Davidson, A. Histamine activates suppressor cells *in vitro*: a coculture technique. *J. Clin. Immunol.* (1981), **1**, 73–79.

2 Goodwin, J. S. & Ceuppens, J. Regulation of the immune response by prostaglandins. *J. Clin. Immunol.* (1983), **3**, 295–315.

3 Rola-Pleszczynski, M. Immunoregulation by leukotrienes and other lipoxygenase metabolites. *Immunol. Today.* (1985), **6**, 302–307.

4 Payan, D. G., McGillis, J. P. & Goetzl, E. J. Neuroimmunology. *Adv. Imunol.* (1986), **39**, 299–323.

5 Chilton, F. H., Ellis, J. M., Olson, S. C. & Wykle, R. L. 1-O-alkyl-2-arachidonyl-*sn*-glycero-3-phosphocholine. A common source of platelet-activating factor and arachidonate in human polymorphonuclear leukocytes. *J. Biol. Chem.* (1984), **259**, 12014–12019.

6 Braquet, P., Touqui, L., Shen, T. Y. & Vargaftig, B. B. Perspectives in platelet-activating factor research. *Pharmacol. Rev.* (1987), **39**, 97–145.

7 Jouvin-Marche, E., Ninio, E., Beauvain, G., Tence, M., Niaudet, P. & Benveniste, J. Biosynthesis of PAF-acether (platelet-activating factor). VII. Precursors of PAF-acether and acetyltransferase activity in human leukocytes. *J. Immunol.* (1984), **133**, 892–898.
8 Bussolino, F., Foa, R., Malavasi, F., Ferrando, M. L. & Camussi, G. Release of platelet-activating factor (PAF)-like material from human lymphoid cell lines. *Exp. Haematol.* (1984), **12**, 688–693.
9 Malavasi, F., Tetta, C., Funaro, A., Bellone, G., Ferrero, E. & Caligaris Cappio, F. F_c receptor triggering induces expression of surface activation antigens and release of platelet-activating factor in large granular lymphocytes. *Proc. Nat. Acad. Sci. (USA)* (1986), **83**, 2443–2447.
10 Rola-Pleszczynski, M., Pignol, B., Pouliot, C. & Braquet, P. Inhibition of human lymphocyte proliferation and interleukin-2 production by platelet-activating factor (PAF-acether): reversal by a specific antagonist: BN52021. *Biochem. Biophys. Res. Commun.* (1987), **142**, 754–760.
11 Pignol, B., Mencia-Huerta, J. M., Braquet, P. & Rola-Pleszczynski, M. Inhibition of IL-2 production and lymphocyte proliferation by platelet-activating factor (PAF-acether) or analogs and its reversal by the specific antagonists BN52020 and BN52021. *Fed. Proc.* (1987), **46**, 6990.
12 Dulioust, A., Vivier, E., Salem, P., Benveniste, J. & Thomas, Y. Immunoregulatory functions of PAF-acether. I. Effect of PAF-acether on CD4+ cell proliferation. *J. Immunol.* (1988), **140**, 240–245.
13 Gebhardt, B. M., Braquet, P., Bazan, H. E. P. & Bazan, N. G. Modulation of *in vitro* immune reactions by platelet-activating factor and a platelet-activating factor antagonist. *Immunopharmacology* (1988), **15**, 11–20.
14 Behrens, T. & Goodwin, J. S. Effect of PAF on B and T cell proliferation. *Prostaglandins* (1987), **34**, 154.
15 Ward, S. G., Lewis, G. P. & Westwick, J. Differential effect of platelet-activating factor receptor antagonists on human T lymphocyte proliferation. *Prostaglandins* (1987), **34**, 149.
16 Pignol, B., Hénane, S., Sorlin, B., Rola-Pleszczynski, M., Mencia-Huerta, J. M. & Braquet, P. Effect of long-term treatment with platelet-activating factor (PAF) on interleukin-1 (IL-1) and interleukin-2 (IL-2) production by rat spleen cells. In Braquet, P. (ed.) *New Trends in Lipid Mediator Research* (1988), Vol. 1, pp. 38–43. Karger, Basle.
17 Rola-Pleszczynski, M. & Turcotte, S. Activation of suppressor lymphocytes and monocytes by PAF-acether. *Prostaglandins* (1987), **34**, 148.
18 Rola-Pleszczynski, M., Pouliot, C., Turcotte, S., Pignol, B., Braquet, P. & Bouvrette, L. Immune regulation by platelet-activating factor. I. Induction of suppressor cell activity in human monocytes and CD8 + and T cells and of helper activity in CD4 + T cells. *J. Immunol.* (1988), **104**, 3547–3552.
19 Lacasse, C. & Rola-Pleszczynski, M. Implication of platelet activating factor (PAF) in immunoregulation by human endothelial cells (HEC). *FASEB J.* (1988), **2**, A1450.
20 Vivier, E., Salem, P., Dulioust, A. *et al.* Immunoregulatory funtions of PAF-acether. II. Decrease of CD2 and CD3 antigen expression. *Eur. J. Immunol.* (1988), **18**, 425–430.
21 Farkas, G., Mandi, Y., Koltai, M. & Braquet, P. Role of PAF in splenic lymphocyte-induced impairment of Langerhans cells. *Prostaglandins* (1987), **34**, 158.
22 Dobozy, A., Hunyadi, J., Kenderessy, A., Csato, M. & Braquet, P. Effects of lipid mediator inhibitors on the UV-B irradiation-induced elevated *Candida albicans* killing activity of human keratinocytes and polymorphonuclear leukocytes. In

Braquet, P. (ed.) *New Trends in Lipid Mediator Research* (1988), Vol. 1, 168–176. Karger, Basle.

23 McDonald, A. J., Moqbel, R., Wardlaw, A. J. & Kay, A. B. Platelet-activating factor (PAF-acether) enhances eosinophil cytotoxicity *in vitro*. *J. Allergy Clin. Immunol.* (1986), **77**, 227.

24 Rola-Pleszczynski, M., Gagnon, L. & Sirois, P. Leukotriene B_4 augments human natural cytotoxic cell activity. *Biochem. Biophys. Res. Commun.* (1983), **113**, 531–537.

25 Gagnon, L., Girard, M., Sullivan, A. K. & Rola-Pleszczynski, M. Augmentation of human natural cytotoxic cell activity by leukotriene B_4 mediated by enhanced effector–target cell binding and increased lytic efficiency. *Cell. Immunol.* (1987), **110**, 243–252.

26 Rola-Pleszczynski, M., Gagnon, L., Bolduc, D. & LeBreton, G. Evidence for the involvement of the thromboxane synthase pathway in human natural cytotoxic cell activity. *J. Immunol.* (1985), **135**, 4114–4119.

27 Rola-Pleszczynski, M. & Turcotte, S. Enhancement of human natural killer cell activity by platelet-activating factor. *Immunobiol. (Supplement)* **3**, 135.

28 Rola-Pleszczynski, M., Turcotte, S., Gagnon, L. *et al.* Enhancement of natural killer (NK) cell activity by platelet-activating factor. In Braquet, P. (ed.) *New Trends in Lipid Mediator Research* (1988), Vol. 1, pp. 89–98. Karger, Basle.

29 Mandi, Y., Farkas, G., Koltai, M., Braquet, P. and Beladi, I. The effect of BN52021, a PAF-acether antagonist, on natural killer activity. In Braquet, P. (ed.) *New Trends Lipid Mediator Research* (1988), Vol. 1, 76–84. Karger, Basle.

30 Foegh, M. & Ramwell, P. PAF and transplant immunology. *Prostaglandins* (1987), **34**, 186.

31 Foegh, M. L., Khirabadi, B. S., Rowles, J. R., Braquet, P. & Ramwell, P. W. Prolongation of cardiac allograft survival with BN52021, a specific antagonist of platelet-activating factor. *Transplantation* (1986), **42**, 86–88.

32 Mulno, J. C., Ruggieri, J. P., Ale, A. & Cejas, H. A. Prolongation of rabbit skin allograft survival with immunosuppression and specific antagonist of platelet-activating factor. *Transplant. Proc.* (1988), **20**, 313–315.

33 Filipponi, F., Michel, A., Guillon, J. M., Braquet, P. & Houssin, D. Prolongation of experimental liver xenograft survival using a PAF antagonist. *Prostaglandins* (1988), **35**, 806.

34 Makowaka, L., Chapman, F., Mazzaferro, V. *et al.* The role of PAF-antagonist in experimental hyperacute rejection. *Prostaglandins* (1988), **35**, 806.

35 Bossé, J., Turcotte, S. & Rola-Pleszczynski, M. Platelet activating factor (PAF) enhances the production of cytotoxic cytokines during natural cell-mediated cytotoxicity. *FASEB J.* (1988), **2**, A415.

36 Hartung, H. P. Acetylglyceryletherphosphorylcholine (platelet-activating factor) mediates heightened metabolic activity in macrophages. Studies on PGE_1, TXA_2, and O_2 production, spreading and the influence of calmodulin inhibitor W-7. *FEBS Lett.* (1983), **160**, 209–212.

37 Ho, Y. S., Lee, W. M. F. & Snyderman, R. Chemoattractant-induced activations of c-*fos* gene expression in human monocytes. *J. Exp. Med.* (1987), **165**, 1524–1538.

38 Homma, H. & Hanahan, D. J. Attenuation of platelet-activating factor (PAF)-induced stimulation of rabbit platelet GTPase by phorbol ester, dibutyryl cAMP, and desensitisation: concomitant effects on PAF receptor binding characteristics. *Arch. Biochem. Biophys.* (1988), **262**, 32–39.

39 Bachelet, M., Adolfs, M. J. P., Masliah, J. *et al.* Interaction between PAF-acether and drugs that stimulate cyclic AMP in guinea-pig alveolar macrophages. *Eur. J. Pharmacol.* (1988), **149**, 73–78.

40 Barzaghi, G. & Mong, S. Platelet-activating factor (PAF) stimulates a phospholipase C (PLC) in differentiated human monocytic leukemia (U-937) cells which results in phosphoinositide (PI) hydrolysis and intracellular calcium mobilization. *Prostaglandins* (1988), **35**, 819.

41 Hopple, S., Meurer, R., Westwick, J. & Macintyre, D. E. PAF-induced Ca^{2+} flux and formation of inositol tris- and tetraisphosphates in U937 cells. *FASEB J.* (1988), **2**, A415.

42 Prpic, V., Uhing, R. J., Weiel, J. E. *et al.* Biochemical and functional responses stimulated by platelet-activating factor in murine peritoneal macrophages. *J. Cell Biol.* (1988), **107**, 363–372.

43 Bussolino, F., Turrini, F., Fischer, E., Alessi, D., Karzatchline, M. D. & Arese, P. PAF enahances erythrophagocyctic activity of human monocytes by the protein kinase C dependent phosphorylation of C36 receptor (CR1). Role of PAF receptor antagonists. *Prostaglandins* (1988), **35**, 803.

44 Pignol, B., Hénane, S., Mencia-Huerta, J. M., Rola-Pleszczynski, M. & Braquet, P. Effect of platelet-activating factor (PAF-acether) and its specific receptor antagonist, BN 52021, on interleukin-1- (IL-1) release and synthesis by rat spleen adherent monocytes. *Prostaglandins* (1987), **33**, 931–939.

45 Barret, M. L., Lewis, G. P., Ward, S. & Westwick, J. Platelet-activating factor induces interleukin-1 production from human adherent macrophages. *Br. J. Pharmacol.* (1987), **90**, 113p.

46 Salem, P., Dulioust, A., Derickz, S., Vivier, E., Benveniste, J. & Thomas, Y. PAF-acether (platelet-activating factor) increases interleukin-1 (IL-1) secretion by human monocytes. *Fed. Proc.* (1987), **46**, 922.

47 Rola-Pleszczynski, M., Gingras, D. & Poubelle, P. PAF-acether enhances the production of tumour necrosis factor (TNF) and interleukin-1 (IL-1) by human monocytes. Submitted for publication (1988).

48 Barthelson, R., Valone, F. H., Debs, R. & Philip, R. Synergy in interleukin-1 (IL-1) release by human monocytes stimulated with platelet-activating factor (PAF) plus gamma interferon (IFN gamma) or tumour necrosis factor (TNF). *FASEB J.* (1988), **2**, A1228.

49 Valone, F. H. & Epstein, L. B. Biphasic platelet-activating factor (PAF) synthesis by human monocytes stimulated with interleukin-1 beta (IL-1), tumour necrosis factor (TNF) or gamma interferon (IFN). *FASEB J.* (1988), **2**, A878.

50 Vercellotti, G. M., Yin, H. Q., Gustabson, K. S., Nelson, R. D. & Jacob, H. S. Platelet-activating factor primes neutrophils responses to agonists: role in promoting neutrophil-mediated endothelial damage. *Blood* (1988), **71**, 1100–1107.

51 Paubert-Braquet, M., Lonchampt, M. O., Klotz, P. & Guilbaud, J. Tumor necrosis factor (TNF) primes platelet-activating factor (PAF)-induced superoxide generation by human neutrophils (PMN): consequences in promoting PMN-mediated endothelial cell (EC) damages. *Prostaglandins* (1988), **35**, 803.

52 Worthen, G. S., Seccombe, J. F., Clay, K. L., Guthrie, L. A. & Johnston, R. B., Jr. The priming of neutrophils by lipopolysaccharide for production of intracellular platelet-activating factor. *J. Immunol.* (1988), **140**, 3553–3559.

53 Rola-Pleszczynski, M., Bossé, J., Bissonnette, E. & Dubois, C. PAF-acether enhances the production of tumor necrosis factor by human and rodent lymphocytes and macrophages. *Prostaglandins* (1988), **35**, 802.

54 Dubois, C., Bissonnette, E. & Rola-Pleszczynski, M. Asbestos fibers and silica particles stimulate rat alveolar macrophages to release TNF; autoregulatory role of leukotriene B_4. *Am. Rev. Resp. Dis.* (1989), **139**, 1257–1264.

55 Rola-Pleszczynski, M. & Lemaire, I. Leukotrienes augment interleukin-1 production by human monocytes. *J. Immunol.* (1985), **135**, 3958–3961.

56 Rola-Pleszczynski, M., Chavaillaz, P. A. & Lemaire, M. Stimulation of interleukin-2 and interferon gamma production by leukotriene B_4 in human lymphocyte cultures. *Prostagl. Leuk. Med.* (1986), **23**, 207–210.
57 Dubois, C., Bissonnette, E. & Rola-Pleszczynski, M. Platelet-activating factor (PAF) stimulates tumor necrosis factor production by alveolar macrophages: prevention by PAF receptor antagonists and lipoxygenase inhibitors. *J. Immunol.* (1989), **143**, in press.
58 Gagnon, L., Fillion, L. G. & Rola-Pleszczynski, M. Enhanced production of tumor necrosis factor (TNF)-alpha by human monocytes exposed to leukotriene B_4. *J. Leuk. Biol.* Submitted for publication (1988).
59 Bonavida, B. & Braquet, P. Effect of platelet-activating factor (PAF) on monocyte activation and production of tumor necrosis factor (TNF). *Prostaglandins* (1988), **35**, 802.

Chapter 14
PAF and the establishment of pregnancy

Christopher O'Neill

Introduction

Until relatively recent times the processes of fertilization and development of the early mammalian embryo have remained rather mysterious events. Progress in steroid and peptide endocrinology and, more recently, the development of diagnostic ultrasound, however, have allowed major advances in our understanding of the control, and monitoring of the status, of gametogenesis in both sexes and the progress of pregnancy once it has been well established.

Folliculogenesis, ovulation and spermatogenesis involve the production of hormones by large numbers of highly differentiated cells, thus the signal (hormone) produced is large and hence easily detected. In the case of fertilization however, we are dealing with only two cells: the single oocyte and the individual spermatozoon which fertilizes it (in some polytocous species, of course, these numbers are higher, e.g. the mouse may routinely produce 20 embryos in some strains). The resulting one-cell embryo (the zygote) is, by definition, entirely undifferentiated. Intuitively then, it seems unlikely that such undifferentiated tissues should secrete significant amounts of hormones.

Following fertilization the human embryo undergoes a number of mitotic divisions so that after 4–6 days it reaches the blastocyst stage (the time to reach the blastocyst stage varies considerably between species). At this stage the embryo has <200 cells. However this is the first stage where clear differentiation of cells occurs. The embryo segregates into two different cell populations, the trophectoderm and the inner cell mass (ICM). Such differentiation suggests that the production of hormones would be more likely to occur by this stage of development. The total number of cells however, in each population is still relatively small. It is also at the blastocyst stage that the embryo ceases to exist in the free-living state and forms an attachment and intimate association with the maternal uterine endometrium. This process is known as 'implantation'. It is soon after implantation that the trophectoderm further differentiates into the trophoblast and rapidly proliferates and becomes invasive. This significant mass of tissue then begins to produce large amounts of secreted hormones. In the human the best example of this is human chorionic gonadotrophin (hCG).

Thus, from the time of fertilization till after implantation, the conceptus, because of its very small mass and its undifferentiated state has until recently been considered not to produce signals that direct or effect, in a significant manner, maternal physiology and because of its small mass and lack of defined structures it has not been visible to imaging techniques such as ultrasound. As a consequence the first week or so of pregnancy has remained undetectable.

This inability to detect or monitor early pregnancy apart from restricting to a very great degree our understanding of its basic physiology has important practical implications. For the clinician, this stage of pregnancy becomes a therapeutic 'black box'. If ovulation is shown to occur, insemination with a normal semen sample takes place and there are no occlusions of the reproductive tract, then pregnancy is expected to occur. When this is not the case the clinician currently has no way of defining the cause of pregnancy failure. This condition, known as 'idiopathic infertility' or 'infertility of unknown cause' is common and in most populations 25% of infertile couples suffer from it. It is frustrating to both clinician and patient since neither an effective treatment nor a rational explanation can be offered.

The development in recent years of fertilization of oocytes and culture of early embryos *in vitro* has provided new insights into this phase of pregnancy. Evidence suggests that fertilization may be a relatively efficient process but that the development of embryos through to the blastocyst stage and implantation is very inefficient. Indeed, estimates in a number of species suggest that failure of pre-implantation embryonic development and implantation may be as high as 35% in otherwise apparently normally fertile females. This represents an enormous loss of efficiency in reproduction.

This high incidence of reproductive failure suggests three obvious practical implications:

1 That a significant cause of idiopathic infertility is likely to be due to embryonic demise prior to implantation and that methods for detecting the presence of the embryo immediately following fertilization are necessary to diagnose this.

2 That even modest improvements in the implantation rate will have a significant influence on the treatment of human infertility and on agricultural production.

3 That further disturbance of implantation may offer the possibilities for new technologies of contraception.

Thus an understanding of the mechanism and signals involved in embryo-maternal communication may play a significant part in developing diagnostic and therapeutic tools for this stage of pregnancy.

Embryonic signals

Apart from the gonadotrophins that are secreted later in pregnancy, there has been proposed a variety of signals produced by the pre-implantation embryo. These include: steroids [1–3], prostaglandins [4,5], leukotrienes [6], histamine [7–9], ovum factor [10], an immunosuppressive factor [11], stage specific proteins [12,13] and platelet activating factor. It is likely that the early embryos of many species produce most or all of these compounds which help to induce and control the inflammation-like properties of early pregnancy without compromising the health of either embryo or mother. Possible roles and the inter-relationship of these mediators have recently been reviewed [14] and here the intention is to concentrate on the role of embryo-derived platelet activating factor in early pregnancy and the likelihood of it fulfilling the clinical diagnostic and therapeutic roles required for the adequate management of early pregnancy (Fig. 14.1).

Embryo-derived PAF

Platelet activating factor, 1-O-alkyl-2-acetyl-*sn*-glycerol-3-phosphocholine (PAF), is an ether phospholipid. The ether phospholipids are ubiquitous, although relatively minor components of animal cells [15]. By contrast, some evolutionary primitive prokaryotes contain relatively higher amounts of ether phospholipids [15]. Thus, to the limited extent that ontogeny recapitulates phylogeny, it may not be surprising that the ether lipid, PAF, should play a significant role in the early development of the embryo. The ether phospholipids have also been found to be elevated in a number of cancer or transformed cell lines. Like the early embryo, such cells can be considered at least partially de-differentiated and the processes of early embryo development and in particular implantation have long been considered to share similarities with neoplastic cell growth.

It first became evident that the early embryo produces PAF by the observation [16] in mice, that splenic contraction and mild, but significant, thrombocytopenia occurred shortly after fertilization and throughout the pre-implantation phase of pregnancy. Appropriate control experiments proved that this was due to platelet activation and was solely dependent upon the presence of the embryo [17]. It was further shown that the human [18,19] and mouse [20] embryos at very early stages of development secreted a soluble platelet-activating factor. Purification and charac-

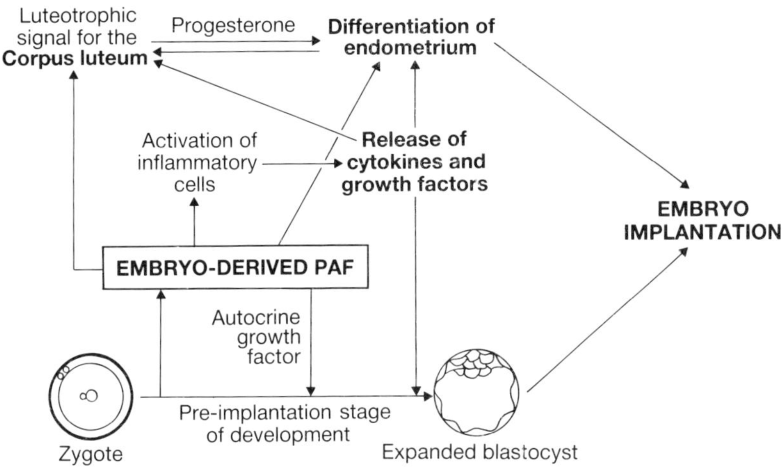

Fig. 14.1 Possible major sites of action of embryo-derived PAF, and the interaction of these functions in support of the establishment of pregnancy. This is not intended to be an exclusive list nor is it meant to show that all uch interactions occur.

terization showed that this agent in both the mouse and the human was homologous with PAF [20,21].

Despite quite high rates of production of PAF by the early embryo [22], it could not be detected in the urine of women soon after successful embryo transfer [23]. This is perhaps not surprising in view of the considerable dilution of embryo-derived PAF which would occur in blood, and also because of the well-known lability of PAF in blood [24,25]. Thus, direct measurement of PAF within body fluids may not be a useful means of monitoring pregnancy. The observation, however, that embryo-derived PAF induced significant maternal thrombocytopenia in a number of species [26] suggested that monitoring maternal platelet count may be a means of diagnosing and monitoring early pregnancy.

A recent study [27] which attempted to validate such alterations as a response to early pregnancy however, showed their response to be quite variable. Patients undergoing *in vitro* fertilization had their peripheral platelet count monitored over the first 10 days following embryo transfer and compared with their platelet count prior to transfer. Of those achieving pregnancy many showed thrombocytopenia throughout the pre-implantation phase with the platelet count returning to pre-ovulatory levels by the time of implantation, while some showed only a transient decrease or no decrease at all. It was apparent from the data however that for those women who failed to show thrombocytopenia there was generally a significant increase in the platelet count observed. It was found that the considerable degree of variability in the response was related to the woman's thrombocrit. A significant negative regression analysis existed between the thrombocrit prior to embryo transfer and the relative change in the peripheral platelet count on the days following embryo transfer. With a larger study it may be possible to construct a nomogram such that, knowing a patient's pre-ovulatory thrombocrit it may be possible to predict with some accuracy the response in the platelet count consistent with early pregnancy. There is however currently insufficient data to determine how reliable such an approach might prove. Alternatively, quantitative detection of the release of platelet specific proteins, such as β-thromboglobulin, or products released from other PAF responsive cells such as polymorphonuclear leukocytes, may serve as a peripheral marker for the release of embryo-derived PAF.

The apparent thrombocytosis in many women in early pregnancy may be due to activation of the thrombopoietic system. Work with experimental animals [28] has shown that severe induction of platelet activation may result in the very rapid onset of thrombopoiesis and in over-compensation with a corresponding significant increase in the peripheral platelet count.

Thus, while the production of embryo-derived PAF caused discernible alterations to maternal physiology in a number of species, the use of such modest changes cannot at this time be used as a reliable means of pregnancy diagnosis.

Production of PAF by the early embryo

Ryan *et al.* [22] undertook a study of the kinetics of production of PAF by embryos. Two-cell mouse embryos in culture produced increasing amounts of PAF for up to 6 h and there was no further increase in PAF production after 24 h. Degenerate embryos failed to produce PAF in culture. After 72 h in culture, two-cell embryos developed to the blastocyst stage. However, a linear reduction in PAF activity was observed for culture media from three consecutive 24 h periods during this period of culture *in vitro*. This appeared to be a factor of *in vitro* culture since morulae and blastocyst embryos (equivalent to a further 48 h and 72 h development, respectively), when freshly collected from the reproductive tract, produced the same level of PAF as two cells. Culture of two-cell embryos in groups of 10–45 for 24 h was carried out and then the amount of PAF determined in a bioassay compared with a standard curve produced by that of a synthetic PAF; 12.8 $\pm$ 1.0 ng PAF/mouse embryo/24 h was found to be produced.

The level of PAF in culture medium is presumably a reflection of the balance between production and catabolism. The relative contributions of these to the loss of PAF activity are not clear at this time. Reduced synthesis may be due to starvation of critical substrates or growth factors *in vitro* or possibly due to a negative feedback of PAF in the culture medium on further embryonic production. Degradation is known to occur by metabolism of PAF to its key intermediate [24,25], lyso-PAF, by the enzyme acetylhydrolase, but its relative activity in the embryo is at this time not known.

It has been known for some time that culture of pre-implantation embryos *in vitro* is detrimental to their subsequent pregnancy potential [29-32], and if PAF is an important embryonic product, then the adverse effect of culture on embryonic PAF production may well be related to the embryos reduced viability.

Similar observations have been made with human embryos produced by *in vitro* fertilization. Using a simple bioassay, it was found that embryos which resulted in pregnancy produced significantly more PAF *in vitro* than did embryos which failed to result in pregnancy following their transfer [18,19,23]. Of a further 85 embryos examined, 43% had a level of PAF that fell in the same range as the embryos that resulted in pregnancy. The production of PAF was related to the type of pharmacological treatment used to induce follicular development, the size and functional characteristics of the follicles from which they originated, the age of the culture medium in which they had developed, and the morphology and cleavage rate of the embryo itself [18].

In a more detailed assessment using a reliable and quantitative bioassay, similar results were observed. The bioassay had a detection limit of 5nM and in double-blind trials on nine separate occasions did not give any false-positive or -negative results. Under these conditions 228 media in which human two-to-four cell embryos had been cultured for 18 h were tested for PAF. A wide range of PAF levels were observed from undetectable to 2700 nM. Of these embryos 121 (53%) gave a concentration significantly greater than the corresponding control culture tube (Table 14.1). The average concentration of PAF in the media in which oocytes

Table 14.1 PAF levels present in human embryos

Parameter	Pregnant	Non-pregnant
Number of patients	30	48
Total number of embryos	94	134
Embryos transferred per patient	3.1	2.8
Number embryos with PAF > control value	55 (58.5%)	66 (49.2%)
PAF concentration (nM) for positive embryos ($\bar{x} \pm$ SE)	295 $\pm$ 107	76 $\pm$ 28
Number of patients with no PAF-positive embryos transferred	4/30 (13.3)	12/46 (26%)

Culture medium in which single human embryos had been incubated for 18h was extracted for PAF and assayed. PAF levels were corrected for the levels seen in a control sample of culture media which had not been exposed to embryos and was extracted in parallel to the test samples. EDPAF = embryo-derived PAF.

had failed to fertilize was 56.6 ± 8.0 nM, not significantly different from the serum containing control culture tubes. The PAF-positive embryos were transferred to 30 patients who became pregnant and to 48 patients who failed to achieve pregnancy. Embryos transferred to women who achieved pregnancy produced more PAF (295 nM) *in vitro* than those transferred to women who failed to achieve pregnancy (75 nM) ($P < 0.03$). The proportion of 'PAF-positive' embryos transferred to pregnant or to non-pregnant women was not different (58.5% versus 49.2%). This suggests that while the production of PAF in itself was not an absolute marker for the capacity of embryos to produce PAF, enhanced production of PAF was associated with pregnancy. This might indicate that a certain minimal production of PAF is required before pregnancy can result and this is consistent with the results of PAF supplementation data to be discussed later. If such a critical lower limit of PAF production exists, its determination must await a more extensive investigation of the correlation between the production of PAF and the subsequent success in cases where only one embryo is transferred. This will take some time and require a multi-centre study since the number of cases in any one *in vitro* fertilization clinic where only one embryo is transferred is small.

Despite the higher amount of PAF produced by embryos resulting in pregnancy, in this trial there was still 13% of patients who became pregnant who had embryos transferred that did not produce PAF. Despite preliminary validation studies using nine different sets of embryo culture medium which failed to detect false-positives or -negatives, this failure to detect PAF in medium from patients who achieved pregnancies was likely to be due to assay failure. In 15% of a large number of culture media containing serum, in which known amounts of synthetic PAF were added, this PAF could not be subsequently detected. Likely reasons for this technical failure might include: (i) enhanced metabolism of PAF prior to extraction; (ii) co-extraction and purification of an inhibitor of the bioassay; and (iii) the binding of PAF to high-affinity binding molecules in serum in some patients but not in others.

Results to date suggest that neither of the first two alternatives provide an explanation. There was no evidence of enhanced activity of acetylhydrolase in any of the culture tubes tested nor was this activity related to any of the endocrine parameters of the patients undergoing treatment. Similarly, there was no evidence for a co-purifying inhibitor of the bioassay, as has recently been reported in another experimental model [33,34]. There is to date little experimental support for high-affinity binding of PAF preventing its detection; however this may be the case. The organic extraction procedure utilized is designed primarily for recovery of PAF from its low-affinity binding to albumin. A number of recent reports suggest specific binding to a number of serum proteins [35,36]. In particular, PAF and lyso-PAF were found to bind to lipoproteins [37]. It is possible that the exaggerated steroid hormone production known to occur in women undergoing *in vitro* fertilization [38–40] might facilitate PAF binding to lipoproteins, since the sex steroids are known to influence the class and type of lipoproteins in blood [41]. Furthermore, serum acetylhydrolase activity is positively correlated with the concentration of low-density lipoproteins and negatively correlated with high density lipoproteins [24,42]. Thus detailed analysis of the PAF carrier molecules may enhance the efficiency of extraction and purification.

While it seems probable that technical factors can account for this false-positive result, one other alternative remains. It may be that at the two-to-four cell stage some embryos which do not yet produce PAF are still capable of resulting in viable pregnancies after transfer. Should this prove to be the case then clearly the use of PAF measurements *in vitro* as a measure of the pregnancy potential of the embryo is of limited value.

The results to date suggest that while PAF is clearly a marker for pregnancy potential and viability of early human embryos it cannot be said at this stage to be an absolute marker. Reduced or absent PAF production is associated with pregnancy failure but at this time there is not a 100% positive association between PAF production and pregnancy. An understanding of the role of PAF in pregnancy may help to define the likely diagnostic potential and limitations of embryo-derived PAF.

The role of embryo-derived PAF in early pregnancy

Direct evidence for the essential role of PAF in the establishment of pregnancy comes from the use of PAF antagonists [43,44]. The administration of a variety of PAF antagonist on days 1–4 of pregnancy in mice (day 1 = day of mating) resulted in highly significant and dose-dependent reductions in the number of embryos undergoing implantation. Similar results have been shown using the rat as a model [45]. In mice the reduction in implantation rate was evident on day 5 of pregnancy by visualizing the implantation sites with Pontamine sky blue dye. Using the PAF antagonist SRI 63-441, it was evident that this contra-gestational action was not due to disruption of the production of the steroid hormones of early pregnancy, progesterone and oestradiol [44].

The effect of the antagonist was not due to embryocidal effects since normal development of two-cell embryos through to the blastocyst stage occurred in the presence of these inhibitors *in vitro* at concentrations that significantly inhibited implantation. Furthermore, blastocysts flushed from the uterus of inhibitor treated mice on day 4 of pregnancy had normal morphology and development [44].

The manner by which PAF exerts this necessary role in pregnancy is not yet entirely clear. Likely maternal sites for its action have been reviewed [46,47] and it is attractive to speculate that the extensive range of cells that PAF is known to activate may play some paracrine role in the establishment of pregnancy. Some recent evidence using PAF antagonists suggest that this may not be the case. Using a broad specificity inhibitor, Iloprost (an analogue of PGI_2), and SRI 63-441 (a PAF receptor antagonist), the dose–response of their anti-platelet actions and their contra-gestational actions showed a poor correlation [44]. While Iloprost had a relatively lower effectiveness against the action of PAF on platelet activation it was considerably more potent in the inhibition of implantation. PAF is known to be a potent mediator of inflammation, inducing peripheral vasodilation and enhanced vasopermeability. However in the

Table 14.2 The contra-gestational and anti-platelet effects of the antagonists Iloprost, WEB 2086, SRI 63-441, SRI 64-412, BN 52021. (From Spinks *et al.* [65])

Inhibitor	Dose giving maximum inhibition of implant (nmol/day)	Dose giving maximum inhibition of platelet aggregation (nM)
Iloprost	5.5	14
WEB 2086	22.0	110
SRI 63-441	60.4	15100
SRI 64-412	117.8	500
BN 52021	23.6	5900

For the contra-gestational study antagonists were administered throughout the pre-implantation period of pregnancy. The anti-platelet effects were evaluated using a platelet aggregation assay as described by Coller *et. al.* [21].

guinea pig, Iloprost potentiated PAF-induced vasopermeability rather than inhibiting it [48]. Furthermore, SRI 63-441 at doses that inhibited implantation did not inhibit the artificially induced deciduoma (increased uterine vasopermeability normally in response to implantation). These results suggest that the actions of PAF on the vasculature are not its crucial role in pregnancy [49].

Of greater significance is the recent observation [47] that for a variety of antagonists tested, the range of contra-gestational doses is narrow and after the effective dose further increases in the amount of drug administered results in a total loss of the functional antagonism of implantation. This was the case for Iloprost, SRI 63-441, WEB 2086, SRI 64-412, and BN 52021 (Table 14.2). This demonstration for a range of chemically-unrelated PAF antagonists compounds is unique to pregnancy and has not previously been reported for any PAF-related condition or test system either *in vitro* or *in vivo*. This suggests that there are features of the action of PAF which are unique to pregnancy and reinforces the likelihood that the maternal cells conventionally associated with the action of PAF (e.g. platelets, leukocytes, or endothelial tissue) are not the primary site of action in pregnancy.

This unique effect of PAF antagonists in early pregnancy suggests a unique target organ; the embryo itself is an intuitively attractive candidate. Indeed, there is now evidence that embryo-derived PAF may play an essential autocrine role in pregnancy.

The production of $^{14}CO_2$ from labelled lactate or glucose was measured to determine whether PAF had a direct effect on embryonic metabolism. Incubation of two-cell embryos in medium supplemented with 1.0 μg PAF/ml resulted in an 18% increase in CO_2 production from lactate. Higher doses resulted in a more variable response. The same dose (1μg/ml) of PAF was responsible for up to a 90% increase in the amount of CO_2 produced from glucose [50]. This was inhibited by the PAF antagonist SRI 63-441 (Ryan & O'Neill, unpublished). Culture of embryos in medium supplemented with PAF did not significantly increase the proportion of embryos developing to the expanded blastocyst stage, however there was a modest ($P < 0.05$) increase in the number of cells in each embryo (72.6 ± 2.7 versus 80.9 ± 4.2).

Cellular mechanisms by which PAF exerts this effect on carbohydrate metabolism have not yet been studied in detail. Its inhibition by the PAF antagonist SRI 63-441 suggests that PAF is acting via membrane receptors although these are yet to be identified on the embryo. In other cell types, PAF binding to cell membranes induces cellular responses following transduction of the signal via membrane guanyl nucleotide regulatory proteins [51–53] promoting generation of inositol triphosphate [54] and diacylglycerol [55]. Inositol triphosphates mobilize calcium [56] and diacylglycerol promotes protein kinase C activity [57]. Protein kinase C may have a role in enhanced carbohydrate metabolism. It effects glucose transfer in adipocytes and glycogenolysis of hepatocytes [58]. In particular, phosphofructokinase may be a substrate for protein kinase C [59]. Phosphofructokinase has been implicated as one of the key regulatory enzymes of early embryonic metabolism [60].

To assess the effect of increasing the available PAF on the pregnancy potential of cultured embryos, expanded blastocysts cultured from the two-cell stage in medium with or without PAF were transferred to pseudopregnant recipients and implantation rates assessed on day 8 of pregnancy [61]. Supplementation of medium with 0.1 μm PAF/ml resulted in a 54% increase in the implantation rate above control levels. By taking into account the between-animal variation, the observed effect could be considered to be due solely to enhanced viability of embryos rather than to any maternal effects following transfer.

These results show that PAF does enhance the viability of embryos as assessed by their capacity to undergo implantation. There is some evidence to suggest that the action of PAF may only be essential at the time of implantation. Administration of the PAF antagonist SRI 63-441 on days 1 and 2 of pregnancy had no significant effect on implantation nor did administration on days 5–8. However administration on days 3 and 4, or 4 alone, suppressed the implantation rate to the same extent as when the drugs were given throughout the entire pre-implantation phase (O'Neill, unpublished). It was noted earlier that PAF antagonists at doses that inhibited implantation did not affect the capacity of mouse embryos to develop *in vitro*, yet PAF antagonists have a different effect on the embryo at the time of implantation *in vitro*.

The pre-implantation mouse embryo grows from the one-cell through to the blastocyst stage in defined culture medium without protein supplementation. Further development and implantation of the embryo requires metabolic activation. This leads to the outgrowth of the trophectoderm onto the substrate and differentiation of the inner cell mass. The metabolic activation can be induced by the provision of either whole serum in the medium or a complex substratum such as reconstituted extracellular matrix. Under either of these conditions the addition of a PAF antagonist inhibited outgrowth in a dose-dependent manner and at doses that did not affect development from the one cell to blastocyst stage [62]. This process is generally recognized to be analogous to implantation [63] and its inhibition *in vitro* by PAF antagonists suggests that the essential role of the PAF in the establishment of pregnancy may be as the autocrine trigger for implantation.

These studies provide a mounting weight of evidence implicating PAF as an essential embryonic mediator for the establishment and maintenance of pregnancy. Its production by the embryo in the first days of pregnancy certainly enhances embryonic metabolism, though the significance of this is yet to be fully defined. However the correlation between embryonic metabolism and subsequent implantation rates suggests that this autocrine control of embryonic metabolic activity has important physiological consequences. An understanding of the pathways of production of PAF by the embryo (be it *de novo*, by a membrane remodelling pathway or a combination of the two) [64,46], is essential for the full understanding of the role and control of pregnancy by PAF. If such evidence for an essential role of PAF in pregnancy is also found in other species, then the potential for the use of PAF as a diagnostic tool in early pregnancy becomes more viable. The enhanced implantation and pregnancy rate induced by the culture of embryos in the presence of exogeneous PAF immediately suggests a potential clinical role in the enhancement of fertility in humans, domestic and endangered exotic species. The observation that a variety of PAF antagonists may inhibit implantation, albeit incompletely, suggests a possible new approach for fertility control.

Acknowledgements

I thank Alaina Ammit, Melanie Collier, Steven Fleming, John Ryan, Douglas M. Saunders and Neil Spinks for their collaboration in many of the studies discussed here and Deborah Gillespie for preparing the manuscript. Some of the work discussed has been performed with the financial assistance of the Australian NH & MRC.

References

1 Wu, J.-T. Metabolism of progesterone by preimplantation mouse blastocysts in culture. *Biol. Reprod.* (1987), **36**, 549–556.

2 Wu, J.-T. & Lin, G. M. The presence of 17β-hydroxysteroid dehydrogenase activity in preimplantation rat and mouse blastocysts. *J. Exp. Zool.* (1982), **220**, 121–124.

3 Dickman, Z., Dey, S. K. & Gupta, J. S. A new concept: control of early pregnancy by steroid hormones originating in the preimplantation embryo. *Vitam. Horm.* (1976), **34**, 215–242.

4 Niimura, S. & Ishida, K. Immunohistochemical demonstration of prostaglandin E_2 in preimplantation mouse embryos. *J. Reprod. Fert.* (1987), **80**, 505–508.

5 Kennedy, T. G. Embryonic signals and the initiation of blastocyst implantation. *Aust. J. Biol. Sci.* (1983), **36**, 531–543.

6 Taylor, C. T., Bolton, V. N., Wilson, C. M. & Collins, W. P. The production of leukotriene B_4 and thromboxane B_2 by human pre-embryos in culture. *Hum. Reprod.* (1988), **3**, (Suppl. 1), Abstract 139.

7 Dey, S. K. Role of histamine in implantation: inhibition of histidine decarboxylase induced delayed implantation in the rabbit. *Biol. Reprod.* (1981), **24**, 867–869.

8 Dey, S. K. & Johnson, D. C. Histamine formation by mouse preimplantation embryos. *J. Reprod. Fert.* (1980), **60**, 457–460.

9 Dey, S. K., Johnson, D. C. & Santos, J. G. Is histamine production by the blastocyst required for implantation in the rabbit? *Biol. Reprod.* (1979), **21**, 1169–1173.

10 Cavanagh, A. C. Production *in vitro* of mouse early pregnancy factor and purification to homogeneity. *J. Reprod. Fert.* (1984), **71**, 581–592.

11 Daya, S. & Clarke, D. A. Immunosuppressive factor produced by human embryos *in vitro*. *New Engl. J. Med.* (1986), **315**, 1551–1552.

12 Nieder, G. L., Weitlauf, H. M. & Suda-Hartman, M. Synthesis and secretion of stage-specific proteins by peri-implantation mouse embryos. *Biol. Reprod.* (1987), **36**, 687-699.

13 Fishel, S. B. & Surani, M. A. H. Evidence for the synthesis and release of a glycoprotein by mouse blastocysts. *J. Reprod. Fert.* (1980), **59**, 181–185.

14 Fleming S., O'Neill C., Collier, M., Spinks, N. R., Ryan, J. P. & Ammit, A. J. The role of embryonic signals in the control of blastocyst implantation. In Yoshinaga, K. (ed.) *Blastocyst Implantation* (1989). *Serono Symposia Publications*. In press.

15 Mangold, H. K. Ether lipids: Relic of the past and promise for the future. *La Rivista delle Sostanze Grasse* (1988), **65**, 349–360.

16 O'Neill, C. Thrombocytopenia is an initial maternal response to fertilization in mice. *J. Reprod. Fert.* (1985), **73**, 567–577.

17 O'Neill, C. Examination of the causes of early pregnancy associated thrombocytopenia in mice. *J. Reprod. Fert.* (1985), **73**, 578–585.

18 O'Neill, C., Gidley-Baird, A. A., Pike, I. L. & Saunders, D. M. A bio-assay for embryo-derived platelet activating factor as a means of assessing quality and pregnancy potential of human embryos. *Fertil. Steril.* (1987), **47**, 969–975.

19 O'Neill, C. & Saunders, D. M. Assessment of embryo quality. *Lancet* (1984), **ii**, 1035.

20 O'Neill, C. Partial characterisation of the embryo-derived platelet activating factor in mice. *J. Reprod. Fert.* (1985), **75**, 375–380.

21 Collier, M., O'Neill, C., Ammit, A. J. & Saunders, D. M. Biochemical and pharmacological characterisation of human embryo-derived platelet activating factor. *Hum. Reprod.* (1988), **8**, 993–998.

22 Ryan, J. P., Spinks, N. R., O'Neill, C., Ammit, A. J. & Wales, R. G. Platelet activating factor (PAF) production by mouse embryos *in vitro* and its effects on embryonic metabolism. *J. Cell. Biochem.* (1989), in press.

23 Saunders, D. M., O'Neill, C., Collier, M. & Ammit, A. J. The identification, quantification and clinical diagnostic use of human embryo-derived platelet-activating factor. In Mizutani, S. & Tomoda, Y. (eds) Placental and endometrial proteins (1988), pp. 395–402. VNU Science Press, The Netherlands.

24 Stafforini, D. M., McIntyre, T. M., Carter, M. E. & Prescott, S. M. Human plasma activating factor acetylhydrolase. Association with lipoprotein particles and role in the degradation of platelet-activating factor. *J. Biol. Chem.* (1987), **262**, 4215–4222.

25 Blank, M. L., Lee, T., Fitzgerald, V. & Snyder, F. A specific acetylhdyrolase for 1-alkyl-2-acetyl-*sn*-glycero-3-phosphocholine (a hypotensive and platelet activating lipid). *J. Biol. Chem.* (1981), **256**, 175–178.

26 O'Neill, C. Embryo derived platelet activating factor; a pre-implantation embryo mediator of maternal recognition of pregnancy. *Domestic Anim. Endocrinol.* (1987), **4**, 69–86.

27 O'Neill, C., Collier, M. & Saunders, D. M. Embryo-derived platelet-activating factor. *Ann. N. Y. Acad. Sci.* (1988), **541**, 398–406.

28 O'Dell, T. T. & Murphy, J. R. Effects of degree of thrombocytopenia on thrombopoietic response. *Blood* (1974), **44**, 147–156.

29 Papaioannou, V. E. & Ebert, K. M. Development of fertilised embryos transferred to oviducts of immature mice. *J. Reprod. Fert.* (1986), **76**, 603–608.

30 Vanderhyden, B. C., Rouleau, A., Walton, E. A. & Armstrong, D. T. Increased mortality during early embryonic development after *in vitro* fertilization of rat oocytes. *J. Reprod. Fert.* (1986), **77**, 401–409.

31 Streffer, C., Van Benningen, D., Mollo, M., Zamboglon, N. & Schulz, S. Kinetics of cell proliferation in the preimplantation mouse embryo *in vivo* and *in vitro*. *Cell Tissue Kinet.* (1980), **13**, 135–143.

32 Bowman, P. & McLaren, A. Cleavage rate of mouse embryos *in vivo* and *in vitro*. *J. Embryol. Exp. Morph.* (1970), **24**, 203–207.

33 Miwa, M., Hill, C., Kumar, R., Sugatani, J., Olson, M. S. & Hanhan B. J. Occurrence of an endogenous inhibitor of platelet-activating factor in rat liver. *J. Biol. Chem.* (1987), **262**, 527–531.

34 Nakayama, R., Yasuda, K. & Saito, K. Existence of endogenous inbibitors of platelet activating factor (PAF) in rat uterus. *J. Biol. Chem.* (1987), **262**, 13 174–13 179.

35 McNamara, P. J., Brouwer, K. R. & Gillespie, M. N. Autocoid binding to serum proteins. Interaction of platelet activating factor (PAF) with human serum alpha-1-acid-glycoprotein. *Biochem. Pharmacol.* (1986), **35**, 621–642.

36 Matsumoto, M. & Miwa, M. Platelet activating factor binding protein in human serum. *Adv. Prost. Thromb. Leuk. Res.* (1985), **15**, 705–706.

37 Benveniste, J., Nunez, D., Dunez, P., Korth, R., Ridault, J. & Fruchart, J. C. Preformed PAF-acether and lyso PAF-acether are bound to blood lipoproteins. *FEBS Lett.* (1988), **226**, 371–376.

38 Gidley-Baird, A. A., O'Neill, C., Sinosich, M. J., Porter, R. N., Pike, I. L. & Saunders, D. M. Failure of implantation in human *in vitro* fertilisation and embryo transfer patients: the effect of altered progesterone/estrogen ratios in humans and mice. *Fert. Steril.* (1986), **45**, 69–74.

39 O'Neill, C., Ferrier, A. J., Vaughan, J., Sinosich, M. J. & Saunders, D. M. Causes of implantation falure following IVF and ET. *Lancet* (1985), **ii**, 615.
40 O'Neill, C., Gidley-Baird, A. A., Pike, I. L., Porter, R. N., Sinosich, M. J. & Saunders, D. M. Maternal blood platelet physiology and luteal phase endocrinology as a means of monitoring pre- and post- implantation embryo viability following *in vitro* fertilisation. *J. IVF ET* (1985), **2**, 59–65.
41 Tikkanen, M. J. & Nikkila, E. A. Regulation of hepatic lipase and serum lipoproteins by sex steroids. *Am. Heart J.* (1987) **113**, 562–567.
42 Osterman, G., Kertscher, H. P., Winkler, L., Schlag, B., Rüshling, K. & Till, U. C. The role of lipoproteins in the degradation of platelet activating factor. *Thromb. Res.* (1986), **44**, 503–514.
43 Spinks, N. R. & O'Neill, C. Embryo-derived platelet activating factor is essential for establishment of pregnancy in the mouse. *Lancet*, (1987), **i**, 106–107.
44 Spinks, N. R. & O'Neill, C. Antagonists of embryo-derived platelet activating factor prevent implantation of mouse embryos. *J. Reprod. Fert.* (1988), **84**, 89–98.
45 Acker, G., Hecquet, F., Etienne, A., Braquet, P. & Mercia-Huerta, J. M. Role of platelet-activating factor (PAF) in the ovoimplantation in the rat: effect of the specific PAF-acether antagonist, BN 52021. *Prostaglandins*, (1988), **35**, 233–241.
46 O'Neill, C., Collier, M., Ryan, J. P. & Spinks, R. N. Embryo-derived platelet activating factor. *J. Reprod. Fert.* (Supplement) (1989), **37**, 19–27.
47 O'Neill, C., Collier, M., Spinks, R. N., Beuk, M., Ryans, J. P. & Ammit, A. J. An autocrine role for PAF in early embryogenesis. In Handley, D. A., Saunders, R., Houlihan, W. & Tomesch, J. (eds) *Platelet Activating Factor in Endotoxin and Immune Disease*, Marcel Dekker, New York, in press.
48 Archer, C. B., Frohlich, C. P., Page, C., Paul, J., Morley, J. & MacDonald, D. M. Synergistic interaction between prostaglandins and PAF-acether in experimental animals and man. *Prostaglandins* (1984), **27**, 495–501.
49 Spinks, N. R. & O'Neill, C. The effects of a specific PAF receptor antagonist (SRI 63441) on some aspects of maternal physiology. *Proc. Aust. Soc. Reprod. Biol.* (1988), **20**, 52.
50 Ryan, J. P., Spinks, N. R., O'Neill, C., Saunders, D. M. & Wales, R. G. Enhanced rates of implantation and increased metabolism of mouse embryos cultured in the presence of platelet activating factor. *Proc. Fert. Soc. Aust.* (1987), **6**, 47.
51 Ng, D. S. & Wong, K. GTP regulation of platelet activating factor binding to human neutrophil membranes. *Biochem. Biophys. Res. Commun.* (1986), **141**, 353–359.
52 Avdonin, P. V., Svitina-Ulitina, I. V. & Kulikov, V. I. Stimulation of high-affinity hormone sensitive GTPase of human platelets by 1-O-alkyl-2-acetyl-*sn*-glyceryl-3-phosphocholine. *Biochem. Biophys. Res. Commun.* (1985), **731**, 307–313.
53 Haslam, R. J., Williams, K. A. & Davidson, M. M. Receptor–effector coupling in platelets: roles of guanine nucleotides. *Adv. Exp. Med. Biol.* (1985), **192**, 265–280.
54 Lapetina, E. G. Platelet-activating factor stimulates the phosphatidylinositol cycle. *J. Biol. Chem.* (1982), **257**, 7314–7317.
55 Braquet, P., Touqui, L., Shen, T. Y. & Vargaftig, B. B. Perspectives in platelet-activating factor in research. *Pharmacol. Rev.* (1987), **39**, 97–145.
56 Berridge, M. J. & Irvine, R. F. Inositol triphosphate, a novel second messenger in cellular signal transduction. *Nature* (1984), **312**, 315–321.
57 Nishizuka, Y. Studies and perspectives of protein kinase C. *Science* (1986), **233**, 305–312.
58 Kirsch, D., Obermaier, B. & Haring, H. U. Phorbol esters enhance basal D-glucose transport but inhibit insulin stimulation of D-glucose transport and insulin binding

in isolated rat adipocytes. *Biochem. Biophys. Res. Commun.* (1985), **128**, 824–832.

59 Hofer, H. W., Schlatter, S. & Graefe, M. Phosphorylation of phosphofructokinase by protein kinase C changes the allosteric properties of the enzyme. *Biochem. Biophys. Res. Commun.* (1985), **129**, 892–897.

60 Barbehenn, E. K., Wales, R. G. & Lowry, O. H. Measurement of metabolites in single preimplantation embryos; a new means to study metabolic control in early embryos. *J. Embryol. Exp. Morph.* (1978), **43**, 29–46.

61 Ryan, J. P., Spinks, N. R., O'Neill, C. & Wales, R. G. Implantation potential and foetal viability of embryos cultured in the presence of platelet activating factor. *Proc. Aust. Soc. Reprod. Biol.* (1988), **20**, 47.

62 O'Neill, C. The role of embryo-derived PAF in implantation. *Proc. Aust. Soc. Reprod. Biol.* (1987), **19**, 16.

63 Bryson, D. L. Development of mouse eggs in diffusion chambers. *Science* (1964), **144**, 1351–1352.

64 Snyder, F. The significance of dual pathways for the biosynthesis of platelet activating factor: 1-alkyl-2-lyso-*sn*-glycero-3-phosphate as a branch point. In Winslow, C. M. & Lee, M. (eds) *New Horizons in Platelet Activating Factor Research* 13–26. John Wiley, Chichester.

65 Spinks, N. R., O'Neill, C., Ryan, J. P., Collier, M. & Ammit, A. J. Antagonists of platelet activating factor (PAF) and their effects on early pregnancy. In Braquet, P. (ed.) *Ginkgolides: Chemistry, Biology, Pharmacology and Clinical Perspectives* (1989), Vol. 2. Prous Publishers, Barcelona, in press.

Chapter 15
PAF and foetal development

John M. Johnston and Noriei Maki

Introduction

The concept that the foetus participates in the process of the initiation of parturition is indeed an old one. In 460–370 BC, Hippocrates suggested that the foetus 'becomes agitated and breaks through the membranes'. This view was subsequently reinforced by W. Harvey in the seventeenth century and Van Deventer in the eighteenth century. Spiegelburg and colleagues in 1882 further recognized the importance of the foetus and suggested that the foetus may provide the signal for uterine activity. All of these postulates would be consistent with the quote attributed to Harvey in 1628 that, 'the assistance of the foetus is chiefly required in the birth, is evident, not in Birds only, which do by their own industry without help of their Parents break up the shell, but also in other Animals' [1,2]. In recent years, this concept has been further supported and some of the molecular events involved in the communication between the foetus and the mother expanded (for reviews see [3–6]). It is hoped that the understanding of the basic mechanisms involved in the initiation of parturition will aid in reducing perinatal mortality and morbidity from the complications of pre-term birth.

Although it is the purpose of this chapter to emphazise the relationship of PAF to foetal development, it is clear that in a number of cell types and tissues PAF metabolism and the arachidonic acid cascade are closely associated. Therefore, the relationship between these two autacoids and the glycerophospholipid that serves as a precursor to these potent second messengers will be emphasized. In this regard, it is important to point out that certain similarities are shared by the events of parturition and the inflammatory response. It was first suggested in the 1970s by Amoroso & Perry [7] and more recently by Mitchell *et al.* [8] that certain similarities are shared by these two biological phenomena. Specific evidence and support of this concept have recently been provided by Romero and colleagues who have suggested that a relationship exists between various autokines and toxins in amniotic fluid and the incidence of pre-term labour [9]. The presence of endotoxin in the amniotic fluid may be associated with the production of various autacoids since it has been established that certain endotoxins will cause the stimulation of prostaglandin formation in several cell types, including macrophages and monocytes [10]. This group of investigators have also reported that certain endotoxins will stimulate prostaglandin E_2 production by human amnion tissue in a dose-dependent manner [11]. Furthermore, there was a higher concentration of endotoxin in the amniotic fluids obtained from women with pre-term labour in comparison to those obtained without pre-term labour [12]. Additional support for the postulate that there is a relationship between various infections and pre-term labour came from the observations that the products of endotoxin action on cells, namely interleukin-1 and tumour necrosis factor were also elevated in the patients having pre-term labour. Interleukin-1 activity was normally present in the amniotic fluid of women during the third trimester, but absent in the mid-trimester [9]. Interleukin-1 will stimulate prostaglandin formation in human amnion and decidual explants. Tumour necrosis factor activity was absent in the amniotic fluid of women without infection but was present under conditions in which infection was present [9]. Production of tumour necrosis factor by at least one of the intra-uterine tissues, namely the decidua, was also reported. It was suggested that pre-term labour can be viewed as an event occurring when the intrauterine or maternal environment is threatening to the well being of the foetus. This is an appealing concept in view of the parallel studies that we will discuss in relation to the association between PAF and eicosanoids to the inflammatory process as well as the initiation of labour. The major emphasis here will be placed on the relationship of PAF to the initiation of labour and its relationship to eicosanoids.

Glycerophospholipids as precursors of the autacoids associated with initiation of parturition

The involvement of lipids in the initiation of parturition was first suggested by Luukkainen & Csapo [13], who reported that the intravenous infusion of a lipid emulsion to pregnant rabbits resulted in an increased responsiveness of rabbit uteri to oxytocin. Ogawa *et al.* [14] and Lanman and co-workers [15,16] later reported that the active component of these emulsions was a phosphatidylcholine containing an essential fatty acid such as linoleic acid or arachidonic acid, in the *sn*-2 position. The importance of arachidonic acid in the initiation of parturition has been demonstrated in a number of species, including the rabbit as reported by Nathanielsz *et al.* [17], the quail by Hertelendy and colleagues [18,19] and in the human by our group [20]. It is well known from the early investigations of Lands & Samuelsson [21] and Vonkeman & van Dorp [22] that arachidonic acid must be released from its esterified form in the glycerophospholipids in order that the arachidonic acid can serve as a precursor for eicosanoids. Karim [23] reported that prostaglandins were present in amniotic fluid and that prostaglandin-rich extracts of amniotic fluid obtained from women in labour increased the intensity of spontaneous contractions of the uterus. The role of prostaglandins in the initiation of parturition has been described recently in detail by Bleasdale & Johnston [4]. In an early investigation it was suggested that the arachidonic acid that was found in increased amounts during labour and served as the precursor of prostanoids was derived from glycerophospholipids in the foetal membranes [20]. Approximately 20% of the total fatty acid of amniochorion was arachidonic acid [24]. When the arachidonic acid was released from amnion tissue obtained from women at term and in labour Okita *et al.* [25] found that in early labour, the arachidonic acid content changed only in the (diacyl)phosphatidylethanolamine and phosphatidylinositol fractions. The decrease in arachidonic acid in each lipid species of amnion was approximately 40%. A decrease of arachidonic acid in these two lipids was also noted in the chorion laeve obtained after the onset of labour. Although most of the arachidonic acid was present in the ethanolamine plasmalogen fraction, a loss in arachidonic acid in this glycerophospholipid was not evident during early labour. The presence of significant amounts of plasmalogen provides the explanation as to why this tissue stains intensely with the plasmal stain as reported by McCoshen *et al.* [26]. (The importance of plasmalogens in relation to PAF metabolism will be discussed below.) No significant decrease in arachidonic acid was also observed in the entire phosphatidylcholine fraction [27]. It should be noted, however, that the ether-containing phosphatidylcholines were not analysed separately in this study. The glycerophospholipid species and the enzymatic basis for the release of arachidonic acid that occurs during parturition in various uterine tissues are illustrated in Fig. 15. 1. Employing defined substrates it was demonstrated that a calcium-dependent phospholipase A_2 activity present in foetal membranes was primarily associated with the microsomal fraction [28]. The enzyme preferentially cleaved phosphatidylethanolamine containing esterified arachidonate in the *sn*-2 position (Fig. 15.1b, **1**). A calcium-independent phospholipase A_2 activity has been recently described in amnion tissue and the relationship of this enzyme to arachidonic acid release and PAF biosynthesis will be discussed below. Phosphatidylinositol was not a substrate for the phospholipase A_2, thus the activity of phospholipase C with a specificity for phosphatidylinositol was examined. It was demon-

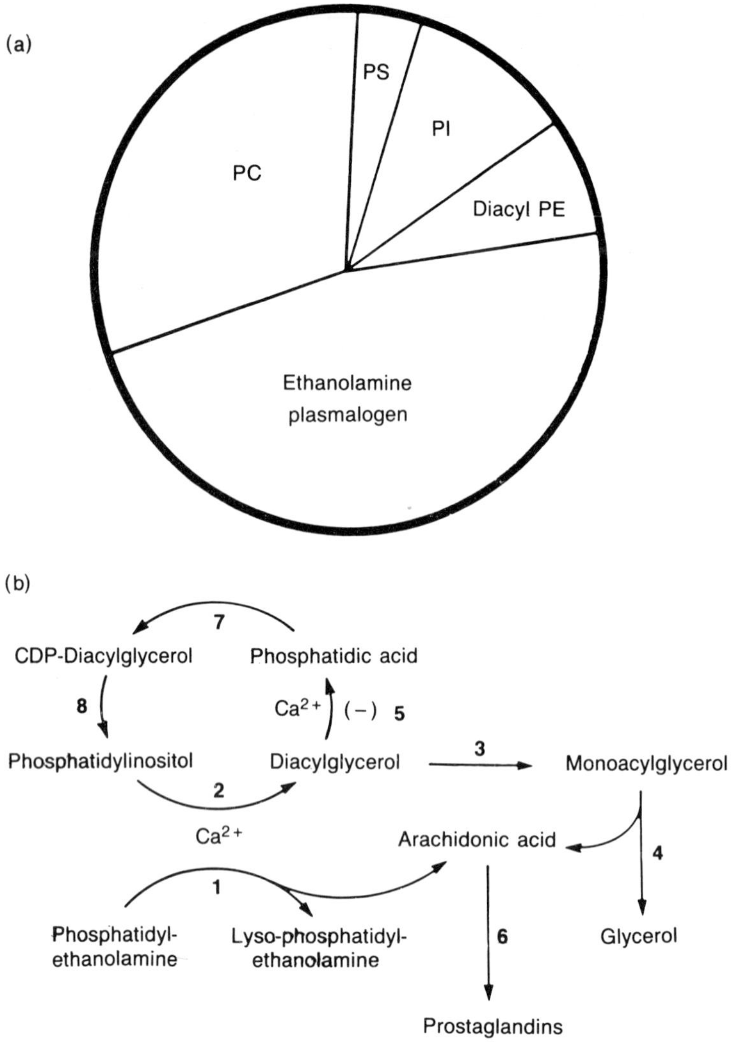

Fig 15.1 (a) Distribution of arachidonate in the glycerophospholipids of amnion obtained at term prior to the onset of labor. PC = phosphatidylcholine, PS = phosphatidylserine, PI = phosphatidylinositol, PE = phosphatidylethanolamine; (b) Enzymatic pathways for the mobilization of arachidonic acid in amnion. Reactions are catalysed by: **(1)** phospholipase A_2; **(2)** phosphatidylinositol-specific phosphlipase C; **(3)** diacylglycerol lipase; **(4)** monoacylglycerol lipase; **(5)** diacylglycerol kinase; **(6)** prostaglandin synthase complex; **(7)** CTP:phosphatidate cytidylyltransferase; **(8)** CDP-diacylglycerol:inositol 3-phosphatidyltransferase. From Bleasdale & Johnston [4].

strated by Di Renzo *et al.* [29] that stoichiometric amounts of inositol phosphate and diacylglycerols were simultaneously released from phosphatidylinositol when phosphatidylinositol was employed as the substrate (**2**). The enzyme was present primarily in the cytosolic fraction and had a specificity for phosphatidylinositol and Ca^{2+} requirement. A diacylglycerol lipase (**3**) and a monoacylglycerol lipase (**4**) were present in the microsomal fraction of the various intra-uterine tissues [30]. It was also demonstrated that diacylglycerols and monoacylglycerols containing arachidonic acid were preferentially hydrolysed. A similar reaction sequence has recently been demonstrated in human platelets by Majerus and colleagues [31]. The diacylglycerols produced in amnion from phosphatidylinositol can also be phosphorylated by a diacylglycerol kinase (**5**), forming phosphatidic acid [32]. The arachidonic acid as catalysed by di- and monoacylglycerol lipases occurred rather than the formation of phosphatidic acid when the diacylglycerol and Ca^{2+} concentrations were elevated.

This model (Fig. 15.1b) provides the enzymatic basis for the selective release of arachidonic acid from (diacyl)phosphatidylethanolamine and phosphatidylinositol that was observed during early labour. A central role for Ca^{2+} in the regulation of activities of these enzymes is evident. Participation of Ca^{2+} in arachidonic acid metabolism and the initiation of parturition has recently been confirmed by the use of specific channel blockers [33]. An increase in various prostanoids in amniotic fluid that parallels the observed increase in free arachidonic acid in this compartment that occurs during early labour has been reported (see [3,4]).

Of interest was the observation that PAF might induce changes in calcium homeostasis as it does in numerous other tissues where PAF has been shown to be active (for review see [34]). Billah & Johnston [35] have isolated and identified PAF in the amniotic fluid obtained from women in active labour (Fig. 15.2). PAF was not detected in the amniotic fluid obtained from women with a similar gestational age but not in labour. These observations were confirmed by Nishihara and colleagues [36] employing GC/MS procedures for identification of PAF. This group of investigators also demonstrated that PAF was a potent agonist of myometrial contraction in the rat. Similar studies have also been reported in the guinea-pig [37] and human [38] myometrium. It was demonstrated that PAF as well as the ionophore A23187 plus Ca^{2+}, stimulated the release of PGE_2 by amnion tissue [39] PAF will also stimulate PGE_2 synthesis 10–20-fold in human amnion cells which have been placed in culture for 5 days (Bleasdale, J. E., unpublished). The concentration of PAF in amnion tissue increased some 20-fold following exposure to Ca^{2+} and the ionophore. Based on this observation, the activities of various enzymes involving PAF and eicosanoid metabolism were further examined in amnion tissue. Initially, PAF biosynthesis via the remodelling

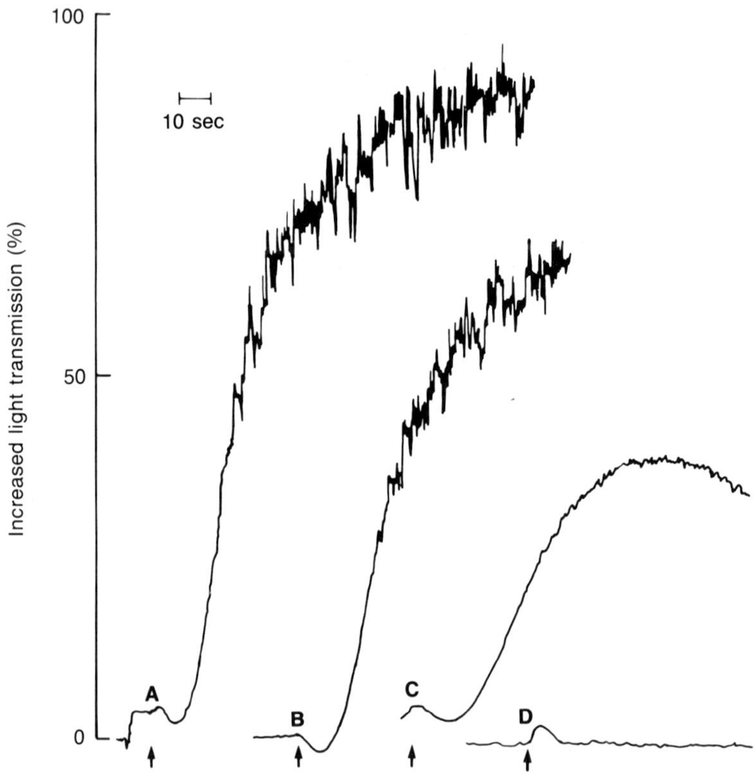

Fig. 15.2 Platelet aggregation in response to amniotic fluid PAF at various concentrations. The phospholipids in the lipid extract of amniotic fluid obtained from women in labour were separated by thin-layer chromatography. Thin-layer areas corresponding to PAF were eluted and the extracts were tested for platelet-aggregating activity. (**A**), (**B**), and (**C**) represent lipid extracts from 10, 5 and 2 ml of amniotic fluid, respectively, and (**D**) represents a lipid extract from 50 ml of amniotic fluid obtained from a woman at term but not in labour. From Billah & Johnston [35].

pathway was investigated. This reaction sequence is illustrated in Fig. 15.3 (**IV–VI**). The activities of lyso-PAF:acetyl-CoA acetyltransferase and PAF acetylhydrolase (reactions **V** and **VI**, respectively), were demonstrated in amnion tissue [40]. The former enzyme was microsomal while the latter was predominantly associated with the cytosolic fraction. Maximal activation of the acetyltransferase was demonstrated at physiological intracellular concentrations of Ca^{2+} (10^{-7} M). No difference in the specific activity of acetylhydrolase was observed in foetal membranes obtained during early gestation or at term before labour. As recently suggested, the activation of acetyltransferase may be catalysed by protein kinase C [41,42]. Protein kinase C activity was previously demonstrated in amnion tissue [43]. In contrast, Gomez-Cambronero and colleagues have suggested that lyso-PAF:acetyl-CoA acetyltransferase is activated by

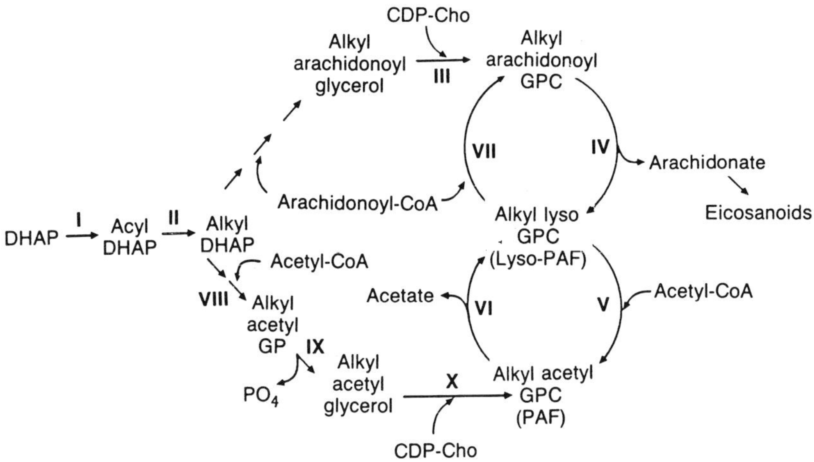

Fig. 15.3 The metabolism of PAF and its inter-relationship to the arachidonic acid cascade. The enzymes of the *de novo* and remodelling pathways of PAF biosynthesis are depicted, as follows: Rx **I**, DHAP:acyl-CoA acyltransferase; Rx **II**, alkyl-DHAP synthetase; Rx **III**, 1-alkyl-2-acyl-glycerol:CDP-choline cholinephosphotransferase (DTT-sensitive); Rx **IV**, phospholipase A_2; Rx **V**, lyso-PAF:acetyl-CoA acetyltransferase; Rx **VI**, PAF-acetylhydrolase; Rx **VII**, 1-alkyl-2-lyso-GPC:acyl-CoA acyltransferase; Rx **VIII**, 1-alkyl-2-lyso-glycero-3-phosphate:acetyl-CoA acetyltransferase; Rx **IX**, 1-alkyl-2-acetyl-glycero-3-phosphate (GP) phosphohydrolase; and Rx **X**, 1-alkyl-2-acetyl-glycerol: CDP-choline cholinephosphotransferase (DTT-insensitive).

the adenylcyclase system [44]. The importance and mechanism of acetyltransferase activation in relation to the synthesis of PAF in relation to labour awaits future investigation. In addition to PAF, the presence of lyso-PAF, and alkyl-acyl-GPC in amnion tissue has also been demonstrated [39].

As previously discussed, the phospholipase A_2 in amnion tissue that preferentially cleaves arachidonoyl-containing phosphatidylethanolamines is regulated by Ca^{2+} [28,40]. The phospholipase A_2 activity in foetal membranes has been re-examined utilizing the alkyl-acyl-glycerophosphocholine (GPC) as a substrate. This compound serves as the precursor of PAF [45,46] by supplying lyso-PAF. Phospholipase A_2 activity was assayed in amnion tissue employing hexadecyl-oleoyl-GPC and palmitoyl-oleoyl-GPC as substrates. The results of this study are shown in Fig. 15.4. As is illustrated, in the absence of added Ca^{2+}, the hydrolysis of the alkyl substrate was 2–6 times higher than that of the diacyl derivative. The hydrolysis of palmitoyl-oleoyl-GPC was stimulated severalfold by the addition of Ca^{2+}, whereas the hydrolysis of hexadecyl-oleoyl-GPC was not. Thus, it appears that at least three phospholipase A_2 activites are present in amnion tissue: (i) a Ca^{2+}-dependent phospholipase A_2 which preferentially utilizes phosphatidylethanolamine containing

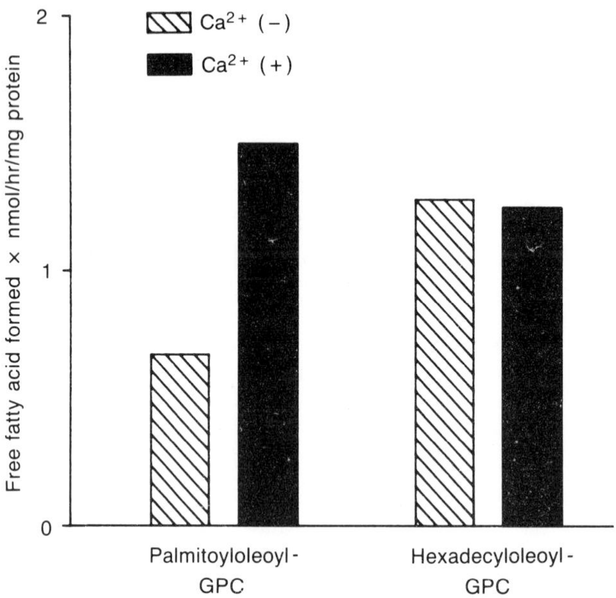

Fig. 15.4 Substrate specificity of the phospholipase A_2 in human amnion microsomes. Radiolabelled substrates utilized were 1-palmitoyl-2-[^{3}H]oleoyl-GPC and 1-*O*-hexadecyl-2-[^{3}H]oleoyl-GPC. Incubations were conducted in the presence of 1 mM EGTA or 1 mM EGTA and 2 mM Ca^{2+}. GPC = glycerophosphocholine.

arachidonic acid [28]; (ii) a Ca^{2+}-independent phospholipase A_2 that catalyses the hydrolysis of substrates containing the alkyl group in the *sn*-1 position [40,45,46]; and (iii) a PAF acetylhydrolase which is Ca^{2+}-independent [40]. The Ca^{2+}-independent phospholipase A_2 may be the enzyme that is utilized to synthesize lyso-PAF which, in turn, can be acetylated by the acetyltransferase in PAF biosynthesis. It was also found that other cell types, such as neutrophils, macrophages, platelets and eosinophils, were enriched with alkyl arachidonoyl-GPC (for review see [47]). The cleavage of these substrates would not only release the lyso-PAF for PAF biosynthesis but also arachidonic acid for eicosanoid synthesis.

Although amnion tissue contains most of the enzymes and substrates that are required for the synthesis of PAF via the remodelling pathway, we were unable to demonstrate any significant release of PAF into the incubation media [35]. It would appear that amnion tissue is not the source of the PAF found in the amniotic fluid. An alternative tissue source might be the foetal lung since 40–50% of the PAF found in the amniotic fluid was associated with the fraction enriched with lamellar bodies (surfactant-containing). Similarly 50% of the lyso-PAF, and >90% of the alkyl-acyl-GPC were present in this fraction [35]. Since the surfactant-containing lamellar bodies found in amniotic fluid originate in the foetal lung, this tissue may be the source of the PAF associated with the lamellar bodies found in amniotic fluid in association with labour.

PAF metabolism in foetal lung

The concentration of PAF, as well as lipid precursors, in foetal rabbit lung and liver tissues from day 21 through to the end of gestation were determined [48] and are shown in Fig. 15.5. In foetal liver, the concentration of PAF did not change significantly throughout the latter stages of

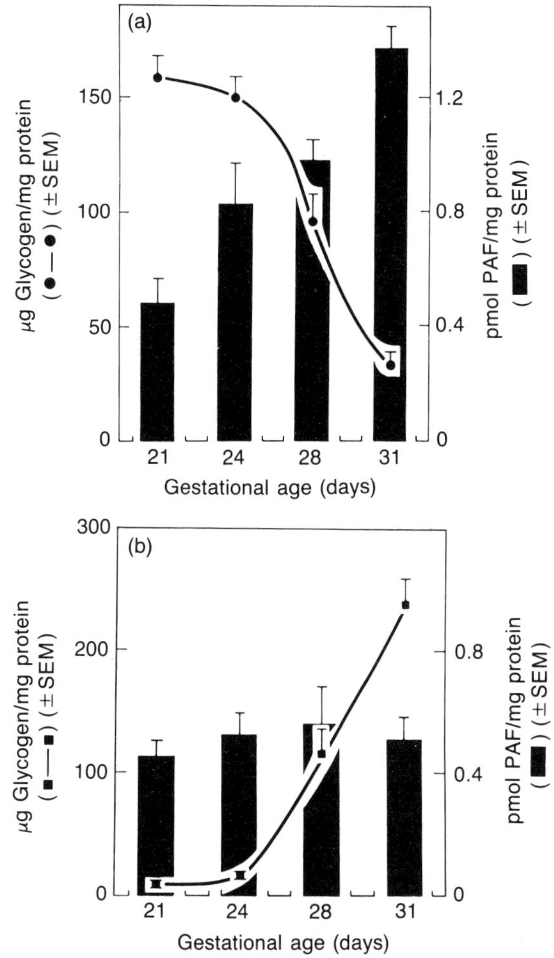

Fig. 15.5 Concentration of PAF and glycogen in (a) foetal rabbit lung and (b) liver as a function of gestational development. Values are the means ± SEM of at least nine separate determinations for lung and five determinations for liver. From Hoffman *et al.* [49].

gestation. The concentration of PAF in foetal rabbit lung was similar to that of foetal liver on day 21 of gestation, but then rapidly increased threefold by day 31. In contrast, the concentration of lyso-PAF and alkylacyl-GPC in foetal lung decreased by 60% between day 21 and day 31 of gestation. A similar increase in PAF concentration was found in human foetal lung tissue in organ culture during a 6-day incubation period [49]. This organ culture system was characterized several years ago by Snyder *et al.* [50,51], and it was demonstrated that the type-II pneumonocytes differentiate into surfactant-producing and secreting cells during a 6–8 day incubation period.

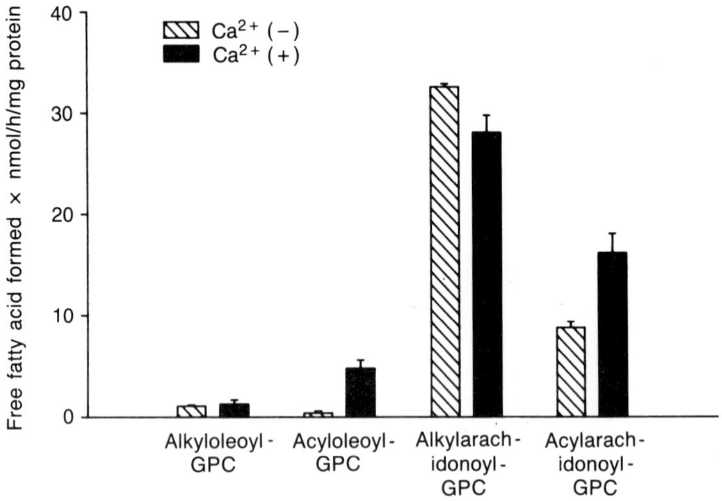

Fig. 15.6 Phospholipase A_2 activity in adult rabbit lung microsomes. Alkyl and acyl groups C_{16}. GPC = glycerophosphocholine.

The enzymes concerned with PAF metabolism in lung tissue were assayed during the latter stages of gestation. The activities of the enzymes involved in the remodelling pathway (Fig. 15.3, **IV**, **V** and **VI**) were assayed. A Ca^{2+} independent phospholipase A_2 with a substrate specificity for alkyl-containing glycerophospholipids similar to that described in amnion tissue was also present in foetal rabbit lung (Fig. 15.6) [45,46]. The activity of this enzyme in day-31 foetal rabbit lung was twice that found in adult tissue. Alkyl-arachidonoyl-GPC was preferentially hydrolysed compared to acyl-arachidonoyl-GPC and both arachidonoyl-containing substrates were cleaved to a greater extent when compared to the alkyloleoyl containing substrate. Again, this phospholipase A_2 may account for the preferential hydrolysis of arachidonoyl-containing alkyl-GPCs in lung and several cell types and account for the simultaneous generation of the precursor of two potent autacoids, namely PAF and eicosanoids. The lyso-PAF: acetyl-CoA acetyltransferase activity in foetal lung was also assayed throughout gestation [48]. The specific activity of acetyltransferase increased threefold in foetal rabbit lung between days 21 and 24 of gestation and remained elevated until birth. Similarly, the activity of this enzyme increased in human foetal lung when this tissue was placed in organ culture for 6 days. Interestingly, the acetyltransferase activity in human and rabbit foetal lung was several orders of magnitude higher than that of foetal kidney or liver and would correlate well with the increased amount of PAF found in lung tissue. In addition to the remodelling pathway, a *de novo* pathway for PAF biosynthesis has been found in several tissues by Snyder [34]. This pathway is illustrated by reactions **I**, **II**, **VIII**, **IX** and **X** of Fig. 15.3. The final reaction to this sequence is catalysed by a specific choline phosphotransferase which employs alkyl-acetylglycerol as the phosphocholine acceptor. The enzyme involved in PAF biosynthesis is insensitive to dithiothreitol treatment as opposed to the enzyme catalysing phosphatidylcholine biosynthesis which is inactivated by this sulfhydryl reagent. The activity of the dithiothreitol-insensitive phosphotransferase increased dramatically in foetal rabbit lung during gestation [52]. No change in the choline phosphotransferase activity involved in phosphatidylcholine biosynthesis was observed in foetal rabbit lung as we reported several years ago [53]. Based on the enzymatic studies for PAF biosynthesis by both the remodelling and *de novo* pathways it was concluded that in foetal rabbit lung there was an increase in the capacity for the synthesis of PAF. These mechanisms could account for the increase in PAF found in foetal lung during the later stages of gestation.

We speculate that the last major organ system to mature in the foetus, namely the foetal lung, produces and secretes surfactant with its associated PAF into the amniotic fluid (Fig. 15.7). As has been previously discussed [39], the PAF interacts with amnion membranes to stimulate the production and release of PGE_2. It is also possible that the PAF may autocatalytically cause an increase in PAF synthesis and release since PAF will increase intracellular Ca^{2+} [54] which in turn is known to increase lyso-PAF:acetylCo-A acetyltransferase activity in both amnion [39] and lung tissues [48]. It has been suggested that a similar autocatalytic synthesis of PAF occurs in neutrophils [55].

PAF catabolism in amnion tissue

Although the major emphasis of this review has concentrated on PAF and its metabolism, it is readily apparent that the formation of PAF and eicosanoid biosynthesis is intimately associated with a number of biological phenomena. These include not only the initiation of parturition (for review see [56]) but the phenomena of implantation, aggregation of

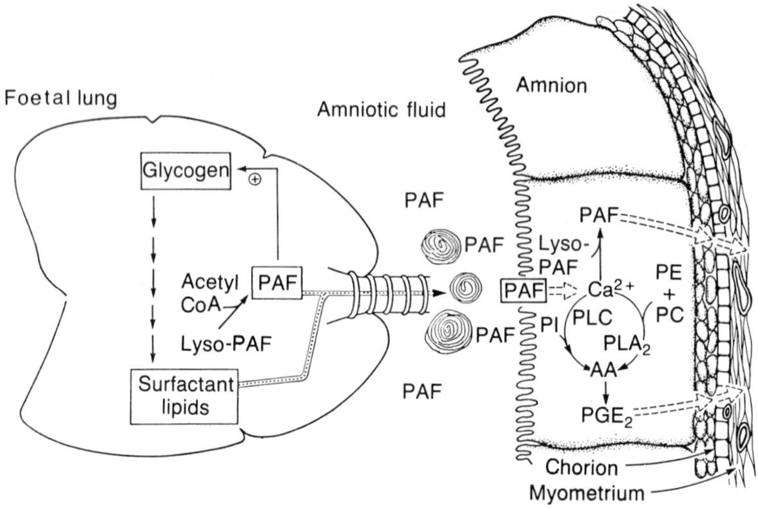

Fig. 15.7 Proposed role of PAF in the initiation of parturition.
PI = phosphatidylinositol; AA = arachidonic acid; PE = phosphatidylethanolamine; PC = phosphatidylcholine; PLC = phospholipase C; and PLA_2 = phospholipase A_2.

certain cells, and various reactions of the inflammatory response. As previously discussed, the relationship between the formation of the two potent autacoids is evident when it is appreciated that the precursors of the arachidonic acid used for eicosanoid formation and lyso-PAF for PAF biosynthesis may be the same. In support of this concept is the recent observation that in many cells and tissues the precursor to both autacoids, namely alkyl-arachidonoyl-GPC is a major phosphatidylcholine species [47].

Based on recent evidence it has been suggested that the plasmalogen derivative of glycerophosphorylethanolamine (GPE) may also be involved in PAF and arachidonic acid metabolism. When a kidney cell line was pre-incubated with either alkyl-labelled lyso-PAF or alkyl-acyl-GPC and subsequently challenged with various stimuli, it was reported that over 30% of the radiolabel was recovered in the ethanolamine phospholipid fraction [57]. Subsequent studies demonstrated that 80% of the radio-labelled PAF or its precursor was present in the ethanolamine plasmalogen fraction. Baker [58] has reported that PAF is primarily converted to the plasmalogen ethanolamine derivative in a macrophage cell line. It would appear that the major degradative pathway may be its conversion to the alkyl ethanolamine derivatives which are, in turn, converted into plasmalogens. The plasmalogens can rapidly be cleaved by a plasmalogenase which is present in many tissues (for review see [59]). As previously discussed, amnion tissue obtained at term and in early labour contains a significant amount of the plasmalogen ethanolamine species (>75% of the total phosphatidylethanolamine fraction at this gestational age). The plasmalogen was also enriched with arachidonic acid [27]. As indicated in Fig. 15.8, when amnion tissue was obtained between 12–17 weeks of gestation almost equal amounts of the plasmalogen and diacyl species of ethanolamine glycerophospholipids were present. As has been discussed, it is suggested that the PAF is secreted by the foetal lung in association with lamellar bodies into the amniotic fluid and accounts for, in part, the presence of PAF in the amniotic fluid during early labour [5]. The PAF in amniotic fluid stimulates the synthesis and release of PGE_2 from amnion tissue as well as the possible further synthesis of PAF by tissue by Ca^{2+}

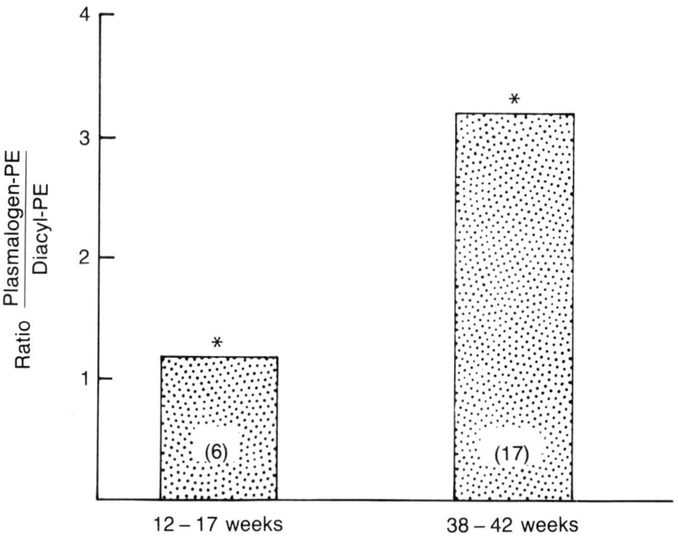

Fig. 15.8 The ratio of plasmalogen phosphatidylethanolamine (PE) to diacyl-PE in amnion from mid (12–17 weeks) and late (38–42 weeks) gestation. The total concentration of ethanolamine glycerophospholipids did not change throughout gestation. *, $P < 0.001$.

activation [40]. In amnion tissue, therefore one might expect an increase in the ethanolamine plasmalogen fraction due to PAF stimulation. As seen in Fig. 15.8 [56], this was indeed the case and the ratio of plasmalogen to diacyl-GPE was increased from 1:1 in early membranes at 12–17 weeks to 3:1 at term (38–42 weeks). No change was found in the total ethanolamine-containing glycerophospholipid in the two gestational age groups. These findings provide further indirect support for the concept that PAF may directly affect amnion tissue followed by its conversion to the ethanolamine-containing plasmalogens. Saito and colleagues [60,61] have provided additional evidence for a role of PAF in reproduction by the demonstration that PAF and inhibitors of PAF are present in whole rat uteri. PAF synthesis has also been demonstrated in endometrium of the rabbit uterus [46] and to cause the release of $PGF_{2\alpha}$ and PGE_2 by human endometrium [62].

PAF in the amniotic fluid of complicated pregnancies

We have recently examined the PAF concentration in the amniotic fluid of women with complicated preganancies as well as that of uncomplicated pregnancies, 'at term and not in labour' and 'in labour' [63]. An eightfold increase in the concentration of PAF was found in the amniotic fluid

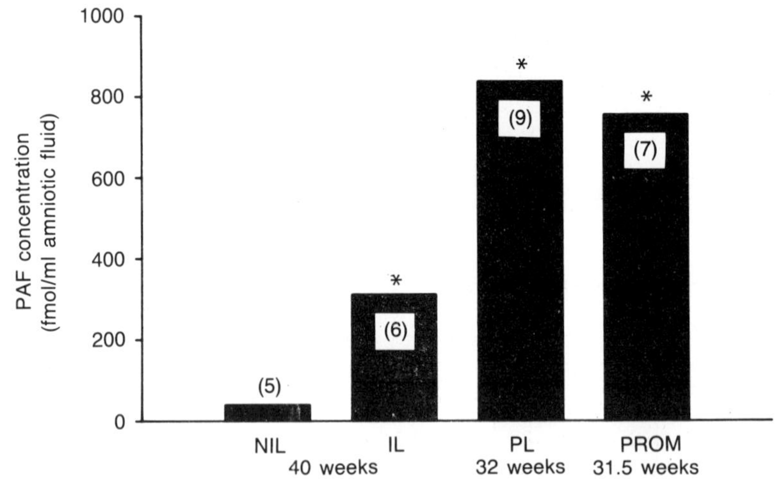

Fig. 15.9 PAF concentration in the amniotic fluid obtained from women at term (40 weeks) who were not in labour (NIL), in labour (IL) and in complicated pregnancies with premature labour (PL) and premature rupture of membranes (PROM). *, $P < 0.05$ versus NIL.

obtained from the 'term in labour' samples compared to that of the 'term, not in labour' samples (<312 versus 40 fmol/ml) confirming our original observations employing the platelet aggregation assay with the serotonin release assay. As is shown in Fig. 15.9, the PAF concentrations in the amniotic fluid of patients with 'premature labour' and 'premature rupture of membranes' were significantly increased. There was a more than 20-fold increase in the concentration of PAF in patients with 'premature labour' (838 fmol/ml). The gestational age of this group of patients was an average 32 weeks. The PAF concentration was also elevated in the group of patients in which there was a 'premature rupture of membranes'. The mean gestational age of this group was 31.5 weeks and the concentration of PAF found in the amniotic fluid was 756 fmol/ml. In the limited number of samples, no difference in the concentration of PAF in amniotic fluid was found in the patients with complicated pregnancies when each group was sub-divided into patients with infection versus the non-infected group. It would appear that the patient population which is destined to have a much higher incidence of premature labour has a significantly higher concentration of PAF in the amniotic fluid. It is also of interest that there may be a decreased incidence of respiratory distress syndrome in the infants delivered from women with premature rupture of membranes [63]. The role of PAF in foetal lung maturation is discussed below. We and others have suggested a role for eicosanoids in the initiation of labour (for review see [4]). Based on these observations, it is suggested that a second potent autacoid, PAF, may also play an important role in the events of labour in both 'at term' and at 'pre-term' population groups [5]. The involvement of multiple factors in such a fundamental process as parturition may be more biologically appealing than the so-called 'trigger concept' which has been suggested by several groups of investigators. It is interesting that PAF and eicosanoids are not only involved in the initiation of parturition, but also have a primary inportance in embryo implantation (see Chapter 14).

PAF in foetal lung maturation

As was discussed, the PAF synthesized in the foetal lung and secreted in association with surfactant may participate in the molecular events in leading to the initiation of parturition. A direct effect of PAF on the maturational process of the foetal lung type-II pneumonocytes may be mediated by facilitating the mobilization of glycogen which is utilized for the synthesis of the glycerophospholipids of surfactant. The effect of PAF on glycogen metabolism was first suggested by Hanahan and colleagues, who observed that PAF at concentrations as low as 2×10^{-10} M rapidly increased glycogenolysis and glucose release in the perfused rat liver (for review see [65]). Considerable evidence has accrued to suggest that during foetal lung maturation the glycogen present in the maturing type-II pneumonocyte provides much of the carbon and energy sources required for the synthesis of the major glycerophospholipid of surfactant, namely disaturated phosphatidylcholine [66,67]. This obtained since the synthesis of the glycerophospholipids may be highly dependent on the endogenous glycogen stores during foetal development because of the low blood supply to the foetal lung [68]. As previously discussed, it has been observed that the concentration of PAF in rabbit foetal lung tissue during the latter stages of gestation [48] and in human foetal lung explants [49] increased during development. It was also found that the specific activity of the regulatory enzyme of the remodelling pathway of PAF biosynthesis was significantly higher in the type-II pneumonocyte than several other lung cell types [48]. The temporal relationship between the increase in

PAF concentration, glycogen breakdown and the synthesis of disaturated phosphatidylcholine in foetal rabbit lung during the latter stages of gestation is illustrated in Fig. 15.10.

In order to directly assess the role of PAF on glycogen metabolism in foetal lung, PAF was injected intra-peritoneally to foetal rabbits on day 24 of gestation and the glycogen content determined in foetal lung and liver after 45 min [69]. Day-24 foetal rabbits were utilized since it was previously demonstrated that the glycogen content is maximal in the type-II cells at this time of foetal development. The glycogen levels found in foetal

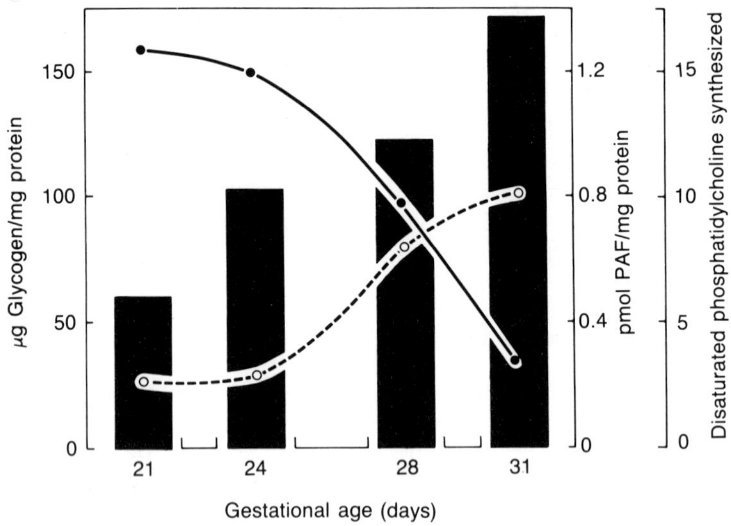

Fig. 15.10 The temporal relationship between PAF concentration (*bars*), glycogen breakdown (●—●) and disaturated phosphatidylcholine biosynthesis (○---○) in foetal rabbit lung during the latter stages of gestation. From Snyder, Johnston & Mendelson [50]. *Third bar*, PAF antagonist SRI 63-441, *fourth bar*, PAF antagonist plus PAF.

lung tissue following various treatments are illustrated in Fig. 15.11a. As is illustrated, a significant decrease in both lung and liver glycogen pools was observed following the injection of PAF compared to the vehicle-injected foetuses. A dose-dependent response to PAF was found at PAF concentrations 10^{-11} M. When either the antagonist SRI 63-441 or PAF antagonist plus PAF was injected, no difference in glycogen breakdown was found compared to controls. Similarly, the injection of the enantiomer of the naturally-occurring L-PAF, namely D-PAF, did not significantly alter the glycogen content of either the foetal lung or liver. The lactate content of foetal lung, liver and plasma of these foetuses were also determined following PAF injection. The results of this study are illustrated in Fig. 15.11b. As can be seen, there was a two to threefold increase of the lactate content in the PAF-injected animals of foetal lung, liver and plasma

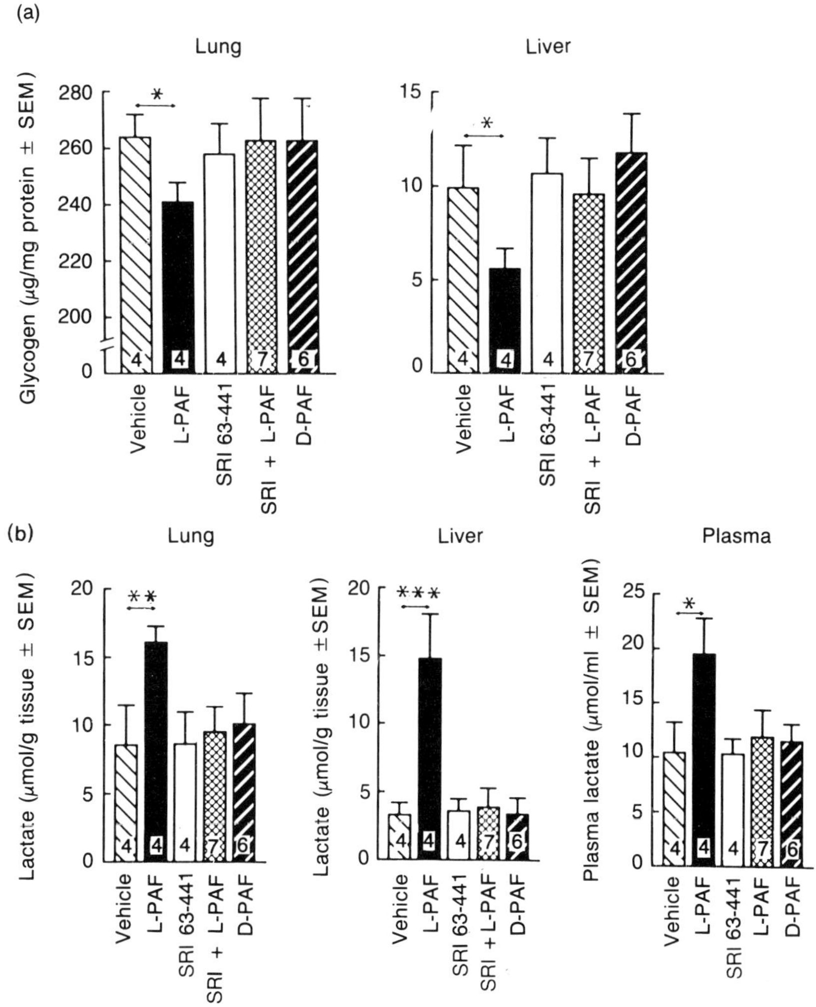

Fig. 15.11 (a) Glycogen content of 24 day rabbit foetal lung and liver 45 min after the injection of L-PAF, SRI 63-441 (PAF receptor antagonist), SRI plus L-PAF or the enantiomeric D-PAF; (b) lactate concentration in lung, liver and plasma 45 min following the injections listed under (a). *, $P < 0.05$; **, $P < 0.025$; and ***, $P < 0.01$.

compared to the vehicle-injected animals. In contrast, no change in lactate was found in the foetuses injected with either the PAF receptor antagonist, the antagonists plus L-PAF, or the enantiomer of PAF, D-PAF. A study has been recently completed in which PAF was administered directly in the vitellin vein of the foetus and the glycogen content of the foetal lung and liver was determined (J. R. Bourbon, D. R. Hoffman & J. M. Johnston, unpublished). In this study, 19.5-day foetal rats were employed and lung glycogen content was determined 24 h following the administration of

2.5 μg of PAF. The foetal lung glycogen content decreased significantly from 362 to 300 μg/glycogen/mg protein after such treatment. Again, no decrease was noted when the enantiomer of PAF was administered. In a series of experiments in which [^{14}C] glucose and PAF were injected simultaneously into the vitellin vein of the foetus, the radioactivity incorporated into the lung glycogen was reduced significantly when compared to control foetuses which had received a vehicle. The assay was completed at 3 h following the administration of PAF and radiolabelled glucose. As a result of these findings, it has been suggested that during foetal development there is a PAF activated glycogen degradation in parallel with the increase in pulmonary PAF concentration. The increased glycogen breakdown would result in an increase in the availability of glycero-3-phosphate and dihydroxyacetone phosphate for the synthesis of the glycerol backbone of the surfactant glycerophospholipid as well as increased levels of acetyl-CoA for palmitoyl-CoA biosynthesis. Both these are required for the synthesis of the major glycerophospholipid of surfactant, namely 1,2-disaturated phosphatidylcholine. The elevated acetyl-CoA may also facilitate a further increase in PAF synthesis since the intracellular concentration of acetyl-CoA in foetal lung tissue is well below the K_m for acetyl-CoA of the lyso-PAF:acetyl-CoA acetyltransferase (approximately 5 μM) (R. Frenkel & J. M. Johnston, unpublished). The importance of PAF during lung development is also suggested by the observations of Kumar & Hanahan [70] and Johnston *et al.* [5] who demonstrated that PAF markedly stimulates the release of surfactant by the type-II pneumonocyte during foetal lung development providing a mechanism to explain the rapid increase of PAF in the amniotic fluid that occurs at the onset of labour.

Metabolism of PAF in maternal plasma

The biochemical mechanisms which are involved in the synthesis and release of PAF and arachidonic acid in various foetal tissues have been described. In addition, a possible relationship between PAF and the stimulation of prostaglandin formation during foetal lung maturation, and the relationship of these events to parturition, have been discussed. The major emphasis of this review of PAF has been concerned with PAF metabolism in foetal tissues. A recent observation concerning the metabolism of PAF in the maternal compartment may hopefully be integrated with the events of parturition and the interactions between the foetal and maternal compartment. It has previously been reported that the activity of PAF acetylhydrolase in plasma is elevated in spontaneously hypertensive rats [71] as well as in a group of white males suffering from hypertension [72]. Indeed, the activity of this enzyme proved to be the so-called 'acid labile factor' present in plasma that was responsible for inactivating the PAF formed during anaphylaxis [73,74]. The activity of PAF acetylhydrolase in maternal blood was assayed in order to see if the capacity to inactivate PAF produced in various foetal tissues would be altered in the rabbit maternal plasma throughout gestation. Inactivation of PAF produced in the foetal compartment prior to its contact to myometrium would be of considerable importance since PAF has been shown to be a potent stimulator of myometrial contraction in a number of species [36–38]. As is illustrated in Fig. 15.12, prior to insemination, the

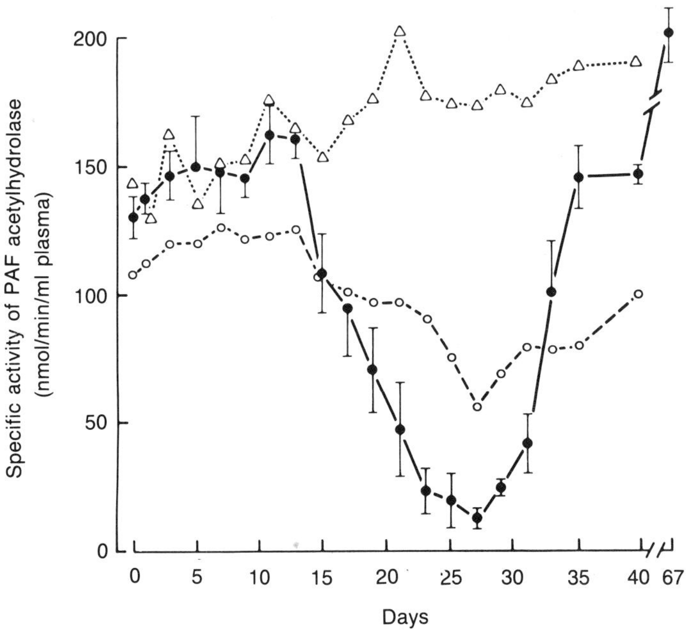

Fig. 15.12 PAF acetylhydrolase activity in rabbit maternal plasma throughout gestation. Rabbits 1, 2 and 3 (●—●) were uncomplicated pregnancies (mean ± SEM) and delivered a total of 20 live and three dead offspring on an average of 31 days of gestation. Rabbit 4 (△---△) was not pregnant. Rabbit 5 (○---○) delivered two dead offspring on day 34 (weight similar to 28 day foetus).

activity of female rabbits was approximately 130 nmol/min/ml plasma [75]. In the first 15 days of pregnancy, the activity increased slightly to 160 nmol/min/ml plasma and commencing on day 15 dramatically dropped to levels of approximately 10 nmol/min/ml plasma between days 23 and 29 of gestation. Following delivery, the activity returned to the pre-pregnancy levels (approximately 150 nmol).

A similar decrease in acetylhydrolase has been found in the human (Johnston, J. M. and Maki, N., unpublished). The mean acetylhydrolase activity was 44 $nmol^{-1} \times ml^{-1}$ plasma in non-pregnant women and de-

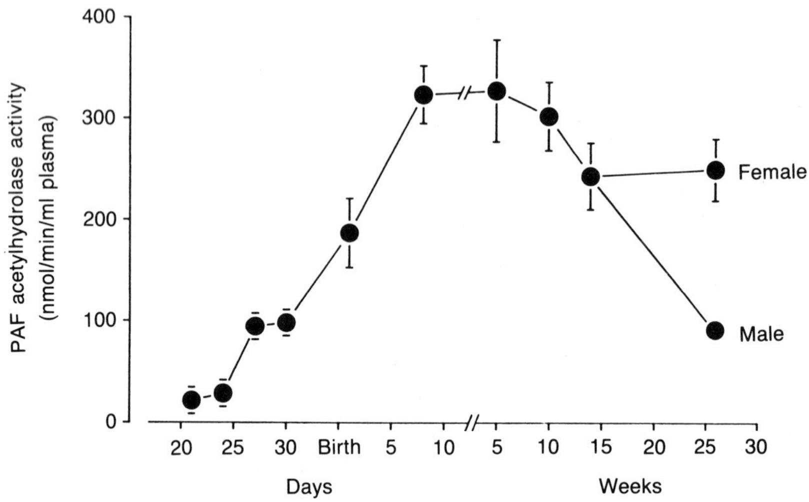

Fig. 15.13 Plasma PAF acetylhydrolase activity (mean $\pm$ SEM) in foetuses, newborn rabbits, and young adult rabbits.

creased to 26 by 32 weeks of gestation. Interestingly, the activity did not decrease in a limited group of patients with pregnancy-induced hypertension. Thus, we speculate, that patients with pregnancy-induced hypertension have a decreased capacity to modulate various pressor agents such as angiotensin II, as a result of the decrease in the concentration of the potent hypotensive agent PAF. We are presently asking the question 'Is PAF the elusive compound that modifies the pressor response during the latter stages of human pregnancy?'

We also analysed the activity of foetal and neonatal rabbit plasma starting on day 21 of gestation (Fig. 15.13). On day 21 of gestation the activity was approximately one-fifth of that found in the maternal circulation. However, during the latter stages of gestation the ratio was reversed and the foetal enzymatic activity was several times higher than that in the corresponding maternal plasma. In the post-natal period the acetylhydrolase activity in the offspring rose to values approximately twice as high as those found in the non-pregnant rabbit or after the cessation of lactation. As a result of these findings, we suggest that the failure to respond physiologically to appropriate antigen challenge [76–78] or to PAF infusion [79] that has been noted in the neonate and young rabbits is due to the high activity of PAF acetylhydrolase in these animals.

Conclusion

It is well established in a number of species that the capacity to synthesize and secrete adequate amounts of lung surfactant is a crucial maturational

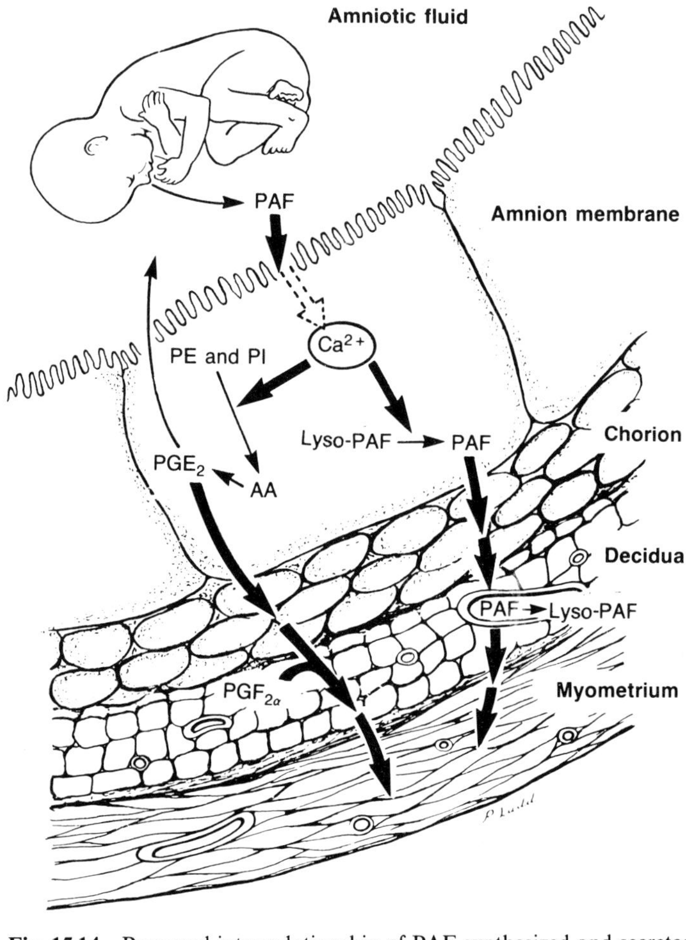

Fig. 15.14 Proposed inter-relationship of PAF synthesized and secreted by the foetal lung into amniotic fluid. The PAF in amniotic fluid stimulates prostaglandin and PAF biosynthesis in amnion tissue (an avascular foetal membrane in the human), possibly by a Ca^{2+} mediated event. Production of PGE_2 and PAF may be further magnified by the stimulation of PGE_2 and PAF in chorion laeve and PGE_2, $PGF_{2\alpha}$ and PAF in decidua vera tissues. Tissue PAF may be inactivated by PAF acetylhydrolase during early and mid gestation due to its high specific activity in maternal plasma. However, late in gestation PAF escapes inactivation in the vascular decidua as a result of the decrease in maternal plasma acetylhydrolase activity.

event in preparing the foetus for post-natal life. It is suggested that PAF is produced in increased amounts by the foetal lung late in gestation and is secreted in association with surfactant into the amniotic fluid as is illustrated in Fig. 15.14. PAF accumulates in the amniotic fluid only when it exceeds the capacity for the hydrolysis by the PAF acetylhydrolase known to be present in the amniotic fluid [35]. PAF also has direct effect on the foetal lung by stimulating glycogenolysis, thus providing both the carbon source and energy for the synthesis of the glycerophospholipids of surfactant needed for the maturation of the foetal lung, and also the secretion of surfactant by the type-II pneumonocyte. The increased PAF found in amniotic fluid stimulates prostaglandin formation and additional PAF biosynthesis in amnion tissue, possibly via a Ca^{2+} mediated event. Ca^{2+} would also activate both the phospholipase A_2 and C activities resulting in the release of arachidonic acid from diaclyphosphatidylethanolamine and phosphatidylinositol, respectively, for prostaglandin biosynthesis which is known to occur in this tissue. Prostaglandin and PAF formation may be further amplified by the autocatalytic stimulation of PGE_2, $PGF_{2\alpha}$ and PAF in chorion laeve and decidua vera tissues. The small amount of PAF produced during the first and second trimesters of pregnancy is prevented from reaching the myometrium due to the high maternal circulating levels of PAF acetylhydrolase. The tissue site of the inactivation is most probably the decidua vera due to the 'lush' blood supply of this tissue. However, late in gestation the increased PAF synthesized in the uterine tissues escapes inactivation by the vascular decidua due to the precipitous decrease in maternal plasma PAF acetylhydrolase activity, thus allowing this potent stimulator of myometrial contraction to reach this smooth muscle and initiate the rhythmical contractions of early labour. It is hoped that both the reported results and future observations will be utilized to ultimately prevent the consequences of an untimely birth which may extend far beyond the neonatal period.

Acknowledgements

J. M. J. gratefully acknowledges the research contributions of his colleagues, Drs T. Okazaki, G. C. Di Renzo, N. Sagawa, M. M. Billah, M. M. Anceschi, C. Ban, D. R. Hoffman, M. J. Angle amd J. E. Bleasdale. Drs Ban, Hoffman and Angle were recipients of Chilton Foundation Fellowships. We are especially appreciative to Dr Janice R. Okita, who carefully performed the experiments on the fatty acid composition of foetal membranes. The proposed function of ethanolamine plasmalogens in relation to the metabolism of PAF is based on these experiments (Fig. 15.8). We also gratefully acknowledge the editorial assistance of Ms Dolly Tutton. Investigations performed in the authors' laboratories were supported by U. S. Public Health Service grants HD13912 and HD11149 and the Robert A. Welch Foundation, Houston, Texas.

References

1 Thorburn, G. D. Physiology and control of parturition. Reflections on the past ideas for the future. *Anim. Reprod.* (1979), **2**, 1–27.

2 Thorburn, G. D. Past and present concepts on the initiation of parturition. In *Ross Conference on Initiation of Parturition: Prevention of Prematurity. Report of the Fourth Ross Conference on Obstetrics Research* (eds) MacDonald, P. C. & Porter, J. C. (1983), pp. 2–11. Ross Laboratories, Columbus, OH.

3 MacDonald, P. C., Porter, J. C., Schwarz, B. E., & Johnston, J. M. Initiation of parturition in the human female. *Semin. Perinatol.* (1978), **2**, 273–286.

4 Bleasdale, J. E. & Johnston, J. M. Prostaglandins and human parturition: regulation of arachidonic acid mobilization. In *Reviews in Perinatal Medicine* (1984), Vol. 5, pp. 151–191. Alan R. Liss, New York.

5 Johnston, J. M., Bleasdale, J. E. & Hoffman, D. R. Functions of PAF in reproduction and development: involvement of PAF in foetal lung maturation and parturition. In Snyder, F. (ed.) *Platelet-Activating Factor and Related Lipid Mediators* (1987), pp. 375–402. Plenum, New York.

6 Bleasdale, J. E. & Di Renzo, G. C. Foetal influence on human parturition. *Foetal Medicine* (1989), **1**, 242–288.

7 Amoroso, E. C. & Perry, J. S. The existence during gestation of an immunological buffer zone at the interface between maternal and foetal tissues. *Philos. Trans. R. Soc. London [B]* (1975), **271**, 343–361.

8 Mitchell, M. D., Strickland, D. M., Brennecke, S. P. & Saeed, S. A. New aspects of arachidonic acid metabolism in human parturition. In *Ross Conference on Initiation of Parturition: Prevention of Prematurity. Report of the Fourth Ross Conference on Obstetrics Research*, (1983), pp. 145–153. Ross Laboratories, Columbus, OH.

9 Romero, R. In McNellis, D. M., Challis, J. R. G., MacDonald, P. C., Nathanielsz P. W. & Roberts, J. M. (eds) *The Onset of Labor: Cellular and Integrative Mechanisms* (1988), pp. 157–160. Perinatology Press, Ithaca, NY.

10 Kurland, J. I. & Brockman, R. Prostaglandin E production by human blood monocytes and mouse peritoneal macrophages. *J. Exp. Med.* (1978), **147**, 952–957.

11 Romero, R., Hobbins, J. C. & Mitchell, M. D. Endotoxin stimulates prostaglandin E_2 biosynthesis by human amnion. *Obstet. Gynecol.* (1988), **71**, 227–228.

12 Romero, R., Roslansky, P., Oyarzun, *et al.* Labor and infection. II. Endotoxic concentration in amniotic fluid correlates with the presence of labor in intraamniotic infections. *Am. J. Obstet. Gynecol.* (1988), **158**, 1044–1049.

13 Luukkainen, T. U. & Csapo, A. I. Induction of premature labor in the rabbit after pre-treatment with phospholipids. *Fert. Steril.* (1963), **14**, 65–72.

14 Ogawa, Y., Herod, L., & Lanman, J. T. Phospholipids and the onset of labor in rabbits. *Gynecol. Invest.* (1970), **1**, 240–248.

15 Lanman, J. T., Herod, L. & Thau, R. Premature induction of labor with dilinoleyl lecithin in rabbits. *Pediatr. Res.* (1972), **6**, 701–704.

16 Lanman, J. T., Herod, L. & Thau, R. Phospholipids and fatty acids in relation to the premature induction of labor in rabbits. *Pediatr. Res.* (1974), **8**, 1–4.

17 Nathanielsz, P. W., Abel, A. & Smith, G. W. Hormonal factors in parturition in the rabbit. In Comline, K. S., Cross, K. W., Dawes, G. S. *et al.* (eds) *Foetal and Neonatal Physiology* (1973), pp. 594–601. Cambridge University Press, Cambridge.

18 Hertelendy, F. Prostaglandin-induced premature oviposition in the coturnix quail. *Prostaglandins* (1972), **2**, 269–279.

19 Hertelendy, F., Yeh, M. & Bielier, H. V. Induction of oviposition in the domestic hen by prostaglandin. *Gen. Comp. Endocrinol*, (1974), **22**, 529–531.

20 MacDonald, P. C., Schultz, F. M., Duenhoelter, J. H. *et al.* Initiation of human parturition I. Mechanism of action of arachidonic acid. *Obstet. Gynecol.* (1974), **44**, 629–636.

21 Lands, W. E. M. & Samuelsson, B. Phospholipid precursors of prostaglandins. *Biochim. Biophys. Acta*, (1968), **164**, 426–429.

22 Vonkeman, H. & van Dorp, D. A. Phospholipid precursors of prostaglandins. *Biochim. Biophys. Acta.* (1968), **168**, 426–432.

23 Karim, S. M. M. Identification of prostaglandins in human amniotic fluid. *J. Obstet. Gynecol. Br. Commonw.* (1966), **73**, 903–908.

24 Schwarz, B. E., Schultz, F. B., MacDonald, P. C. & Johnston, J. M. Initiation of human parturition III. Fetal membrane content of prostaglandin E_2 and $F_{2\alpha}$ precursor. *Obstet. Gynecol.* (1975), **46**, 564–568.

25 Okita, J. R., MacDonald, P. C. & Johnston, J. M. Mobilization of arachidonic acid from specific glycerophospholipids of human fetal membranes during early labor. *J. Biol. Chem.* (1982), **257**, 14 029–14 034.

26 McCoshen, J. A., Tomita, K., Fernandez, C. & Tyson, J. E. Specific cells of human amnion selectively localize prolactin. *J. Clin. Endocrinol. Metab.* (1982), **55**, 166–169.

27 Okita, J. R. *Alterations in the Arachidonic Acid Content of Specific Glycerophospholipids of Amnion and Chorin Laeve During Human Parturition* (1981). Ph.D. Dissertation., The University of Texas Health Science Center at Dallas.

28 Okazaki, T., Okita, J. R., MacDonald, P. C. & Johnston, J. M. Initiation of human parturition: X. Substrate specificity of phospholipase A_2 in human fetal membanes. *Am. J. Obstet. Gynecol.* (1978), **130**, 432–438.

29 Di Renzo, G. C., Johnston, J. M., Okazaki, T., Okita, J. R., MacDonald, P. C. & Bleasdale, J. E. Phosphatidylinositol-specific phospholipase C in fetal membranes and uterine decidua. *J. Clin. Invest.* (1981), **67**, 847–856.

30 Okazaki, T., Sagawa, N., Bleasdale, J. E., Okita, J. R. MacDonald, P. C. & Johnston, J. M. Initiation of human parturition: XIII. phospholipase C, phospholipase A_2, and diacylglycerol lipase activities in fetal membranes and decidua vera tissues from early and late gestation. *Biol. Reprod.* (1981), **25**, 103–109.

31 Majerus, P. M., Prescott, S. M., Hofmann, S. L. Neufeld, E. J., Wilson, D. B. Uptake and release of arachidonate by platelets. In Samuelsson, B., Paoletti, R., Ramwell, P. (eds), *Advances in Prostaglandin, Thromboxane, and Leukotriene Research* Vol. VII, (1983), pp. 45–52. Raven Press, New York

32 Sagawa, N., Okazaki, T., MacDonald, P. C. & Johnston, J. M. Regulation of diacylglycerol metabolism and arachidonic acid release in human amniotic tissue. *J. Biol. Chem.* (1982), **257**, 8158–8162.

33 Olson, D. M., Opavsky, M. A. & Challis, J. R. G. Prostaglandin synthesis by human amnion is dependent upon extracellular Ca^{2+}. *Can. J. Physiol. Pharmacol* (1983), **61**, 1089–1092.

34 Snyder, F. Enzymatic pathways for platelet-activating factor, related alkyl glycerolipids, and their precursors. In Snyder, F. (ed.) *Platelet-Activating Factor and Related Lipid Mediators* (1987), pp. 89–113. Plenum, New York.

35 Billah, M. M. & Johnston, J. J. Identification of phospholipid platelet-activating factor (1-O-alkyl-2-acetyl-*sn*-3-phosphocholine) in human amniotic fluid and urine. *Biochem. Biophys. Res. Commun.* (1983), **113**, 51–58.

36 Nishihara, J., Ishibashi, T., Imai, Y. & Muramatsu, T. Mass spectrometric evidence for the presence of platelet-activating factor (1-O-alkyl-2-acetyl-*sn*-glycero-3-phosphocholine) in human amniotic fluid during labour. *Lipids* (1984), **19**, 907–910.

37 Montrucchio, G., Alloatti, G., Tetta, C., Roffinello, C., Emanuelli, G. & Camussi, G. *In vitro* contractile effect of platelet-activating factor on guinea pig myometrium *Prostaglandins* (1986), **32**, 539–554.

38 Tetta, G., Montrucchio, G., Alloatti, G. *et al.* Platelet-activating factor contracts human myometrium *in vitro. Proc. Soc. Exp. Biol. Med.* (1986), **186**, 376–381.

39 Billah, M. M., Di Renzo, G. C., Ban, C. *et al.* Platelet-activating factor metabolism in

human amnion and the responses of this tissue to extracellular platelet-activating factor. *Prostaglandins* (1985), **30**, 841–850.

40 Ban, C., Billah, M. M., Truong, C. T. & Johnston, J. M. Metabolism of platelet-activating factor PAF (1-O-alkyl-2-acetyl-*sn*-glycero-3-phosphocholine) in human fetal membranes and decidua vera. *Arch. Biochem. Biophys.* (1986), **246**, 9–18.

41 Lenihan, D. J. & Lee, T.-C. Regulation of platelet-activating factor synthesis: modulation of 1-alkyl-2-lyso-*sn*-glycero-3-phosphocholine:acetyl-CoA acetyltransferase by phosphorylation and dephosphorylation in rat spleen microsomes. *Biochem. Biophys. Res. Commun.* (1984), **120**, 834–839.

42 Ninio, E., Mencia-Huerta, J. M., Heymans, F. & Benveniste, J. Biosynthesis of platelet-activating factor. I. Evidence for an acetyl-transferase activity in murine macrophages. *Biochim. Biophys. Acta.* (1982), **710**, 23–31.

43 Okazaki, T., Ban, C. & Johnston, J. M. The identification and characterization of protein kinase C activity in fetal membranes. *Arch. Biochem. Biophys.* (1984), **229**, 27–32.

44 Gomez-Cambronero, J., Velasco, S., Sanchez Crespo, M., Vivanco, F. & Mato, J. M. Partial purification and characterization of 1-alkyl-2-lyso-*sn*-glycero-3-phosphocholine:acetyl-CoA acetyltransferase from rat spleen. *Biochem. J.* (1986), **237**, 439–445.

45 Angle, M. J. & Johnston, J. M. The biosynthesis of lysoPAF: A phospholipase with specificity for alkyl-acyl-GPC. In *Second International Conference on PAF, Gatlinburg, TN* (1986), p.47.

46 Angle, M. J., Paltauf, F. & Johnston, J. M. Selective hydrolysis of 1-O-alkyl-2-arachidonoyl-glycerophospholipids by phospholipase A_2 in rabbit lung. *Biochim. Biophys. Acta.* (1988), **962**, 234–240.

47 Sugiura, T. & Waku, K. Composition of alkyl ether-linked phospholipids in mammalian tissues. In: Snyder, F. (ed.) *Platelet-Activating Factor and Related Lipid Mediators* (1987), pp. 55–88. Plenum, New York.

48 Hoffman, D. R., Truong, C. T. & Johnston, J. M. Metabolism and function of platelet-activating factor in rabbit fetal lung development *Biochim. Biophys. Acta.* (1986), **879**, 88–96.

49 Hoffman, D. R., Truong, C. T. & Johnston, J. M. The role of platelet-activating factor in human fetal lung maturation and the initiation of parturition. *Am. J. Obstet. Gynecol.* (1986), **155**, 50–75.

50 Snyder, F. Johnston, J. M. & Mendelson, C. R. Differentiation of type II cells in human fetal lung *in vitro*. *Cell Tissue Res.* (1981), **220**, 17–25.

51 Snyder, J. M., Mendelson, C. R. & Johnston, J. M. The morphology of lung development in the human fetus. In: Nelson, G. (ed.) *Pulmonary Development and Transition from Intrauterine to Extrauterine Life* (1985), pp. 19–46. Marcel Dekker, New York.

52 Hoffman, D. R., Bateman, M. & Johnston, J. M. Synthesis of platelet-activating factor by cholinephosphotransferase in developing fetal rabbit lung. *Lipids* (1988), **23**, 96–100.

53 Schultz, F. M., Jimenez, J. M., MacDonald, P. C. & Johnston, J. M. Fetal lung maturation: I. Phosphatidic acid phosphohydrolase in rabbit lung. *Gynecol. Invest.* (1974), **5**, 222–229.

54 Snyder, F. Chemical and biochemical aspects of platelet activating factor: a novel class of acetylated ether linked choline phospholipids. *Med. Res. Rev.* (1985), **5**, 107–140.

55 Doebber, T. W. & Wu, M. S. Platelet-activating factor (PAF) stimulates the PAF-synthesizing enzyme acetyl-CoA:alkyl-*sn*-glycero-3-phosphocholine-O-acetyltrans-

ferase and PAF synthesis in neutrophils. *Proc. Nat. Acad. Sci. (USA)*, (1987), **84**, 7557–7561.

56 Johnston, J. M., Maki, N., Angle, M. J. & Hoffman, D. R. Regulation of the arachidonic acid cascade and PAF metabolism in reproductive tissues. In Mitchell, M. D. (ed.) *Eicosanoids in Reproduction* (1989). CRC Uniscience Press. In press.

57 Daniel, L. W., Waite, M. & Wykle, R. L. A novel mechanism of diglyceride formation. *J. Biol. Chem.* (1986) **261**, 9128–9132.

58 Baker, R. C. 1-O-Alkyl-1-enly-2-acyl-GPE (ethanolamine plasmalogen) is the end ether lipid metabolite of platelet activating factor. *FASEB. J.* (1988), **3**, A1377.

59 Horrocks, L. A. & Sharma, M. Plasmalogens and O-alkyl-glycerophospholipids. In Hawthorne J. N. & Ansell, G. B. (eds) *Phospholipids* (1982), pp. 51–54. Elsevier Biomedical Press, Amsterdam.

60 Yasuda, K., Satouchi, K. & Saito, K. Platelet-activating factor in normal rat uterus. *Biochem. Biophys. Res. Commun.* (1986), **138**, 1231–1236.

61 Nakayama, R., Yasuda, K. & Saito, K. Existence of endogenous inhibitors of platelet-activating factor (PAF) with PAF in rat uterus. *J. Biol. Chem.* (1987) **262**, 13 174–13 179.

62 Smith, S. K. & Kelly, R. W. Effect of platelet-activating factor in the release of $PGF_{2\alpha}$ and PGE_2 by separated cells of human endometrium. *J. Reprod. Fert.* (1988), **82**, 271–276.

63 Hoffman, D. R., Romero, R. & Johnston, J. M. Detection of platelet-activating factor in the amniotic fluid of complicated pregnancies (1989), *Am. J. Obstet. Gynecol.* In press.

64 Sell, E. J. & Harris, T. R. Association of premature rupture of membranes with idiopathic respiratory distress syndrome. *Obstet. Gynecol.* (1977), **49**, 167–169.

65 Hanahan, D. J. Platelet activating factor: a biologically active phosphoglyceride. *Ann. Rev. Biochem.* (1986), **55**, 483–509.

66 Maniscalco, W. M., Wilson, C. M., Gross, I., Gobran, L., Rooney, S. A. & Warshaw, J. B. Development of glycogen and phospholipid metabolism in fetal and newborn rat lung. *Biochim. Biophys. Acta.* (1978), **530**, 333–346.

67 Boubon, J. R., Rieutort, M., Engle, M. J. & Farrell, P. M. Utilization of glycogen for phospholipid synthesis in fetal rat lung. *Biochem. Biophys. Acta.* (1982), **712**, 382–389.

68 Rudolph, A. M., Itskouitz, J., Iwamoto, H., Reuss, M. L. & Heymann, M. A. Fetal cardiovascular responses to stress. *Semin. Perinatol.* (1981), **5**, 109–120.

69 Hoffman, D. R., White, R. G., Angle, M. J., Maki, N. & Johnston, J. M. Platelet-activating factor induces glycogen degradation in fetal rabbit lung *in utero. J. Biol. Chem.* (1988), **263**, 9316–9319.

70 Kumar, R. & Hanahan, D. J. Diversity of the biological aspects in specific cells and tissues. In Snyder, F. (ed.) *Platelet-Activating Factor and Related Lipid Mediators* (1987), pp. 239–254. Plenum, New York.

71 Blank, M. L., Hall, M. N., Cress, E. A. & Snyder, F. Inactivation of 1-alkyl-2-acetyl-*sn*-glycero-3-phosphocholine by a plasma acetylhydrolase: higher activities in hypertensive rats. *Biochem. Biophys, Res. Commun.* (1983), **113**, 666–671.

72 Crook, J. E., Mroczkowski, P. J., Cress, E. E., Blank, M. L. & Snyder, F. Serum platelet-activating factor acetylhydrolase activity in white and black essential hypertensive patients. *Circulation* (1986), **74**, 329. (Abstract).

73 Farr, R. S., Cox, C. P., Wardlow, M. J. & Jorgensen, R. Preliminary studies of an acid-labile factor (ALF) in human sera that inactivates platelet-activating factor (PAF). *Clin. Immunol. Immunopathol.* (1980), **15**, 318–330.

74 Farr, R. S. Wardlow, M. L., Cox, C. P., Meng, K. E. & Greene, D. E. Human serum acid-labile factor is an acylhydrolase that inactivates platelet-activating factor. *Fed.*

Proc. (1983), **42**, 3120–2122.
75 Maki, N., Hoffman, D. R. & Johnston, J. M. PAF (platelet-activating factor) acetylhydrolase activities in maternal, fetal, and newborn rabbit plasma during pregnancy and lactation. *Proc. Nat. Acad. Sci (USA)* (1988), **85**, 728–732.
76 Binaghi, R. A., Oettgen, H. F. & Benacerraf, B. Anaphylactic antibody in the young rat. *Int. Arch. Allergy Appl. Immunol.* (1966), **29**, 105–111.
77 Hargis, B. J. & Malkeil, S. Production of hypersensitivity in the neonatal mouse. *J. Immunol.* (1970), **104**, 942–949.
78 Meng, A. L., Pinckard, R. N. & Halonen, M. Ontogeny of the release and reactivity to the mediators of IgE-induced acute allergic reactions in the rabbit: the homologous PCA reaction. *J. Immunol.* (1973), **110**, 1554–1561.
79 Angle, M. J., Pinckard, R. N., Showell, H. J. & McManus, L. M. Ontogeny of the responsiveness to intravenous platelet-activating factor. *Lab. Invest.* (1987), **57**, 321–328.

Index